INTEGRATIVE HEALTH PROMOTION

CONCEPTUAL BASES FOR NURSING PRACTICE

Second Edition

Susan Kun Leddy, PhD, RN

Professor Emerita, School of Nursing
Widener University
Chester, Pennsylvania

JONES AND BARTLETT PUBLISHERS
Sudbury, Massachusetts

BOSTO ... ORE

World Headquarters
Jones and Bartlett Publishers
40 Tall Pine Drive
Sudbury, MA 01776
978-443-5000
info@jbpub.com
www.jbpub.com

Jones and Bartlett Publishers
 Canada
6339 Ormindale Way
Mississauga, Ontario
L5V 1J2

Jones and Bartlett Publishers
 International
Barb House, Barb Mews
London W6 7PA
UK

Jones and Bartlett's books and products are available through most bookstores and online booksellers. To contact Jones and Bartlett Publishers directly, call 800-832-0034, fax 978-443-8000, or visit our website, www.jbpub.com.

Substantial discounts on bulk quantities of Jones and Bartlett's publications are available to corporations, professional associations, and other qualified organizations. For details and specific discount information, contact the special sales department at Jones and Bartlett via the above contact information or send an email to specialsales@jbpub.com.

Library of Congress Cataloging-in-Publication Data
Leddy, Susan.
  Integrative health promotion : conceptual bases for nursing practice / by Susan Kun Leddy.— 2nd ed.
     p. ; cm.
  Includes bibliographical references and index.
  ISBN 0-7637-3840-9
  1. Holistic nursing. 2. Health promotion. 3. Alternative medicine.
  [DNLM: 1. Health Promotion—methods. 2. Holistic Nursing. 3. Health Behavior. 4. Holistic Health.
  5. Nursing Theory. WY 86.5 L472i 2005] I. Title.
  RT42.L38 2005
  610.73—dc22

                              2005024306

Production Credits
Acquisitions Editor: Kevin Sullivan
Associate Editor: Amy Sibley
Production Director: Amy Rose
Production Editor: Renée Sekerak
Production Assistant: Rachel Rossi
Marketing Manager: Emily Ekle
Manufacturing and Inventory Coordinator: Amy Bacus
Cover Design: Kristin E. Ohlin
Printing and Binding: Malloy Incorporated
Cover Printing: Malloy Incorporated

Printed in the United States of America
09 08 07 06 05   10 9 8 7 6 5 4 3 2 1

Dedication

To Debbie, Erin, and Katie, with all my love.

Contents

About the Author

Susan Kun Leddy earned a bachelor of science in nursing from Skidmore College, Saratoga, New York in 1960, a master of science in nursing (teaching medical-surgical nursing) from Boston University in 1965, a doctor of philosophy (nursing science) from New York University in 1973, and did post-doctoral work at Harvard University (1985) and the University of Pennsylvania (1996–98).

Dr. Leddy initially taught in diploma schools of nursing for four years and then in the baccalaureate program at Columbia University before completing doctoral work. She was then one of four founding faculty for the RN-BSN program at Pace University. In 1976, after a year as an NLN consultant, she was asked to do a feasibility study and then write the proposal to the State of New York for a new RN-BSN program at Mercy College. She became the first chairperson of the program (Mae Pepper was the first faculty member), which opened in 1977.

Dr. Leddy left Mercy College in 1981 to first become dean of the School of Nursing, and then dean of the reconstituted College of Health Sciences, at the University of Wyoming. In 1988, she became dean of the School of Nursing at Widener University, Chester, Pennsylvania, returning to graduate teaching there in 1993. She is now professor emerita in the School of Nursing.

In addition to authoring *Integrative Health Promotion: Conceptual Bases for Nursing Practice*, Dr. Leddy is the co-author with Lucy Hood of *Conceptual Bases of Professional Nursing*, 6th edition, copyright 2006; *Health Promotion: Mobilizing Human Strengths to Promote Wellness*, copyright 2006; and is working on a manuscript, *Nursing Knowledge and Nursing Science*, with Jacqueline Fawcett. She has authored numerous periodical publications.

Dr. Leddy has two daughters, Deborah and Erin. Deborah is a student of veterinary medicine at the University of Pennsylvania, and Erin is a graduate student in the social work program at West Chester University. Dr. Leddy's granddaughter, Katie, was born October 12, 2001.

Dr. Leddy is an avid traveler, and especially enjoys traveling to exotic places. She also knits, quilts, weaves (a little), and dabbles in watercolor painting and creative writing.

Preface

I believe that the promotion of health is the core of professional nursing knowledge and practice. Given this belief, I have been dismayed and frustrated by the overwhelming emphasis on disease and illness in most nursing educational programs. It is my hope that this book will serve as an exemplar of health promotion content that should be taught, particularly in graduate programs.

I have attempted to present a coherent synthesis of numerous, disparate literatures. *Chapter 1: Health, Health Promotion, and Healing*, lays out a conceptual "map" for the book, clarifying the critical differences between the "disease perspective" dominant in the biomedical, epidemiological, and public health literatures, and the "person perspective", which appears in nursing and alternative/complementary medical literatures. This edition, where all chapters have been updated, presents theory and practical strategies from both perspectives, toward the goal of integrative practice.

The content in Chapter 2, in my opinion, is of vital importance for nursing practice, yet almost completely absent from the nursing literature. It is my long-standing and heartfelt belief that nurses and clients need to utilize strengths as resources to address client weaknesses. Additionally, nurses must stop trying to be the expert who solves all problems, and, instead, practice within an egalitarian model with power and expertise shared with the client.

As in practically all other areas of scientific knowledge, definitive research evidence to support health promotion practice is just not available. Abstracts of research are presented throughout the book, and the "state of the art" is reviewed wherever possible. However, the very limited evidence derived from well designed research continues to be of concern. Additionally, the health promotion literature is largely atheoretical. I have attempted to present what theory/models I could find. Theory-based scholarship is critically needed to advance the science.

My rationale in organizing the book has been to present the conceptual bases of health promotion in Section I, followed by several chapters in Sections II and III that address primarily either the disease or person worldview. The chapters in Section IV apply the conceptual content from both worldviews to nursing practice.

Integrative health promotion is a vision. It is my sincere hope that by presenting a glimpse of what might be, that this book will further a reality of knowledge-based health promotion practice as an essential and substantial component of professional nursing.

Susan Kun Leddy, PhD, RN

CONCEPTUAL BASES OF HEALTH PROMOTION

Section I, *Conceptual Bases of Health Promotion*, includes seven chapters that provide a contextual exploration of the meaning of health promotion and healing in a variety of health belief systems, health strengths models and theories, and cultures. This section also includes chapters on legal and ethical influences and health promotion, and integrative approaches to client assessment. Chapter 1, *Health, Health Promotion, and Healing*, differentiates between health protection (the prevention of disease risk factors and disease), health promotion (facilitating health-related lifestyle changes), and healing to promote wholeness, integration, harmony, and, therefore, health. The disease and the person world views, and their implications for beliefs about health, are compared and contrasted. In Chapter 2, *Health Strengths*, the theory of healthiness is discussed as are its various concepts. It is proposed that strengths serve as resources to promote health and healing. In Chapter 3, *The Meaning of Health: Health Care Belief Systems*, a number of lay, community-based (Cuanderismo and Shamanism), and professional (Western biomedicine and traditional—including Chinese, Ayurveda, and naturopathic and homeopathic medicines) health care belief systems are described, so that the student can appreciate the diversity of belief systems that provide a context for integrative nursing. Chapter 4, *The Meaning of Health: Models and Theories*, presents 11 models or theories that can guide the promotion of health and healing in nursing practice. Chapter 5, *The Meaning of Health: Cultural Influences*, explores the influence on health promotion of indigenous cultural beliefs of Asian Americans (Vietnamese Americans), Appalachians, Hispanics (Mexican Americans), African Americans, and Native Americans, and concludes with a presentation of multiple characteristics, influences, and practices that should be considered in multicultural health promotion planning. Chapter 6, *Ethical and Legal Influences on Health Promotion*, presents issues of power and empowerment, preferential valuing among the ethical principles of autonomy, nonmaleficence, beneficence, and justice, and a non-traditional model for professional ethics. The chapter concludes with a review of licensing issues, negligence, electronic transmittal of health information, and implications of food and drug regulation, with special considerations for integrative health promotion. Chapter 7, *Beyond Physical Assessment*, reviews guidelines for risk and disease screening, presents numerous frameworks for the assessment of healthiness, and discusses integrative techniques (tongue and pulse assessment) to broaden the database from which the client and nurse develop a health promotion plan.

HEALTH, HEALTH PROMOTION, AND HEALING

Acknowledgment: Parts of this chapter were previously published in Leddy, S. (1998). *Leddy & Pepper's Conceptual bases of professional nursing* (4th ed.). Philadelphia: Lippincott.

Abstract

This chapter presents a conceptual framework for integrative health promotion. Distinctions among health protection, health promotion, and healing are discussed within two worldviews of health, the disease and the person perspectives. Health protection and health promotion are considered to be consistent with the disease perspective. The dominant approach to "health" in the literature is health protection, which focuses attention on the prevention of disease risk factors and disease. Health promotion focuses on facilitating individual health-related lifestyle changes. In contrast, healing and holistic nursing are considered to be consistent with the person perspective. Facilitating healing to promote wholeness, integration, and harmony is the desired primary emphasis of holistic nursing. Integrative health promotion is based on a healing philosophy, and utilizes both health protection/promotion strategies and holistic, non-invasive therapeutic nursing modalities to facilitate the health of individuals, families, and communities, both locally and globally.

Learning Outcomes

By the end of the chapter the student should be able to:

- Compare and contrast the disease and person perspectives of health
- Discuss health protection and disease risk prevention

■ Describe elements of behavioral, ecological, and policy approaches to health promotion

■ Discuss selected conceptual or theoretical approaches to healing

■ Describe roles for nurses to facilitate healing

■ Describe selected characteristics of holistic nursing

■ Describe elements of integrative nursing

Basic philosophic assumptions about the nature of reality, including human beings and the human-environment relationship, are referred to as paradigms or worldviews. In different worldviews, the meaning of health can vary significantly. Different interpretations of the meaning of health are associated with different interpretations of the meaning of health promotion. The author has synthesized two contrasting paradigms of health from the literature, labeled the disease and the person worldviews. It is proposed that health protection (avoidance of risk) and health promotion (lifestyle change) are consistent with the disease worldview, whereas healing is consistent with the person perspective. This chapter will explore the different meanings of health, health promotion, and healing, eventually proposing a combination of strategies from both worldviews.

The Disease Perspective of Health

In the disease perspective of health, the human being is usually conceptualized as a whole, comprised of parts. The internal environment of the human being is regarded as a composite of distinct biological, psychological, and spiritual components. Human beings are physically separated by boundaries from the external environment. Thus, the human being interacts with a physically separate environment, which is viewed as a context. The human being is *in* the environment. Therefore, a composite of distinct areas such as biological, ecological, social, cultural, economic, and political components interact to form the total environment. Human and environmental interactions are linear and result in quantifiable cause and effect changes. Although both human being and environment may be affected by change, unidirectional change is the usual mode of analysis. For example, in nursing, the impact of the environment on the human being's health is of interest, and, in ecology, the impact of the human on environmental conditions is relevant.

"Normal" human functioning is perceived to be homeostatic, that is, operating within a relatively narrow range of balance or stability. The environment contains stressors that act on a person and to which a person must react. The environment acts on the individual through stressors, and in reacting to the stressors, internal stability of the individual is upset. Change, although acknowledged to be inevitable, is considered to be a threat. The threat may involve disease, illness, or sickness, affecting well-being and health.

IDEAS OF HEALTH CONSISTENT WITH THE DISEASE PERSPECTIVE

Health

Health is difficult to define. In many definitions, physiologic and psychological components of health are dichotomized. Other subconcepts that might be included in definitions of health include environmental and social influences, freedom from pain or disease, optimum capability, ability to adapt, purposeful direction and meaning in life, and sense of well-being. In this book, within the disease perspective, health has been defined as a state or condition of integrity of functioning (functional capacity and ability) and perceived well-being (feeling well). This definition is consistent with one perspective of the dictionary derivation of *hoelth* (from Old English) as sound, and *hale*, meaning strength. As a result, a person is able to:

- Function adequately (can be objectively observed)
- Adapt adequately to the environment
- Feel well (as subjectively assessed)

Within the disease perspective, more or less health is viewed as a state of being. Health may be dichotomized into wellness and illness, or viewed as a continuum from an ideal state of high-level wellness to terminal illness and death. When conceptualized on a continuum, the absence of disease defines health. Normal health status is viewed as a standard of adequacy to access capabilities for role or task performance. Disease is dysfunction, the human experience of disease is illness, and behavioral dysfunctions due to health problems are sickness.

Disease

Disease is a medical term. It is a "dysfunction of the body" (Benner et al., 1996, p. 45), and a deviation from clearly established norms. The objective of the physician is to classify observable changes in body structure or function (signs) into a recognizable clinical syndrome. A correct label, or diagnosis, implies disease course and duration, communicability, prognosis, and appropriate treatment. Medical intervention is aimed at curing the disease. Part of nursing intervention supports and promotes the medical regimen through, among other things, administering treatments, encouraging rest, and evaluating the effectiveness of interventions.

Historically, diseases were believed to be due to one agent, which in a sufficient dose, caused certain predictable signs and symptoms. Increasingly, however, a variety of factors related to the person (host), agent, and environment have been viewed as being interrelated in the cause and effective treatment of disease. For example, genetic factors, stress, and poor air quality have all been implicated in the development of asthma. All of the interrelationships must be considered in determining a plan for care.

Illness

Illness is a subjective feeling of being unhealthy that may or may not be related to disease. A person may have a disease without feeling ill and may feel ill in the absence of disease. For example, a person may have hypertension (a disease) controlled with medication, diet, and exercise. This person may have no symptoms and no illness. Another person may have pain and feel ill, but may not have an identifiable disease. What is important is how the person feels and what he or she does because of those feelings.

Nursing interventions focus on the client's responses to symptoms. In contrast, medical care focuses on efforts to label (diagnose) and treat the symptoms. When a person's illness is accepted by society, and thus given legitimacy, it is considered "sickness."

Sickness

Twaddle, a medical sociologist, defined sickness as "a status, a social entity usually associated with disease or illness, although it may occur independently of them" (1977, p. 97). Once the person is defined as sick, various dependent behaviors are condoned that otherwise might be considered unacceptable. The nurse's role is to assist until the person is able to independently reassume responsibility for decision-making.

Well-Being

Well-being is a subjective perception of vitality and feeling well that is a component of health within the disease perspective. It is a variable state that can be described objectively, experienced, and measured. Experienced at the lowest degrees, a person might feel ill. Experienced at the highest levels, a person would perceive maximum satisfaction, understanding, and feelings of contribution. Thus, well-being status can be plotted on a continuum, as shown in Figure 1-1.

Smith (1981, p. 47), in a now classic work, presented four models of health consistent with the disease perspective that, initially, were viewed as forming a scale—a progressive expansion of the idea of health. Subsequent research, however, has indicated that many people hold beliefs from all four models of health concurrently. Smith's four models of health are the clinical model, the role performance model, the adaptive model, and the eudaimonistic model.

The clinical model is the narrowest view. People are seen as physiologic systems with interrelated functions. Health is identified as the absence of signs and symptoms of medically defined disease or disability; persons are healthy if they are not ill. Thus, health might be defined as a "state of not being sick" (Ardell, 1979, p. 18) or as a "relatively passive state of freedom from illness… a condition of relative homeostasis" (Dunn, 1977, p. 7). Much of our present health care delivery system is set up to deal with disease and illness after it occurs, based on this model of health. In the clinical model of health, the opposite end of the continuum from health is disease.

Next on the scale is the idea of health as role performance. This model adds social and psychological standards to the concept of health. The critical criterion of health is the person's ability to fulfill roles in society with the maximum (e.g., best, highest) expected performance. Persons are healthy if they are able to work. If a person is unable to perform their expected roles, this inability can mean illness even if the individual appears clinically healthy. For example, "somatic health is… the state of optimum capacity for the elective performance of valued tasks" (Parsons, 1958, p. 168). In the role performance model of health, the opposite end of the continuum from health is sickness.

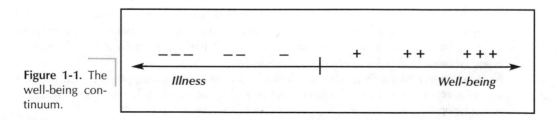

Figure 1-1. The well-being continuum.

Incorporating the clinical and role performance models is the adaptive model. Health is perceived as a condition in which the person can engage in effective interaction with the physical and social environment. The adaptive meaning of health is related to the ability to adjust; persons are healthy if they are able to cope. There is an indication of growth and change in this model. For example, McWilliams, Stewart, Brown, Desai, and Coderre define health as the "individual's ability to realize aspirations, satisfy needs, and respond positively to the challenges of the environment" (1996, p. 1), and Roy and Andrews define health as "a state and a process of being and becoming an integrated and whole human being" (1999, p. 54). In the adaptive model of health, the opposite end of the continuum from health is illness.

Smith (1981) considers the eudaimonistic model to be the most comprehensive conception of health. In this model, health is a condition of actualization or realization of the person's potential. For example, human health is "the actualization of inherent and acquired human potential" (Pender, Murdaugh, & Parsons, 2002, p. 22). Health "transcends biological fitness. It is primarily a measure of each person's ability to do what he wants to do and become what he wants to become" (Dubos, 1978, p. 74). In the eudaimonistic model, health is dichotomized, with being well at the opposite end of the continuum from disabling illness. Woods and colleagues (1992) identified characteristics consistent with the eudaimonistic meaning of health, including having goals, positive self-concept, positive body image, social involvement, positive mood, harmony, energy, healthy lifeways, creativity, and rational thinking.

HEALTH PROTECTION AND DISEASE RISK PREVENTION

Pender and colleagues (2002, p. 7) describe health protection as "motivated by a desire to actively avoid illness, detect it early, or maintain functioning within the constraints of illness." According to Pender (2002), health protection is illness or injury specific, "avoidance" motivated, and seeks to prevent insults to health and well-being.

From the perspective of the disciplines of medicine, public health, and epidemiology, disease is the dominant approach to "health." If health is defined as the absence of disease, then the emphasis becomes the prevention of disease risk factors and disease. Health protection behavior is defined as actions designed to avoid or ward off threats to health (Kulbok et al., 1997). Health protection (interchangeably used with illness prevention) activities "are those that protect a person from a specific harm."

Health protection strategies consist of preventative activities and are categorized into three levels of prevention (Hravnak, 1998, p. 284). In a now classic work, Clark and Leavell (1965) defined the primary, secondary, and tertiary levels of prevention.

Primary prevention takes place before there are symptoms of disease, with a focus on promotion of general health or protection against disease or environmental influences. Therefore, primary prevention includes generalized health promotion as well as specific protection against disease.

Secondary prevention occurs as soon as disease symptoms are identified. The focus is on early diagnosis and prompt and adequate treatment to prevent complications and limit disability. Secondary prevention emphasizes early diagnosis and prompt intervention to stop or control the disease process and reduce disability.

Tertiary prevention occurs within chronic disease. Rehabilitation is intended to restore the client to an optimal level of functioning within the constraints of any disability.

In the biomedical conception of health, the emphasis in all three categories of prevention is on disease. Even primary prevention is focused on the reduction of the risk of incidence of diseases or disorders. However, prevention of specific diseases does not deal with the basic causes of the health problem.

Risk connotes danger, hazard or peril, chance, fate, or luck, but is based on the scientific notion of probability. To reduce disease risk, primary prevention is often based on epidemiological data. Epidemiology, as a discipline, focuses on how diseases originate and spread in populations. Specifically, epidemiology examines the relationships between physiological, psychological, social, and environmental events, and the incidences (new cases) and prevalence (total number of cases) of diseases. Determination of a causal relationship between a risk factor and a disease is based on retrospective (case control) and prospective (cohort) studies, using 5 criteria: strength (relative risk), specificity, temporal relationship, coherence (biological sense and dose response relationship), and preventive clinical trials (Winett, 1995).

Epidemiological data should serve as a basis for understanding risk factors associated with disease and for the modification of such factors. It is important to remember that disease risk factors often represent an interaction of agent, host, and environmental factors, and that relative risk is related to the strength of association between a risk factor and rates of morbidity and mortality.

Being diagnosed as having disease risks poses challenges for people who have to translate population characteristics into personal meaning; cope with ambiguity; interpret the possibility of illness in the absence of symptoms; remain vigilant; and possibly attempt risk reduction (Kavanagh & Broom, 1998). In addition, being labeled at risk presents the individual with a very ambiguous situation. Because risk is based on statistical probability in a population, if action is taken by an individual to try to reduce his or her risk, there can be no clear confidence in the extent of personal vulnerability or the ultimate effectiveness of the remedial action.

A healthy lifestyle has become almost synonymous with a lifestyle characterized by risk evasion or risk reduction. Although "by increasing anxiety regarding disease, accidents and other adverse events, the risk epidemic enhances both health care dependence and health care consumption....fear of disease continues to be the most effective tool for lifestyle changes" (Forde, 1998, pp. 1155-1156). Risks imposed by others, such as environmental agents, include: 1) natural and synthetic toxic chemicals; 2) pollution with radiation and nuclear waste; 3) physical objects; 4) pathogenic organisms; and 5) substances used as nutrients.

The United States' health care system remains primarily disease- and disease risk-oriented. The major portion of national expenditures for medical care goes for the cure and control of illness; relatively little is spent for prevention and health education, even though health promotion programs are associated with lower levels of workplace absenteeism and health care costs (Aldana, 2001). Even efforts toward prevention and health education are illness-oriented. For example, children are taught to brush their teeth to avoid cavities (not because the mouth will feel, look, taste, and smell better) and to dress warmly so they will not "catch a cold" (rather than so that they will feel better).

The national preoccupation with disease risk is evident in *Healthy People 2010*, published in 2000 by the U.S. Department of Health and Human Services. This report describes national objectives for health promotion and disease prevention, including two overarching goals to be achieved by the year 2010 (pp. 8-16):

- Increase quality and years of healthy life
- Eliminate health disparities

Focus areas (with a total of 467 objectives) have been proposed in 28 categories and are listed in Box 1-1.

Box 1-1

Healthy People 2010 Focus Areas

- Access to quality health services
- Arthritis, osteoporosis, and chronic back conditions
- Cancer
- Chronic kidney disease
- Diabetes
- Disability and secondary conditions
- Educational and community-based programs
- Environmental health
- Family planning
- Food safety
- Health communication
- Heart disease and stroke
- HIV
- Immunization and infectious diseases
- Injury and violence prevention
- Maternal, infant, and child health
- Medical product safety
- Mental health and mental disorders
- Nutrition and overweight
- Occupational safety and health
- Oral health
- Physical activity and fitness
- Public health infrastructure
- Respiratory diseases
- Sexually transmitted diseases
- Substance abuse
- Tobacco use
- Vision and hearing

Disease prevention and health promotion differ in whether the main emphasis is on resistance to movement toward the negative (disability), or in movement toward the positive (well-being) (Breslow, 1999).

HEALTH PROMOTION

The Cumulative Index of Nursing and Allied Health Literature (CINAHL) describes health promotion as "the process of fostering awareness, influencing attitudes, and identifying alternatives so that individuals can make informed choices and change their behavior to achieve an optimum level of physical and mental health, and improve their physical and social environment" (CINAHL, 1992, p. 118). Pender et al., (2002, p. 7) suggests that "health promotion is motivated by the desire to increase well-being and actualize human health potential." According to Pender and colleagues (2002), health promotion is not illness, or injury, specific, is "approach" motivated, and seeks to expand positive potential for health.

There are a number of different approaches to health promotion. The medical approach emphasizes correcting problems or disease through treatment and prevention of risks. However, "medical pain relief and medical reduction of symptoms are not typically accomplished by enhancing health....Most medications or medical treatments do not actually restore or fully heal our natural ability to sustain a high level of well-being" (Jahnke, 1997, p. 5). The individual (behavioral) approach focuses on secondary and primary prevention to improve health status through lifestyle and behavior changes of individuals, the socioenvironmental approach addresses psychological, social, and environmental aspects of health, so that health becomes a means of empowerment (Hartrick, 1998; Robertson & Minkler, 1994), and the societal approach focuses on broader health promotion policy.

The Individual (Behavioral) Approach

Smith & Orleans (2004) describe five levels of health promotion. They are:

1. Basic biological processes (e.g., the physiology of nicotine addition)

2. Individual psychological processes (e.g., stages of change)

3. Family and social group processes (e.g., social support)

4. Larger social, cultural, and environmental factors (e.g., access to safe settings for exercise)

5. Institutional and public policy factors (e.g., taxes on tobacco)

Health promotion is often focused on the *individual*, as in the following definitions:

1. "The process of enabling people to increase control over, and to improve, their health" (World Health Organization, 1986).

2. "Any actions or behaviors taken by individuals to improve or promote well-being or health" (Kulbok et al., 1997, pp. 13-14).

3. "Health promotion is behavior motivated by the desire to increase well-being and actualize human health potential" (Pender et al., 2002, p. 7).

4. Health promotion "consists of activities directed toward increasing the level of well-being and actualizing the health potential of people, families, communities, and society" (Hravnak, 1998, p. 284).

Some sources relate health promotion for individuals to health education. In the literature, health education is the label frequently used to refer to individual (lifestyle) and structural (fiscal or ecological) health promotion elements, whereas health promotion is the term used for the broader, structural aspect, in which education plays a part (Benson & Latter, 1998; Huff & Kline, 1999). Health promotion emerged out of health education and designates a broader level of outcomes than does health education. However, health education is considered a primary approach for achieving health promotion outcomes.

Health education has been defined as "any planned combination of learning experiences designed to predispose, enable, and reinforce voluntary behavior conducive to health in individuals, groups, or communities" (Green & Kreuter, 1991, p. 432). From this perspective, nursing intervention should focus on helping clients to gain health-related knowledge, attitudes, and practices associated with achieving specific health-related behavior. Breckon, Harvey, and Lancaster (1994) identified the following characteristics of health education:

- Involves changing habits and attitudes

- Individual responsibility

- Information dispensing

- Planned change

- Community advocacy

The Nurse's Role in Promoting the Health of Individuals

"The [nurse] is not the person who stands back, assesses, plans, and evaluates, but a facilitator who teaches clients how to self-assess, decide on wellness goals, plan on actions to meet those goals, and self-evaluate success" (Clark, 1996, p. 1). Emphasizing the individual approach to health promotion, Clark (1996), Gillis (1995), and Hravnak (1998) propose that the nurses' roles in health promotion should be focused on promoting lifestyle changes rather than specific behavior changes, and empowering clients to increase their control over determinants of health and well-being. Other nursing roles in health promotion are listed in Box 1-2.

Box 1-2

Nursing Roles in Health Promotion of Individuals

- Direct client's attention to positive cues when health-promoting behaviors occur

- Promote positive self-esteem and self-efficacy

- Assist clients to understand the determinants of health

- Decrease illness-related reoccurences and prevent complications, reduce re-admissions or office visits, and improve cost effectiveness

- Create environments conducive to health

- Be sensitive to the variety of physical, cultural, social, and ecological dimensions involved in promoting health lifestyles

- Be an effective role model for wellness

- Facilitate consistent client involvement in the assessment, implementation, and evaluation of health promotion goals

- Teach clients to perceive life experiences as manageable and meaningful by increasing self-responsibility and commitment to self-care

continued

BOX 1-2 CONTINUED

- Teach and facilitate client self-care strategies to enhance fitness, nutritional status, stress management, positive relationship building, coherent belief systems, and their environment

- Facilitate client creative problem solving to enhance health

- Facilitate client assertive behavior

- Maximize functional status

- Teach clients effective communication skills

- Assist clients to differentiate themselves from the practitioner and significant others

- Facilitate richness of client social supports

- Facilitate effective learner, family, and work role behaviors in clients

- Integrate family members and caregivers into the plan, and support those with caregiver burden

- Document nursing's contribution to reduced costs (Anderson, 1997)

Health promotion practice requires the nurse to adopt a "consumer" model rather than the traditional "professional" model. In this shift in thinking, the emphasis is on the empowerment of the client instead of the professional expertise of the nurse and other health care specialists (Gillis, 1995). Traditionally, the professional has tended to be authoritarian, prescriptive, persuasive, and a generalized information giver from an "expert" to an "ignorant" lay person. "We know best," is the covert, if not overt, philosophy of most health professionals. However, the role of the professional is shifting to that of consultant, advocate, mediator, and supporter. In the new paradigm, the professional is empowering, client-centered, and uses a collaborative approach (partnership). In addition, O'Neill (1997) emphasizes that it is crucial that more attention be paid by nurses to the "collective, political, and environmental dimensions of their role" (p. 175).

The Socioenvironmental (Ecological) Approach

Although the emphasis of much American health education/promotion is focused on individual lifestyle change, there is more emphasis on the environment, and an ecological perspective, in other countries. A socioenvironmental or ecological view emphasizes the interconnectedness of lifestyle and environmental matters when health is being considered with the person in balance with the family, community, and environment. Ecological analyses include multiple physical, social, and cultural dimensions of the environment (Stokols, 1996).

Box 1-3

Suggested Nursing Approaches Consistent with the Socioenvironmental View

- Shift from person-focused to environmentally based and community-oriented health promotion.

- Identify various physical and social conditions within environments that can affect physiologic, emotional, and/or social well-being.

- Use comprehensive approaches that integrate psychological, organizational, cultural, community planning, and regulatory perspectives.

- Recognize that "people-environment transactions are characterized by cycles of mutual influence" (Stokols, 1996, p. 286). Be aware of the dynamic interplay among personal and situational factors affecting the client.

- Recognize the fit (or lack of fit) between the client's biological, behavioral, and sociocultural needs and the environmental resources available to them.

- Integrate knowledge from different disciplines.

- Coordinate among the various persons and groups involved with the client.

Source: Adapted from Stokols, D. (1996). Translating social ecological theory into guidelines for community health promotion. *American Journal of Health Promotion, 10,* 282-298.

Nursing approaches emphasize the dynamic interplay between situational and personal factors. Nursing approaches consistent with the socioenvironmental view are listed in Box 1-3.

Whereas the socioenvironmental approach focuses on the interaction of individual, family, community, and the environment, the societal approach focuses on broader health promotion policy.

The Societal (Policy) Approach

Health promotion can be defined in broader societal terms as:

"Any planned combination of educational, political, regulatory, and organizational supports for actions and conditions of living conducive to the health of individuals, groups, or communities" (Green & Kreuter, 1991, p. 432).

"Concern about the creation of living conditions in which a person's experience of health is increased... A health promotion program can improve health without necessarily reducing the prevalence of disease or specific risk factors" (Hartrick, 1998, p. 219).

"Health promotion may be defined as follows: Health promotion is the [political] process by which the ecologically-driven socio-political-economic determinants of health are addressed as they impact on individuals and the communities within which they interact" (Whitehead, 2004, p. 314).

Explicit in these definitions is the need for interventions to stimulate, establish, and sustain an appropriate combination of educational, organizational, and political supports needed to create environments that are conducive to adopting and maintaining a healthful personal lifestyle (O'Neill, 1997). In addition, Kemper (1992) stresses the need to consider broad societal issues that affect health, fearing that the current focus of health promotion on employed and insured groups ignores whole segments of our society. He emphasizes that the broader issues of education, employment, environment, crime, and social support must be addressed if we are to have a healthy society.

Concepts of empowerment, equity, collaboration, and participation are means or methods of achieving health promotion. Figure 1-2 displays a possible structure for health promotion with a multiplicity of intervention levels.

According to Whitehead (2004, p. 315), the attributes of health promotion can be summarized as:

- The need and desire to develop and implement community-driven health reform based on social action, social cohesion, and social capital;

- The willingness of communities to become empowered and self-reliant in determining collective health needs and priorities

- The attainment of health gain as a fundamental priority and shared social objective of community action;

- The active development of public health policy by communities as it applies to those communities.

Kemper (1992, p. 174) describes three elements that are emphasized in societal approaches to health promotion:

1. *Equity.* "In the world view of health promotion, the goal of equal access to health carries more importance than optimizing each person's individual health. The WHO emphasizes providing basic health services to all people before moving on to the more sophisticated needs of subgroups.... The universal perception is that large portions of the American population do not have access to basic health resources."

2. *Power.* "The focus of health promotion is social action for health. The goal is to give people a voice in changing unhealthy environments."

3. *Scope.* "Good housing, safe transportation, basic education, good food supplies, and strong social relationships are within the domain of health promotion."

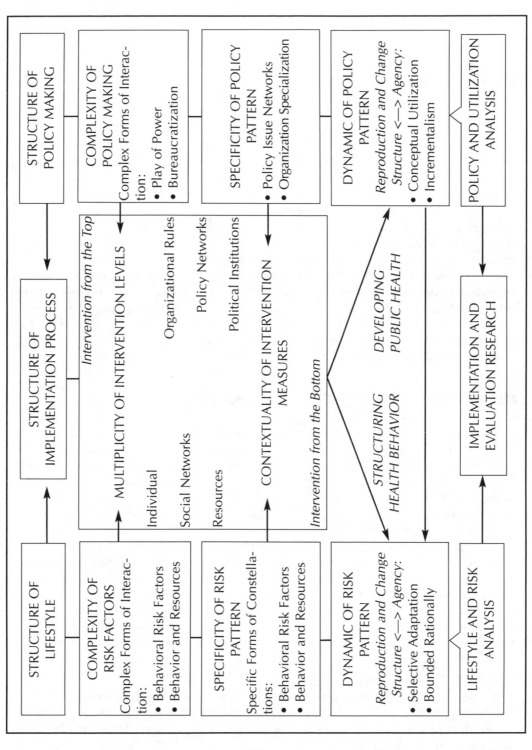

Figure 1-2. A possible structure for health promotion (reprinted from *Soc Sci Med, 41*, Rutten, A. The implementation of health promotion: A new structural perspective, pp. 1627-1637. © 1995, with permission from Elsevier Science).

The most significant shift in conceptualization and emphasis in health promotion has been "from teaching people how to manage their health [individual/behavioral orientation] to a more socially embedded approach that capitalizes on the inherent capacity of community members to establish their own goals, strategies and priorities for health....a socioecological, community development approach to community health" (Whitehead, 2004, p. 316).

Policy making is not characterized by overall rationality or systematic planning. In fact, "policy making may be more accurately described as a process of 'muddling through'" (Rutten, 1995, p. 1632). One concern is the political opposition of those in power with a vested interest in the status quo. To be successful in changing policy, policy advocates try to persuade and negotiate with those in power to find mutually acceptable compromises. One strategy for muddling through involves making only incremental changes that do not vary very much from existing policies (Rutten, 1995).

Despite these political realities, nurses can promote healthy public policy by engaging in widespread public consultation with the public and important policy makers in order to develop a supportive environment for any possible health promotion interventions. One objective should be to strengthen community action through self-help groups, community projects, and neighborhood and community development. It is also essential that personal skills in obtaining information and resources be fostered, so people can manage and control their own activities. Health services may need to be reoriented, and advocacy mechanisms established in order to provide needed services. Chapter 11, *Empowering Community Health*, includes an in-depth discussion of nursing actions to promote societal health.

The Person Perspective of Health

In the person perspective of health, the human being is considered to be a unitary, indivisible whole. The human, although distinct, is embedded in and is, therefore, *of* the environment. Humans can be distinguished within but not separated from the environment. Thus, environment, as a whole, is viewed as co-existent with the human being. The human being and the environment participate (Leddy, 1995) in mutual process associated with unpredictable and nonlinear changes. Change is inevitable and provides an opportunity for growth toward increased complexity.

In this perspective, the goal for a person is to develop his or her potential toward increased diversity. With the emphasis on the process of becoming, health is viewed as a synthesis of manifestations of an underlying pattern reflecting the whole of the human being. Pattern manifestations characterize the whole human being and are not differentiated into good or bad, healthy or not healthy, or better or worse dichotomies. The emphasis for nursing knowledge development and practice is on appreciation of changing pattern manifestations, facilitation of self-healing, and deliberate environmental manipulation to promote growth.

Ideas of Health Consistent with the Integration Perspective

Health within the person perspective is defined by the author as "the pattern of human-environment participation." This definition is consistent with another perspective of the dictionary derivation of health (from Old English) as *hal*, or whole. According to this definition, the purposes of health are to:

- Enable the individual to enfold or unfold in the process of becoming

- Construct meaning

- Use choices to participate in change

In the person perspective, health is viewed as encompassing both disease and nondisease (Newman, 1994). Disease can be considered "a manifestation of health...a meaningful aspect of health" (Newman, 1994, p. 5) and "a meaningful aspect of the whole" (p. 7). Illness and wellness are viewed as a single process of ups and downs that are manifestations of varying degrees of organization and disorganization. Disputing that death is the antithesis of health, Newman (1994) maintains that disease and nondisease are not opposites, but rather are complementary facets of health, a unitary process. Illness, like wellness, simply represents a pattern of life at a particular moment. The tension characteristic of disease throws one off balance, which promotes growth toward a new level of evolving capacities, diversity, and complexity.

Within this perspective, disease and nondisease are aspects of the unitary phenomenon of health. Both disease and nondisease are viewed as manifestations of person-environment mutual process and both represent the underlying pattern of energy. Given this perspective, disease can be viewed as an integrating factor, "[and] can help people see themselves and their interactions with others more clearly" (Newman, 1994, p. 27). Viewing disease this way permits the nurse to focus on the transforming potential of disease rather than on the disabling outcomes of disease. Health is an evolving or emerging process, a forward movement with mutual person-environment patterns.

Within the person perspective, health can be conceptualized as an actively continuing process that involves initiative, ability to assume responsibility for health, value judgments, and integration of the total person. It is dynamic and evolving, a fluid process rather than an actual state. Thus, health is difficult to quantify for objective evaluation. Nurses try to help clients promote growth toward their potential by focusing on strengths, acknowledging needs for support, and by collaborating with clients. A client's goals and feelings are major determinants of nursing intervention. These ideas of health are basic to the concept of healing.

Healing

Definitions of Healing

In this chapter, the previous discussions of disease prevention and the multiple forms of health promotion (biomedical, behavioral, socioenvironmental, and societal) have been consistent with conceptions of health within the disease perspective of health. In contrast, healing is proposed as consistent with conceptions of health within the person paradigm. For example, definitions of healing emphasize the relationship of healing to wholeness as follows:

1. "To be healed is to be whole" (Quinn, 1997, p. 1). "The root of the word heal is the Anglo-Saxon word *haelan*, which means to be or to become whole.... Wholeness, or harmony of body-mind-spirit, may thus be thought of as a dynamic process of being in right relationship." (Harmony is a synonym for connection. Synonyms for connection are relationship, congruity, and unification.) "When true healing occurs, relationship is re-established—relationship to and within self, to others, with one's purpose" (Quinn, 1989, p. 553).

2. Healing is "the return of the integrity and wholeness of the natural state of an individual" (McKivergin, 1997, p. 17).

3. "Healing is an experiential, energy-requiring process in which space is created through a caring relationship in a process of expanding consciousness and results in a sense of wholeness, integration, balance, and transformation, and which can never be fully known" (Wendler, 1996, p. 836).

4. "Heal is the activity of becoming whole" (Kritek, 1997, p. 11).

5. "Healing is the innate, intelligent, and purposeful response of a disordered system to initiate reordering. It is a process which moves toward order and integration of the whole person" (McCabe, 1998, p. 42).

Cunningham (2001, p. 220) differentiates spontaneous healing from assisted healing. Spontaneous healing occurs without deliberate intervention "by the subject's mind or by others." In contrast, assisted healing involves some kind of intervention, either externally assisted (drugs or procedures) or internally assisted, which "describes the deliberate invoking, by the [client], of potentials of his or her own mind and spirit, to facilitate healing."

Healing is not the same as curing. "Curing... refers to the elimination of the signs and symptoms of disease.... Diseases may be cured, but people require healing. In addition, individuals who will never be cured may, in fact, be healed" (Quinn, 1989, pp. 553, 555).

Outcomes of Healing

"Outcomes reflect a change in a person's awareness, perception, behavior, and relationship to self, Creator, other, and creation" (McKivergin, 1997, p. 24). McKivergin describes a number of possible healing outcomes, as follows:

1. Whole person outcomes

   - *Physical.* Decreased pain, enhanced wound healing, increased energy.
   - *Emotional.* Enhanced ability to feel, to name feelings, and to express oneself.
   - *Intellectual.* Perceptual reframing of an experience that influences the belief structure, attitudes, and ways of thinking about life; healing of a painful memory; increased enthusiasm and expression of self; expansion of consciousness.
   - *Social.* Improved relationship with self, self-esteem, improved self-concept; deeper connection with others and understanding of the reciprocal nature of relationships.
   - *Spiritual.* Deeper sense of connectedness with all of life, self, Creator, creation; enhanced meaning regarding a life event; forgiveness of self or others.
   - *Vocational.* Identification of and alignment with life's purpose and path of expression; improved excitement and creativity in work.
   - *Environmental.* Harmony with nature and inherent healing rhythms; recognition of meaning and metaphor in the symbols of the earth.

2. Ability to cope outcomes
   - Enhanced recognition of the impact of stress on life.
   - Access to relaxation response, ability to maintain a flow state.
   - Decreased exhibition of self-destructive behavior.

3. Sense of well-being and quality of life outcomes
   - Increased happiness.
   - Life satisfaction.
   - Sense of security.

4. Functional capacity outcomes
   - Increased ability to care for self.
   - Move.
   - Have less pain.

5. System related outcomes
   - Greater sense of freedom and openness.
   - Establishment of healthy boundaries.
   - Connectedness.
   - Willingness to change and become less defined by external parameters.

Roles for Nurses in Healing

Healing requires a different view of the role of the nurse. "Care has become synonymous with the provision of things and procedures... The assumption made is that since the patient got well after the intervention, that he or she got well because of the intervention... The techniques, the interventions per se, are totally besides the point, they are irrelevant" (Quinn, 1989, pp. 554-555).

A number of authors argue that healing is an innate capacity of the person, which the nurse facilitates (Kritek, 1997; Nightingale, 1859; Quinn, 1989; Wells-Federman, 1998). "Healing within professional nursing acknowledges the human condition not so much as something to be denied, transcended, or controlled, but something to be honored and addressed constructively in active mutuality with the patient" (Kritek, 1997, p. 23). A nurse as an instrument of healing is "one who offers unconditional presence and helps remove the barriers to the healing process; one who creates the space and opportunity for another to feel safe" (McKivergin, 1997, p. 17).

Quinn (1992) describes two different theoretical perspectives of the nurse-client-environment process:

1. The nurse in the environment of the client. "Following appraisal and alteration of the physical environment, the holistic nurse in the environment might then turn attention to the use of particular healing modalities to assist in patterning a more healing environment for the client" (p. 27).

2. The nurse as the environment of the client. "The nurse turns toward her or his understanding of the 'nurse-self' as an energetic, vibrational field, integral with the client's environment" (p. 27).

Regardless of the nurse's perspective, activities to facilitate healing include:

- Removing barriers to the healing process.

- Participating in creating environments that will support healing.

- Facilitating wholeness in others through an interaction based on a mutuality of purpose.

- "Knowingly participate[ing] in the web of interconnectedness toward repatterning and healing for ourselves and for others through the intentional use of our own consciousness…[where] the nurse's consciousness becomes a tuning fork, resonating at a healing frequency" (Quinn, pp. 28, 29). This includes repatterning one's consciousness so it is experienced as unified, harmonious, peaceful, and ordered.

- Allowing healing to emerge. The best instrument for the assessment of whether healing is happening is the subjective knowing of both client and nurse.

- Attending to the meaning of disease for the client.

- Establishing a healing relationship. This involves mobilizing hope for the nurse as well as the client, identifying positive achievements, using healing rituals and symbols, being enthusiastic, committed, encouraging, and attentive, having positive regard and high expectations for improvement (*Integrative Medicine Consult*, 1999). Certain characteristics of nurse healers help to facilitate the effective meeting of roles.

Characteristics of Nurse Healers

McKivergin (1997) proposes a number of characteristics of nurse healers. One cluster of characteristics of nurse healers is related to awareness that self-healing is a continual process, requiring recognition of personal strengths and weaknesses, openness to self-discovery, and an awareness of present and future steps in personal growth. Another cluster of characteristics of nurse healers relates to being in a healthy, centered, and energetic place themselves so that they have enough personal energy to serve as an instrument of healing to another. According to McKivergin (1997), the ability of nurses to model self-care and healthy ways of protecting themselves may include such strategies as:

- Giving and receiving only love

- Praying for protection of the Creator

- Visualizing white light surrounding self and other

- Establishing healthy boundaries

Nurse healers are aware that a nurse's presence is as important as his or her technical skills. They engage in active listening, empowering clients to recognize that they can cope with life processes. Time with clients is perceived as an opportunity to serve and share with them. Insights are shared without imposing personal values and beliefs. Through respect and love for clients, regardless of who and how they are, nurse healers are able to guide the client in discovering creative options. There is a nonjudgmental acceptance of what clients say, and recognition that clients know the best life choices for themselves.

In addition, nurse healers act with intention. "Intentionality involves the projection of awareness, with purpose and efficacy" (Schlitz, 1995, p. 120). But, a number of questions about intentionality persist, including how a person's intentions interact with their body's natural capacity to heal itself, the roles of rapport, anticipation, hope, and belief in communication of intentionality, and the processes by which distant healers heal?

Conceptual and Theoretical Approaches to Healing

The literature describes a number of healing process concepts and theories. Examples include therapeutic capacity, right relationship, integration, the endogenous healing process, and therapeutic landscapes. Each of these approaches emphasizes a different aspect that contributes to healing.

Therapeutic Capacity. Working within the health protection perspective, many nurses perceive their role as "doing battle" with the disease process on behalf of the client, getting the problem solved, but not necessarily responding to the needs of the client (Waters & Daubenmire, 1997). In contrast, the concept of therapeutic capacity proposes that the essence of nursing lies in creating a healing environment and in engaging the client's consciousness in the healing process. "Therapeutic capacity has three dimensions: clinical interventions, caring dynamics, and transpersonal efficacy... defined as the ability to create a shared corridor of consciousness that facilitates the [client's] endogenous healing process... [client] and nurse 'connect'" (Waters & Daubenmire, 1997, pp. 60-61).

Right Relationship. Quinn (1997) has described right relationship as "any pattern of organization within the system that supports, encourages, allows, or generates actualization and self-transcendence" (p. 2). The emergence of right relationship:

- Increases coherence of the whole system.

- Decreases chaos or disorder in the whole.

- Maximizes free energy in the whole.

- Maximizes freedom, autonomy, and choice in the whole.

- Increases the capacity for creative unfolding of the whole.

Integration. "Self-reintegration is defined as a self-creation process whereby individuals develop new capabilities by reorganizing the self and the environment so that there is a meaning and purpose in living that transcends the stressful experience. It is the inner journey toward wholeness and fulfillment" (Rosenow, 1997, p. 505). Quinn (1997) suggests that people have an innate tendency toward wholeness, autonomy, self-actualization, and ultimately self-transcendence, and a drive toward belonging, being a part of something larger, connecting, and interdependency. Integration restores a greater sense of control, order, and harmony (Medich et al., 1997). Through the bringing together of parts of a whole in the healing process, movement is mobilized toward actualizing health potentials and well-being.

Even illness can be thought of as a rite of passage through which a person moves from one phase of life into another. Rites of passage have three phases—separation, transition, and return:

- *Separation.* A feeling of vulnerability acts as a trigger for the person to change or separate from old ways of being or doing. Responding to the challenge involves the person's active participation in recovery.

- *Transition.* During this phase, a person may need time alone, experience unusual states of consciousness, rehearse activities, and/or gather information. Social support through information giving, feedback, and encouragement, and/or demonstrations of caring by family, friends, or health care professionals and the recognition of improvement can facilitate progress through this phase.

- *Return.* The challenges and connections of reentry occur after the healing work (or ritual) is finished and the person goes back to daily life activities (Achterberg, Dossey, & Kolkmeier, 1994). Transformation reflects a new state of being (Medich, Stuart, & Chase, 1997).

According to Rosenow (1997), the main characteristics that shape a person's journey through life are the search for meaning and for fulfillment. Hope, self-control, purpose, competence, devotion, affiliation, production, and renunciation are psychosocial resources or inner strengths that contribute to a person's perception of well-being. Some defining characteristics within the self-reintegration process are:

- Adjustment.

- Self-responsibility. "A state where an individual develops a desire and tendency for self-direction and determinism. It is the belief that one is reliable, trustworthy, and accountable" (p. 505).

- Returning to a normal lifestyle.

- Affirmation of attitudes. "Developing an attitude in order to replace negative ideas with positive ideas that can assist in maximizing one's potential after the illness. This process allows individuals to 1) reframe the illness to a health challenge; 2) reorder their values or standards; and 3) reclaim life satisfaction" (p. 505).

- Obtaining a higher quality of life or well-being. An ongoing journey of self-creation toward a higher potential of functioning (p. 505).

Integrated resource concepts that promote reintegration include:

- Hope or inner strength. Expansion of energy toward wellness. Dimensions of hope include optimism, courage, meaning in life, attainable goals, personal attributes, peace, and energy (p. 507).

- Growth toward health or sense of direction.

- Personal control or competence.

- Social support and networks or affiliation.

The Endogenous Healing Process. According to Scandrett-Hibdon (1996), healing is mentioned in professional literature in limited ways, focusing primarily on the healer, healing techniques, and wound healing. Healing involves individuals in their own process. In other words, only clients can heal themselves. Six separate elements occurring in healing have been observed in which individuals move from disharmonious to harmonious patterns. These elements, which comprise the endogenous healing process, include (1996, pp. 18-21):

- *Awareness*. The alerting mechanism that cues people to events within their internal and external environments. Unless a person is aware of an issue, it cannot be addressed for change.

- *Appraisal*. The person explores and evaluates what awareness has brought to consciousness, assigns meaning to the disruption or cues, and makes comparisons with previous experiences.

- *Choosing*. From appraisal emerges a sense of clarity with which one can choose and set goals to handle disharmony.

- *Acceptance*. Might be considered to be a further aspect of choosing. In the process of "letting go," or deciding to accept, tension is released and relaxation occurs. Three characteristics of acceptance are: (1) giving in to what is occurring, (2) letting go or ceasing to fix the disturbance, and (3) surrendering or passing responsibility of control to another.

- *Alignment*. The energy shifts toward the goal of healing.

- *Outcome*. A sense of being in harmony and experiencing a sense of wholeness, characterized by physical and psychological comfort, vitality, and a sense of peace and well-being.

Therapeutic Landscapes. Therapeutic landscapes are "those changing places, settings, situations, locales, and milieus that encompass both the physical and psychological environments associated with treatment or healing" (Williams, 1998, p. 1193). A landscape may also include environments of the mind through imagery and visualization. A strong sense of place can have a therapeutic effect. For example, a long-standing relationship with a certain place can facilitate feelings of self-identity, security and direction. In contrast, the "spatial separateness and isolation" found in uncaring or hostile environments such as hospitals, reduce an individual's feeling of control.

Watson (1999, p. 248) discusses "caring-healing architecture" as a "healing space" where there is "an attention to body, mind, and spirit as one." Some of the elements such an environment might incorporate include:

- Noise control and therapeutic use of music

- Concern for air quality and use of aromatherapy

- Thermal comfort

- Privacy

- Lighting and use of color

- Views of nature

- Textural variety

- Concern for aesthetics including the use of art

As Watson (1999, p. 257) points out, "in spite of Nightingale's attention to environment, and in spite of the nursing metaparadigm including environment as part of its subject matter and practice focus, nursing has not systematically heeded this domain in practice."

Table 1-1

Comparisons Between Health Protection, Health Promotion, and Healing

	HEALTH PROTECTION	HEALTH PROMOTION	HEALING
FOCUS	Actions designed to avoid or ward off threats to health	Actions and supports to improve or promote well-being or health	A sense of wholeness, integration, and harmony in which connections are re-established to and within self, and to others, and with one's purpose
KEY CONCEPTS	Relative risk (probability of anger) Levels of prevention: • Primary • Secondary • Tertiary	Lifestyle behaviors Individual responsibility Planned change Empowerment	Relationships (connections) Presence Nurse as facilitating environment Noninvasive therapies
DISCIPLINES	Medicine Public health Epidemiology	Health education Nursing Social work	Holistic nursing Integrative health promotion Physical and occupational therapy

Selected distinctions between health protection, health promotion, and healing are presented in Table 1-1.

Holistic Nursing Practice

Traditionally nurses have practiced according to the beliefs and values of the biomedical system's disease world view. (See Chapter 3 for a discussion of the beliefs and values of the biomedical system). Holistic nursing is not a system of nursing practice, but is characterized by person worldview philosophical values and therapies that contrast with the conventional way of conceptualizing and practicing professional nursing. For example, in holistic nursing, the client is viewed as a whole in mutual process with the environment. The emphasis of care, in active partnership with the client, is on mobilizing strengths to reduce vulnerabilities. Dossey (1999, p. 322) describes holistic nursing as "a philosophy and a model that integrates concepts of presence, healing, and holism." Additionally, according to the American Holistic Nurses' Association (AHNA, 1993), "holistic practice draws on nursing knowledge, theories, expertise, and intuition to guide nurses in becoming therapeutic partners with clients in strengthening the clients' responses to facilitate the healing process and achieve wholeness."

The healing relationship is discussed in depth in Chapter 10. And, noninvasive therapies are discussed extensively in all of Section IV. Selected characteristics of holistic nursing are presented in Box 1-4.

Box 1-4

Selected Characteristics of Holistic Nursing

- The person is viewed as a whole (bio-psycho-social-spiritual aspects) and in mutual process with the environment.
- The focus of nursing is on promoting self-healing by the client.
- Nursing emphasizes presence and mutuality in relationship with the client.
- The client is actively involved and empowered in a partnership with the nurse.
- The client's strengths are mobilized to reduce vulnerabilities.
- Each person is different and, therefore, care must be individualized.
- Noninvasive therapies are used to pattern a healing environment.
- Outcomes include increased well-being, quality of life, and growth of the client and the nurse toward a new level of evolving capacities, diversity, and complexity.

Advantages of Holistic Nursing Practice to Promote Healing

Noninvasive therapeutic modalities often enhance the well-being of individuals without the risks of drugs and other invasive therapies. Although they are not, in themselves, curative, holistic interventions stimulate the healing response. Individuals can learn and use many mind-body healing modalities independently. This empowers people to heal themselves more effectively and to independently enhance their quality of life. Empowerment means that the nurse "provide[s] people with the chance to be involved in their own care, to make vital decisions about their own health, to be touched at deep emotional levels, and to be changed psychologically in the process" (Berman & Larson, 1994, p. 35).

The nurse helps clients to access their own healing capacities. "Nurses offer the gift of walking with a person so that he or she is not alone at the crossroads of healing.... It is possible to cultivate the skill of becoming an instrument and sensing the open door through which healing can emerge.... As nurses offer partnership in the journey of healing, they offer new insights, ways of coping, and a release from the bondage of fear and pain" (McKivergin, 1997, p. 24).

Use of noninvasive therapeutic interventions also fosters professional autonomy, and has financial efficacy, often reducing or containing the cost of care. Holistic interventions are appropriately employed and evaluated by nurses in partnership with clients, in contrast to the limited autonomy for both nurse and client often found in a hospital setting. "The inpatient care system favors the [client] becoming a recipient of care rather than an agent of self-care" (Hravnak, 1998, p. 285).

Integrative Health Promotion

Integrative health promotion is based on a combination of a healing philosophy and the utilization of both health protection/promotion strategies and holistic, noninvasive therapeutic nursing modalities to facilitate the health of individuals, families, and communities, locally and globally. Integrative health promotion for nursing practice proposes utilization of the content of health protection and promotion strategies (disease worldview) within the healing processes that characterize the person worldview of health. This is consistent with the suggestion that worldviews can be viewed "as different ways of perceiving reality, rather than as views of differing realities" (Leddy, 2000, p. 227). Both content and process are recognized as aspects of reality. As a result, research findings about behavior change strategies implementing primary, secondary, or tertiary prevention to reduce health risk and promote health can be incorporated within a philosophy and an approach to nursing practice that emphasizes the processes of healing and holistic nursing. This combination has been labeled here as integrative nursing.

Healing is considered an innate capacity of the person in a healing philosophy. Therefore, the role of the nurse is to facilitate healing by removing barriers to the healing process and participate in creating an environment that will support healing (Quinn, 1992). A healing relationship, based on presence and mutuality, is central to fulfillment of the nurse's role. Healing must emerge rather than result from specific interventions. This shifts the nurse's emphasis from doing to being.

In integrative health promotion, the professional nurse and client enter a partnership, in which the nurse consults with the client to empower the client for self-healing. The focus is on mobilizing client strengths, to reduce vulnerability due to environmental risks and lifestyle behaviors, and to foster growth and meaning. Health is viewed as a process rather than cure of disease. Care is individualized, based on theory and reflective thought, but also directed toward environmental and policy contexts that support health.

Viewing the client as a whole in mutual process with the natural and social environment emphasizes strategies to promote health patterning. A number of noninvasive therapeutic strategies or modalities (discussed in this book) can be taught to clients. Prevention of risk, lifestyle behavior change strategies, and holistic modalities may be utilized by clients to enhance healing. Therefore, the nurses' ability to help clients to select and perform relevant strategies or modalities is relevant to integrative health promotion in all practice settings. It is important that nurses actualize their essential role in health promotion within acute care settings as well as with ambulatory clients in community settings. In addition, it is important that nurses assume a much more active role in promoting the health of communities, both locally and globally.

Chapter Key Points

- Both the disease and the person worldviews of health have important implications for practice and nursing science.

- Disease, illness, sickness, health status, role performance, and wellness are concepts associated with the disease perspective of health.

- Pattern, increased diversity, unitary, and becoming are concepts associated with the person perspective of health.

- Health promotion activities need to be applied at behavioral (individual), ecological (environmental), and policy (societal) levels.

- Health protection, as a medical approach, emphasizes the prevention of disease risk factors and disease.

- In the medical approach to "health," the emphasis is on disease in primary, secondary, and tertiary prevention.

- Holistic nursing emphasizes the whole person, individualized care, and an empowering partnership with the client that is based on mutuality and presence, in order to promote self-healing and growth.

- The facilitation of healing toward wholeness, harmony, and therefore health of nurses and clients, is the essence of holistic nursing.

- Integrative health promotion is based on a healing philosophy and utilizes both health protection/promotion strategies and holistic, noninvasive therapeutic nursing modalities to facilitate the health of individuals, families, and communities, locally and globally.

References

Achterberg, J., Dossey, B., & Kolkmeier, L. (1994). *Rituals of healing: Using imagery for health and wellness.* New York: Bantam.

Aldana, S. G. (2001). Financial impact of health promotion programs: A comprehensive review of the literature. *American Journal of Health Promotion, 15,* 296-320.

American Holistic Nurses' Association (1993). *Description of holistic nursing.* Flagstaff, AZ: American Holistic Nurses' Association.

Anderson, C. A. (1997). The economics of health promotion. *Nurs Outlook, 45,* 105-106.

Ardell, D. B. (1979). The nature and implications of high level wellness, or why "normal health" is in a rather sorry state of existence. *Health Values, 3,* 17-24.

Benner, P., Tanner, C. A., & Chesla, C. A. (1996). *Expertise in nursing practice: Caring, clinical judgment and ethics.* New York: Springer.

Benson, A., & Latter, S. (1998). Implementing health promoting nursing: The integration of interpersonal skills and health promotion. *J Adv Nurs, 27*, 100-107.

Berman, B. M., & Larson, D. B. (Eds.). (1994). *Alternative medicine: Expanding medical horizons.* Washington, DC: U.S. Government Printing Office.

Breckon, D. J., Harvey, J. R., & Lancaster, R. B. (1994). *Community health education: Settings, roles and skills for the 21st century* (3rd ed.). Gaithersburg, MD: Aspen.

Breslow, L. (1999). From disease prevention to health promotion. *JAMA, 281*, 1030-1033.

Clark, C. C. (1996). *Wellness practitioner* (2nd ed.). New York: Springer.

Clark, E. G., & Leavell, H. R. (1965). Levels of application of preventive medicine. In H. Leavell, & A. E. Clark (Eds.), *Preventive medicine for doctors in the community* (3rd ed., pp. 14-38). New York: McGraw-Hill.

Cumulative Index to Nursing and Allied Health Literature (1992). Glendale, CA: CINAHL Information Systems.

Cunningham, A. (2001). Healing through the mind: Extending out theories, research, and clinical practice. *Adv Mind Body Med, 17*, 214-227.

Delaney, F. (1994). Nursing and health promotion: Conceptual concerns. *J Adv Nurs, 20*, 828-835.

Dossey, B. (1999). Holistic nursing. In W. B. Jonas, & J. S. Levin (Eds.), *Essentials of complementary and alternative medicine* (pp. 322-339). Philadelphia: Lippincott Williams & Wilkins.

Dubos, R. (1978, January). Health and creative adaptation. *Human Nature, 1*, 74-82.

Dunn, H. L. (1977, January/February). What high-level wellness means. *Health Values, 1*, 9-16.

Forde, O. L. (1998). Is imposing risk awareness cultural imperialism? *Soc Sci Med, 47*, 1155-1159.

Gillis, A. (1995). Exploring nursing outcomes for health promotion. *Nursing Forum, 30*, 5-12.

Green, L. W., & Kreuter, M. W. (1991). *Health promotion planning: An educational and environmental approach.* Mountain View, CA: Mayfield Press.

Hartrick, G. (1998). Developing health promoting practices: A transformative process. *Nurs Outlook, 46*, 219-225.

Hravnak, M. (1998). Is there a health promotion and protection foundation to the practice of acute care nurse practitioners? *AACN Clinical Issues, 9*, 283-289.

Huff, R. M., & Kline, M. V. (1999). *Promoting health in multicultural populations: A handbook for practitioners.* Thousand Oaks, CA: Sage.

Integrative Medicine Consult. (1999). Boston, MA: Interactive Medicine Communications.

Jahnke, R. (1997). *The healer within: The four essential self-care methods for creating optimal health.* San Francisco: Harper Collins.

Kavanagh, A. M., & Broom, D. H. (1998). Embodied risk: My body, myself? *Soc Sci Med, 46*, 437-444.

Kemper, D. W. (1992). Is health promotion in America misdirected? An international conference report. *American Journal of Health Promotion, 6*, 174.

Kritek, P. B. (Ed.). (1997). *Reflections on healing: A central nursing construct.* New York: National League for Nursing.

Kulbok, P. A., Baldwin, J., Cox, C., & Duffy, R. (1997). Advancing discourse on health promotion: Beyond mainstream thinking. *Advances in Nursing Science, 20*(1), 12-20.

Leddy, S. K. (1995). Measuring mutual process: Development and psychometric testing of the Person-Environment Participation Scale. *Visions: Journal of Rogerian Nursing Science, 3,* 20-31.

Leddy, S. K. (2000). Toward a complementary perspective on worldviews. *Nursing Science Quarterly, 13,* 225-233.

McCabe, P. (1998). Revealing common ground: Comparing themes in traditional natural medicine and holistic nursing. *Australian Journal of Holistic Nursing, 5,* 41-46.

McKivergin, M. (1997). The nurse as an instrument of healing. In B. M. Dossey (Ed.), *Core curriculum for holistic nursing.* Gaithersburg, MD: Aspen

McWilliams, C. L., Stewart, M., Brown, J., Desai, K., & Coderre, P. (1996). Creating health with chronic illness. *Advances in Nursing Science, 18,* 1-15.

Medich, C. J., Stuart, E., & Chase, S. K. (1997). Healing through integration: Promoting wellness in cardiac rehabilitation. *J Cardiovasc Nurs, 11,* 10-26.

Newman, M. A. (1994). *Health as expanding consciousness* (2nd ed.). St Louis: Mosby.

Nightingale, F. (1859). *Notes on nursing: What it is, and what it is not.* London: Harrison & Sons.

O'Neill, M. (1997). Health promotion: Issues for the year 2000. *Canadian Journal of Nursing Research, 29,* 71-77.

Parsons, T. (1958). Definitions of health and illness in light of American values and social structure. In E. G. Jaco (Ed.), *Patients, physicians, and illness,* pp. 120-144. Glencoe, IL: The Free Press.

Pender, N. J. (1990). Expressing health through lifestyle patterns. *Nursing Science Quarterly, 3,* 115-122.

Pender, N. J., Murdaugh, C. L., & Parsons, M. A. (2002). *Health promotion in nursing practice* (4th ed.). Upper Saddle River, NJ: Prentice Hall.

Quinn, J. F. (1989). On healing, wholeness, and the Haelan effect. *Nursing and Health Care, 10,* 553-556.

Quinn, J. F. (1992). Holding sacred space: The nurse as healing environment. *Holistic Nursing Practice, 6,* 26-36.

Quinn, J. F. (1997). Healing: A model for an integrative health care system. *Advanced Practice Quarterly, 3*(1), 1-7.

Robertson, A., & Minkler, M. (1994). New health promotion movement: A critical examination. *Health Education Quarterly, 21,* 295-312.

Rosenow, D. J. (1997). Some core components of healing: A theory of self-reintegration: A journey within oneself. In P. B. Kritek (Ed.), *Reflections on healing: A central nursing construct* (pp. 500-517). New York: National League for Nursing.

Roy, S. C., & Andrews, H. A. (1999). *The Roy adaptation model* (2nd ed.). Stamford, CT: Appleton & Lange.

Rutten, A. (1995). The implementation of health promotion: A new structural perspective. *Soc Sci Med, 41,* 1627-1637.

Scandrett-Hibdon, S. (1996). The history of energy-oriented healing. In D. Hover-Kramer, *Healing touch: A resource for health care professionals* (pp. 18-21). Albany, NY: Delmar.

Schlitz, M. (1995). Intentionality in healing: Mapping the integration of body, mind, and spirit. *Altern Ther Heatlh Med,* , 119-120.

Smith, J. A. (1981). The idea of health. A philosophic inquiry. *Advances in Nursing Science, 3,* 43-50.

Smith, T. W., & Orleans, C. T. (2004). Prevention and health promotion: Decodes of progress, new challenges, and an emerging agenda. *Health Psychology, 23,* 126-131.

Stokols, D. (1996). Translating social ecological theory into guidelines for community health promotion. *American Journal of Health Promotion, 10,* 282-298.

Twaddle, A. C. (1977). *A sociology of health.* St. Louis: Mosby.

U.S. Department of Health and Human Services. (2000). *Healthy people 2010.* Washington, DC: U.S. Government Printing Office.

Waters, P. J., & Daubenmire, M. J. (1997). Therapeutic capacity: The critical variance in nursing practice. In P. B. Kritek (Ed.), *Reflections on healing: A central nursing construct* (pp. 56-68). New York: National League for Nursing.

Watson, J. (1999). *Postmodern nursing and beyond.* Edinburgh, UK: Churchill Livingstone.

Wells-Federman, C. L. (1998). Awakening the nurse healer within (pp. 108-122). In C. Guzzetta (Ed.), *Essential readings in holistic nursing.* Gaithersburg, MD: Aspen.

Wendler, M. C. (1996). Understanding healing: A conceptual analysis. *J Adv Nurs, 24,* 836-842.

Whitehead, D. (2004). Health promotion and health education: Advancing the concepts. *Journal of Advanced Nursing, 47,* 311-320.

Williams, A. (1998). Therapeutic landscapes in holistic medicine. *Soc Sci Med, 46,* 1193-1203.

Winett, R. A. (1995). A framework for health promotion and disease prevention programs. *Am Psychol, 50,* 341-350.

Woods, N. F., Laffrey, S., Duffy, M., Lentz, M. J., Mitchell, E. S., Taylor, D., et al. (1988). Being healthy: Women's images. *Advances in Nursing Science, 11,* 36-46.

World Health Organization. (1986). *The Ottawa charter for health promotion.* Ottawa, Canada: WHO, Canadian Public Health Association, and Health & Welfare.

HEALTH STRENGTHS

Abstract

The chapter begins with a brief review of conceptual approaches to health and illness and a description of a strengths approach to health promotion. The healthiness theory (Leddy, 1996) that forms the structure for this book is then introduced. Aspects and concepts of the theory are described, and measurement and empirical research results are reviewed.

Learning Outcomes

By the end of the chapter the student should be able to:

- Describe two models of health in terms of their different views of change
- Identify five advantages of a strengths approach to health promotion
- Understand how a strengths approach affects the nurse–client relationship
- Explain the aspects and concepts that compose the healthiness theory
- Briefly describe the characteristics of each of the concepts in the healthiness theory and possible interventions that would foster healthiness

The Strengths Perspective

The dominant model of "health" focuses on negatively conceived states such as illness, sickness, and disease. Health may be dichotomized into wellness and illness, or viewed as a continuum from an ideal state of high-level wellness to terminal illness and death. When viewed on a continuum, the absence of disease defines health. From the viewpoint that "normal" human functioning operates within a relatively narrow range of balance or stability (homeostasis), human and environmental interactions pose potential threats to health.

Alternatively, as in this book, health can be perceived as a single process of ups and downs, in which disease and nondisease are viewed as complementary facets of health. Illness, like wellness, simply represents a pattern of life at a particular moment. This text primarily focuses on promoting strengths and positive manifestations such as well-being, harmony, and growth. In this model, change is inevitable and provides an opportunity for growth and the development of potential toward increased complexity. The emphasis for nursing knowledge development and practice is on appreciation of changing pattern manifestations, facilitation of self-healing, and deliberate environmental manipulation to promote growth.

However, although the focus in this book is on the promotion of positive resources for health, this is not meant to imply that the "negative side," comprising responses to threats and stressors, is unimportant (Held, 2004). Both positive and negative responses that occur in person–environment mutual processes function dialectically (growth occurs through synchronizing the contradictions and paradoxes that exist between complementary opposing views). Examples of such opposing views are happiness/sorrow, gains/losses, and yin/yang, in which positive/negative are not absolute states but depend on the perspective of the person. However, given that so much of the literature focuses on the negative, to provide balance, a positive perspective and positive resources are emphasized in this book.

Health promotion focuses on positive health, and its main aim is the building of strengths, competencies, and resources. Human strengths are resources for health. By identifying, acknowledging, concentrating on, and increasing strengths and environmental resources, it is believed that individuals can be helped to improve human functioning and well-being. This requires a shift in perspective to a practice that is perspective based, that focuses on strengths and solutions, and that is based on "proactive constructionist tendencies rather than reaction, coping, and repair" (Nakamura & Csikszentmihalyi, 2003, p. 262). Implicitly promoting a proactive and positive approach, the First International Conference on Health Promotion (held in 1986 in Ottawa, Canada) outlined five levels of action: (1) building public health policy, (2) creating supportive environments, (3) strengthening community action, (4) developing personal skills, and (5) reorienting the health system (WHO, 1986). This book will emphasize the development of personal skills.

Evidence indicates that depression and anxiety can be prevented and good social relationships can be promoted by teaching people when to use strengths, rather than focusing exclusively on repairing damage (Seligman, 2002). Feeling good can make people more optimistic, resilient, and socially connected. Positive beliefs may be tied to physiological changes by positive affect. Positive beliefs may also be connected to physical disease by promoting health through better health behaviors, conscientious application of positive health habits, and appropriate use of health services.

Positive functioning incorporates self-acceptance, personal growth, purpose in life, environmental mastery, autonomy, and positive relations with others including social coherence, actualization, integration, acceptance, and contribution (Keyes & Lopez, 2002). Examples of other positive attributes include courage, interpersonal skill, rationality, insight, optimism, authenticity, perseverance, realism, capacity for pleasure, future-mindedness, personal responsibility, and purpose. Interpersonal or relational attributes include patience, empathy, compassion, cooperation, tolerance, appreciation of diversity, understanding, and forgiveness (Aspinwall & Staudinger, 2003).

Implications of a strengths perspective include a significant alteration in how health professionals think about clients and their families with whom they work, how they think about themselves as professionals, the nature of the knowledge base for practice, and the process of nursing practice itself. What is needed is an egalitarian, collaborative working relationship in a practice based on strengths and solutions (Blundo, 2001). Intentional interventions can foster a client's anticipation of future contingencies, reflection on capability to cope, the ability to elicit and use information, flexibility to change her or his perspective on a problem and plan a course of action, and self-regulation (Aspinwall & Staudinger, 2003; Caprara & Cervone, 2003). Pruning, the giving up of the unattainable, and persevering rather than giving up, are also helpful qualities that can be nurtured. Promoting these outcomes requires the nurse to understand developmental, material, and social contexts that are promoting or debilitating for human strengths.

The Theory of Healthiness

The Theory of Healthiness forms the structural basis for this book. In this theory, health is conceptualized as a dynamically changing life process that manifests the pattern of the unitary human being. One manifestation of health pattern is healthiness, which is defined as a measurable process characterized by mutual process among perceived purpose, connections, and the power to achieve goals. "Healthiness reflects a human being's perceived involvement in shaping change experienced in living. Therefore, healthiness is a resource that influences the ongoing patterning reflected in health" (Leddy, 1997, p. 49).

Purpose, the human being's attribution of significance and direction to the dynamic pattern of human–environment mutual process (participation), was initially conceived to incorporate the dimensions of (1) *meaningfulness* as connections (defined as having rewarding relationships with others) and the characterization of an aspect of the present or the desired future as having meaning, import, or value; and (2) *ends*, defined as goals that a person aims to reach or accomplish. However, when this descriptive theory was empirically tested using the Leddy Healthiness Scale (LHS) (Leddy, 1996), factor analysis separated the connections items into a third concept, which was labeled *connections*. The revised theory is depicted in Figure 2-1.

The theory proposes that by actively channeling energy, the human being gains *power*, which is the perceived ability to direct energy toward the achievement of goals. Power was conceived to incorporate the dimensions of *challenge*, which is perceived opportunity, excitement, curiosity, and/or involvement in change toward meaningful goals; *confidence*, which is

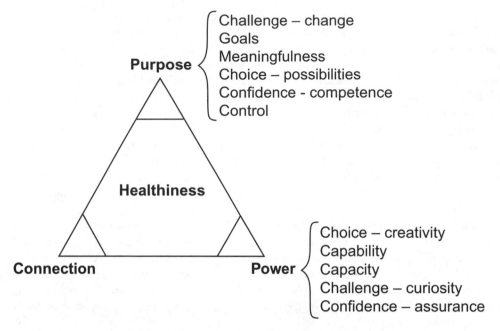

Figure 2-1. Empirically derived components of healthiness (© Copyright by Susan Kun Leddy, 2005. Permission to use granted by the copyright holder).

an assurance of the ability to successfully overcome obstacles to achieve goals; *capacity*, which is a perceived quantity of available energy; *choice*, the perceived freedom and creativity to select from among alternatives (possibilities) for action; *capability to function*, the perceived ability to work, play, and carry out activities of daily living; and *control*, which is the perceived ability to influence the rate, amount, and/or predictability of change.

MEANINGFULNESS

Meaning indicates both the comprehension of words, concepts, or an experience, and an appreciation of the significance of what is understood or perceived by the individual or group. "Meaning-as-comprehensibility refers to the extent to which the event makes sense, or fits with one's view of the world (e.g., as just, controllable, and nonrandom) whereas meaning-as-significance refers to the value or worth of the event for one's life" (Davis, Nolen-Hoeksema, & Larson, 1998, p. 562). *Meaning-as-comprehensibility* assumes that there is order in the universe, and that the distribution of negative and positive events are explainable. *Meaning-as-significance* is a motivational dimension that has to do with life goals and purpose (Park & Folkman, 1998). *Meaning* described in terms of *purpose* refers to beliefs that organize, justify, and direct a person's striving. Accordingly, goals (the other concept that, with meaning, comprise purpose in the healthiness theory) constitute a central element of a person's meaning system.

Meaning is constructed or created by people. Frankl (1978) wrote persuasively that people need to perceive life as making sense in serving some worthy purpose. When meaning is created from experience, life is given a sense of coherence as well as purpose (King, 2004). Three commonly accepted defining characteristics of meaning are purpose (the present has meaning because of the connection with future events), value (provides a sense of goodness or positiveness to life and can provide a justification for a particular course of action), and personal worth (Baumeister & Vohs, 1998). When an outcome perspective is adopted, *meaning* is viewed as coming from extrinsic things that a person wishes to accomplish or have. In contrast, when a process-oriented perspective is used, it helps a person to understand why life experiences are significant and meaningful (King, 2004).

The literature describes two different types of meaning: specific meanings *in* life (situational meaning) and the ultimate meaning *of* life (existential meaning). Situational meaning can be created through cognitive appraisal in daily engagement, commitment, and the pursuit of life goals. Situational meaning can include finding an explanation for an occurrence (sense-making) or finding meaning (meaning-making) by trying to understand why a threatening event happened, what impact it has had, and reappraising to find a positive aspect in a negative event (Schwarzer & Knoll, 2003). Behavior is likely to be motivated in direct relation to how important the individual considers the beliefs, goals, or commitments that are harmed, threatened, or challenged in a given situation (Park & Folkman, 1998).

In contrast, existential (global) meaning is an abstract, generalized sense that may be discovered through religious beliefs, philosophical reflections, and psychological reflection (Wong, 1998). Wong describes existential meaning as "the need for order and coherence in the midst of chaos, the need for personal significance and self-worth in the face of entropy and death, the need for positive meanings in spite of the negative life events that often overwhelm" (p. 396).

Life meaning can be categorized into achievement/work, relationships/intimacy, self-transcendence/generativity, and religion/spirituality domains. Generativity is related to strivings that involve creating, giving of oneself to others, or having an influence on future generations. These kinds of activities seem to result in higher levels of life satisfaction and positive affect (Emmons, 2003). Spirituality includes the desire to establish a relationship with a transcendent dimension of reality. Intimacy, generativity, and spirituality provide intrinsic rewards for goal activity, particularly compared to strivings for power or self-sufficiency (Emmons, 2003).

Schwarzer & Taubert (2002) suggest that cognitive, motivational, affective, relational, and personal dimensions are involved in the conceptualization of a meaningful life. The cognitive dimension includes a belief that there is an ultimate purpose in life, moral laws, and an afterlife. Consequently, the individual pursues worthwhile goals, seeks to actualize his or her potential, and strives toward personal growth, all of which are examples of the motivational dimension. As part of the affective dimension, the individual feels content with the person he or she is and what he or she is doing, feels fulfilled about what he or she has accomplished, and feels satisfied with life. Reflective of the relational dimension, the individual is sincere and honest with others, has a number of good friends, and brings happiness to others. The personal dimension is exemplified by a liking of challenge, acceptance of his or her limitations, and a healthy self-concept.

GOALS

Much of the literature on goals is based on expectancy–value models of motivation. These models suggest that effort requires sufficient confidence in the eventual attainment of a goal (expectancy), and also a goal that matters enough (value) (Carver & Scheier, 2003). Thus, a sense of optimism leads to confidence about successful outcomes; this results in persistence of effort to accomplish goals.

"To be lived well, life must have purpose" (Ryff & Singer, 1998, p. 216). Goals structure life and add purpose. Goals can reflect core values, are associated with projects and pursuits that give meaning and dignity to daily existence, compensate for inferiority feelings, provide meaning in the present and promote hope for the future, and facilitate the realization of an individual's potential. Purpose in life and personal growth are not only contributors to health, but in fact are characteristic features of health (Griffith & Graham, 2004; Ryff & Singer, 1998).

Goals are actions, end states, or values that people see as either desirable or undesirable. A goal that matters gives a person a reason to act. By giving meaning and purpose to people's lives, goals energize and direct activities and determine the direction, intensity, and duration of action. Commitment is "the belief that the goal is important and the belief that one can achieve or make progress toward it" (Locke, 2003, p. 305). Self-enhancement goals include strivings for achievement, agency, and power. Group-enhancement goals include affiliation, intimacy, communion, relatedness, and interpersonal connection. Global-enhancement goals include protecting the environment, improving the quality of life of all people, and eradicating crime and warfare (Schmuck & Sheldon, 2001).

Values are achieved by pursuing goals. People pursue multiple values and thus multiple goals in life, but priorities of values are critical to managing one's life, both in the short range and in the long range (Locke, 2003). However, in the absence of emotion, values would be experienced as dry, abstract, and intellectual. By providing energy, emotions provide an impetus to action. They also serve as a reward for successful action and an inducement to avoid actions that cause pain or suffering. "Emotional intensity reflects subconscious perceived value, threat, or achievement as well as the value in one's value hierarchy" (Locke, 2003, p. 302).

The highest task performance is attained when performance goals are both specific and difficult (Locke, 2003). The discrepancy between input and reference value determines approach or avoidance goals. Approach goals reduce discrepancy while avoidance goals increase differences. Goals can be differentiated on the basis of level of abstraction from concrete to abstract, and vary in importance, with higher levels usually more important. Additionally goals can be described as intrinsic or extrinsic in origin.

Although people are inclined toward activity and integration, they are vulnerable to passivity. Motivation is a critical variable in producing and maintaining change (Ryan & Deci, 2000). Intrinsic motivation is an inherent tendency to seek out novelty and challenges; to extend and exercise one's capacities; to explore, learn, and achieve personal growth, happiness, and meaningful relationships; and to make a contribution to society (Bauer & McAdams, 2004; Ryan & Deci, 2000). Tangible rewards, threats, deadlines, directives, pressured evaluations, and imposed goals diminish intrinsic motivation, while choice, acknowledgement of feelings, and opportunities for self-direction enhance intrinsic motivation by increasing feelings of autonomy. In contrast, external regulation by individuals or groups has been associated with less demonstrated interest, valuing, and effort toward achievement; a concern for money, status, possessions, and physical appearance; and a tendency to disown responsibility for negative outcomes (Bauer & McAdams, 2004).

CONNECTIONS

Connectedness occurs when a person is actively involved with another person (interpersonal), object, group (social), or environment (natural or man-made), and that involvement promotes a sense of comfort, well-being, and reduced anxiety (Hagerty, Lynch-Sauer, Patusky, & Bouwsema, 1993). All things have a unique connectedness that becomes the "respectful, responsible, trusting, and spiritual operative intention between nurse and client" (Lowe, 2002, p. 6). Connectedness occurs through the dynamics of an interdependent and interrelated relationship.

One concept used interchangeably with connection is relatedness. *Relatedness* refers to an individual's involvement with other people, groups, or the natural environment (Patusky, 2002). Feeling cared for, as expressed in liking and concern, are critical to feeling comfortable, secure, and being willing to be self-expressive or responsive in a relationship (Reis, 2001). Relatedness expresses an individual's worldview beyond his or her own sense of self, involving connection and commitment to an outside entity (other humans or a spiritual being) or the environment (natural, physical, or social) (Hanley & Abell, 2002). The substance of the relationship in terms of mutuality and reciprocity, not just its usefulness, is important toward the goals of fulfillment and self-actualization. Creative and artistic expression are inherently relational as are relationships with the natural world and spiritual forces.

Although interaction is a single social event, which may occur between related or unrelated individuals, involvement requires the dedication of time or resources within a relationship (Ryan & Solky, 1996) and usually reflects validation. *Validation* refers to "appreciation for one's dispositions, beliefs, or life circumstances. It contributes to intimacy and meaningful interaction by suggesting that the other values and respects the emotional core of the self" (Reis, 2001, p. 80). A shared informational base of understanding (getting the facts straight) facilitates relatedness.

Additionally, autonomy support is a concept that is important for relatedness in cultures that emphasize an individualist focus. The need for autonomy refers to the human desire to have one's behavior determined by the self, to be capable of action, self-expressive, and spontaneous in action. Autonomy support refers to the ability to assume another's perspective and to facilitate self-initiated expression and action. Autonomy support thus typically involves authentic acknowledgement of the other person's perceptions, acceptance of their feelings, and a lack of attempts to control the other's experience and behavior (Ryan & Solky, 1996). Autonomy support facilitates development, expression, and integration of the self and buffers one from negative outcomes during distress. Consequently, outcomes include increasing self-esteem, self-confidence, feelings of capability and competence, vitality, and feelings of connectedness with others. Autonomy support is needed for social contacts to enhance psychological well-being (Ryan & Solky, 1996).

Patusky (2002) describes a nested ecological approach consisting of four levels of relatedness: the macrosystem (societal beliefs), ecosystem (groups that affect the immediate setting, e.g., work), microsystem (family unit), and ontogenetic (individual development). Within each level, four states of relatedness have been identified: connectedness (comfortable involvement), disconnectedness, parallelism, and enmeshment. Competencies that were associated with these states included synchrony, sense of belonging, reciprocity, and mutuality (Patusky, 2002).

A relationship is an enduring association and an ongoing connection between two persons in which the bond has a sense of history and some awareness of the nature of the relationship; the participants influence each other's thoughts, feelings, and behavior; and they expect to interact again in the future (Reis, 2001). Relationships that heal, soothe, foster growth, facilitate health, and provide satisfactions are essential to a sense of well-being (Ryan & Solky, 1996). The capacity for authentic contact draws out and supports real feelings, sensibilities, and choices, providing a sense of support and nurturance (Ryan & Solky, 1996). Consequently, a sense of belonging is experienced when a person perceives a "fit" with another person, group, or environment, and he or she feels valued, needed, and important within relationships (Hagerty & Patusky, 2003).

Relationships have three domains of impact: the affective, the cognitive, and the behavioral. In the affective domain the question is: How do people feel about each other? In the cognitive domain the question is: what thoughts do people think about each other? And, in the behavioral domain the question is: how do people treat each other? (Kenny, 1994).

CAPABILITY

The concept *capability* is defined as the global belief that one has the ability to achieve desired goals. "Broader and more general dispositional measures are usually better suited for predicting more general patterns of behavior or outcomes that arise across multiple contexts" (Smith, Wallston, & Smith, 1995, p. 52). Similar to the concept of agency, or self-agency, the person views himself or herself as capable of shaping motives, behavior, and future possibilities. Capability is therefore influenced by choice, control, and confidence in the ability to accomplish goals. However, in contrast to the concept of competence, capability does not indicate skill or proficiency in a task. Capability has no action component.

Capability requires confidence, creativity, general cognitive (intellectual) and communication abilities, and specialized knowledge for performance in a particular content area. Other, more general abilities include oral and written mastery of one's own language and at least one foreign language, as well as the following abilities:

- mathematical knowledge

- reading competence for rapid acquisition and concrete processing of written information

- media competence

- independent learning strategies

- social competencies

- divergent thinking, critical judgments, and self-criticism.

In contrast, self-efficacy is related to perceived capability (*can* is a judgment of capability) in specific situations. Bandura (1997) claims that self-efficacy should be assessed at the optimal level of specificity that corresponds to the specific task being assessed and the domain of functioning being analyzed. Self-efficacy also includes an action component, as in feeling capable to perform a specific task. "Self-efficacy is not a personality trait, but a temporary and easy to influence characteristic that is strictly situation- and task-related" (van der Bijl & Shortridge-Baggett, 2001, p. 190).

CONTROL

Personal control consists of personal and environmental beliefs and expectations about how the environment can be effectively shaped and altered so that positive events can be brought about and negative events avoided (Peterson & Stunkard, 1989; Ross & Sastry, 1999). The concept of control is closely related to other concepts that make up *power* in the healthiness theory, specifically choice, confidence, and capability. Personal control may be activated only in the course of meeting challenge.

Perceived control is "the expectation of having the power to participate in making decisions in order to obtain desirable consequences and a sense of personal competence in a given situation" (Rodin, 1990, p. 4). Consequently, the person has a feeling that he or she is influential enough (rather than helpless) to make decisions and affect outcomes. The person also has a perception of himself or herself as having a definite influence on a structured and responsive environment through the exercise of imagination, knowledge, skill, and choice.

In addition to the outcome expectancy (contingency beliefs) described above, perceived control has been understood by Grob (2000) as a composite with an expectation of efficacy (competence beliefs), and the importance to the person of the domains in which perceived control can operate (control expectancy). "The expectancy component refers to generalized cognitive estimates of the amount of control one possesses, whereas the appraisal component refers to the valuation or perceived importance of the situation at stake" (p. 333).

Skinner (1996) suggests that constructs of control include agent–ends relations such as perceived control, personal control, and sense of control; agent–means relations such as capability, beliefs about agency and capacity, and self-efficacy; and means–ends relations such as locus of control, attributions, and responsibility.

The sense of personal control is learned. It is a generalized expectation that events and circumstances in an individual's life depend on personal choices and actions. Individuals with high levels of control use persistence and attention to address problems and are more likely to take action when difficulties arise. In contrast, low levels of control undermine the individual's will and motivation to cope actively with problems (Sastry & Ross, 1998). Intellectual, emotional, behavioral, and physiological vigor in the face of challenging situations and events is associated with high personal control (Peterson & Stunkard, 1989).

Although perceived control is a cognitive appraisal of "the perceived ability to significantly alter events" (Skinner, 1996, p. 549) and includes expectations of having the power to participate in making decisions in a given situation in order to obtain desirable consequences and a sense of personal competence (Rodin, 1990), perception may not be congruent with objective data. Objective or actual control is the demonstrated ability to regulate or influence the attainment, maintenance, or avoidance of intended outcomes through selective responses (Grob, 2000; Rodin, 1990). Objective control involves the actual ability to regulate or influence intended outcomes (Rodin, 1990). One's degree of influence of actual personal control may be affected by chance, luck, fate, or powerful others. Ideally, perceived control is related to actual control.

Belief about control can be a cognitive appraisal in a specific context (situational), or a general, global, dispositional belief (Lazarus & Folkman, 1984). Situational control appraisals are domain specific, based on the valuing of various domains (e.g., health, work, etc.), similar to self-efficacy, and involve the person's beliefs that he or she can shape and influence a particular person–environment process. Situational control is socially transmitted and thus based on a socially structured view of the individual as multidimensional and amenable to relearning and change. Control can also be classified as global. A global sense of control involves "a belief that in general individuals are able to control the conditions of their lives" (Pearlin & Paoli, 2003). Global control is more than an average of goal-specific manifestations and is related to long-term outcomes.

Perceived control involves the judgment that one can obtain desired outcomes and avoid undesirable ones (Thompson, 2002). A potentially negative event is not as stressful when it is accompanied by a belief in personal control. Perceived control is associated with positive emotions, leads to active problem solving, reduces anxiety in the form of stress, and buffers against negative psychological responses (Thompson, 2002). Perceived control consists of two parts: locus of control and self-efficacy (Thompson, 2002). Making progress toward goals is an important source of perceived control and general well-being.

Control does not have to be realistic to be beneficial. Illusion of control (events that are objectively random) has a positive effect on various types of behavior. "Perception of control is often enough to reduce stress, increase motivation, and encourage performance" (Peterson & Stunkard, 1989, p. 820). This occurs through (1) self-fulfilling prophecies that perceptually diminish the magnitude of threats and reduce barriers to taking actions capable of overcoming the threat; (2) alliances with groups and collectives; (3) social support; (4) appeals to higher powers; and (5) negotiation.

A balanced sense of control may foster adaptive planning, as individuals with too high a sense of control may not plan due to a false sense of security, and individuals with too low a sense of control may not plan because they assume they cannot have any influence over the outcome (Clark-Plaskie & Lachman, 1999).

CHOICE

Choice means more than its commonsense implication of making conscious decisions. Choice is motivational rather than cognitive, and is not synonymous with decision making. Freedom has to do with the extent to which a person is his own master, with decisions depending on him- or herself and not on external forces or circumstances. "Freedom is quintessentially concerned with the absence of restraint and interference by others" (Sen, 1988, p. 273). Deprivation of freedom can be considered a deprivation of power.

This is a freedom *to* rather than freedom *from*, and it involves noninterference, meaning that no constraints are imposed on an individual in the exercise of his or her liberty. The individual must make a voluntary, intuitive, and spontaneous choice free from undue influence or coercion. Freedom is not a property or something an individual possesses, but a relationship between agents (Bavetta & Del Seta, 2001).

An individual's decisions depend on the individual to the extent that there are alternatives to choose from. Greater freedom of choice designates "an increased flexibility, a widened spectrum of possible responses to inner and outer stimuli, and an expanded universe of psychological possibilities" (Abend, 2001, p. 3). Thus, freedom is viewed as variety, nonrestrict-edness in choice, and freedom from constraints (Bavetta & Del Seta, 2001). Availability of opportunities reflects a certain degree of freedom.

The value of choice is that it will lead to something (Suzuki, 2002, p. 126). "Choice is not just about being able to choose between a bottle of wine and a banana. It is rather about one's choice of what bottle of wine to buy being totally unrestricted and autonomous" (Bavetta & Del Seta, 2001, p. 220). However, an individual may be unable to enlarge his or her effective liberty if the options available are similar to alternatives already available. Increased alternatives also lead to increased preference. Choice is assumed to go in the direction of the alternative that is perceived to be more attractive.

For example, in a multichoice task study, a student's preference for an alternative depended on opportunity of choice, reinforcement, efficacy of choice, and the number of alternatives. Undistinguishable options, when one has no reason to choose one option rather than another, provide another kind of choice that seems to not be very significant. Choiceful accommodation gives a realistic sense of what is possible (Deci & Ryan, 1985).

CHALLENGE

The literature refers to *challenge* exclusively from within a perspective of stress and coping. Stress is relational in nature, arising from some sort of transaction between the individual and the environment. Stress therefore arises from a judgment that particular demands exceed resources for dealing with them and thus affect one's sense of well-being. Initially, through primary appraisal, a person judges what is at stake. Secondary appraisal then, is concerned with the controllability of the situation. When a situation is appraised as an opportunity for self-growth and coping strategies available to manage the demands are identified, the stress is perceived in terms of challenge (Drach-Zahavy & Erez, 2002).

A disposition toward challenge is expressed as the belief that change rather than stability is normal in life and that anticipation of change is an interesting incentive to growth rather than a threat to security (Kobasa, Maddi, & Kahn, 1982). Challenge occurs when the situation relates to goals, and environmental demands are appraised as within the person's resources or ability to cope. A challenge response is associated with a positive affect or low negative affect and efficient or organized mobilization of physiological resources (Tomaka, Blascovich, Kibler, & Ernst, 1997). Feeling positive about a demanding encounter is a hallmark of feeling challenged (Lazarus & Folkman, 1984) and is reflected in the pleasurable emotions accompanying challenge. "Challenge is experienced when there is an opportunity for self-growth with available coping strategies" (Drach-Zahavy & Erez, 2002, p. 667).

Cognitive appraisal processes intervene between the initial perception and subsequent experience of a potentially stressful situation (Tomaka et al., 1997). "Challenge will lead to attempts to transform oneself and thereby grow rather than conserve and protect what one can of the previous existence" (Kobasa et al., 1982, p. 170). The challenged person feels more confident, less emotionally overwhelmed, and more capable of drawing on available resources than the person who is inhibited or blocked by their response to appraised threat (Lazarus & Folkman, 1984). Challenge appraisals focus on the potential for gain or growth, and they are characterized by pleasurable emotions such as eagerness, excitement, and exhilaration. In contrast, threat focuses on potential harms and is characterized by negative emotions such as fear, anxiety, and anger. Threat appraisal may be a consequence of adequate strengths that could buffer stress. In other words, a strong reservoir of strength could increase an individual's appraisal of potential stressors as challenge rather than threat. However, perception of inequalities, that life has been unfair, and lower socioeconomic standing decrease the odds of having positive psychological experiences.

People who strive to accomplish difficult goals when task complexity is high may perceive their goal as a challenge rather than a threat, leading to high levels of performance (Drach-Zahavy & Erez, 2002). Complex tasks differ from simple tasks in terms of the number of performance components (component complexity), such as the number of acts to perform or the amount of information to remember; coordination required to complete the task (coordinating complexity); and changes in the potential predictability of acts and information cues (dynamic complexity). Effective performance of complex tasks depends on the amount of effort exerted in the task and the development of relevant strategies. "A challenge requires stretching one's abilities, in order to try something new (Deci & Ryan, 1985). The emotions of enjoyment and excitement represent the rewards.

Threat and challenge are not necessarily poles of a single continuum and thus mutually exclusive (Lazarus & Folkman, 1984). Challenge and threat appraisals have their own distinct patterns of coping, with challenge leading to a vigilant coping pattern. Associations have been found between challenge and opportunities for success and social rewards such as recognition and praise, mastery, learning, and personal growth (Skinner & Brewer, 2002), and:

- positive emotions such as happiness and hope and challenge cognitions such as expectation of favorable performance, certainty of performance level, perceptions of increased control, and anticipation of effort
- hope–challenge emotions and perceptions of increased problem-focused coping opportunities and optimistic expectations
- challenge emotions and appraisals of effort and interest such as feeling confident, hopeful, or eager (Skinner & Brewer, 2002)

CONFIDENCE

Confidence is a strong, generalized positive belief or certainty about oneself. Confidence leads to increased persistence and perseverance toward goals. The confident person is sure of him- or herself. Confidence is closely related to self-image and the cognitive decision-making process behind taking action (Kear, 2000). Consequently, in the literature, confidence is implicit in discussions of self-concept and self-esteem. Confidence is associated with sureness in belief about self and is an antecedent to control. In contrast, beliefs about ability to act in a specific context to accomplish anything one sets out to do are more closely associated with capability. Confidence facilitates and may mediate capability.

Self-confidence helps to buffer performance anxiety. Hanton, Mellalieu, and Hall (2004) found that in the absence of self-confidence, increases in competitive anxiety intensity were perceived as outside of the performer's control and debilitating to performance. Under conditions of high self-confidence, increases in symptoms were reported to lead to positive perceptions of control and facilitative interpretations. To protect against debilitating interpretations of competitive anxiety, performers reported the use of cognitive management strategies including mental rehearsal, thought stopping, and positive self-talk.

CAPACITY

A unitary perspective of energy includes the concept of a (1) universal essence composed of particles and waves, and three interchangeable facets: *matter*, which is the potential for structure and identity; *information*, which is the potential for coordination and pattern; and *energy*, which is the potential for process, movement, and change; (2) the concept of a field as a nonobservable domain of influence; (3) a pattern; (4) the oscillation of waves, which determines frequency, amplitude, and resonance of energy; (5) synchronization; and (6) conscious focusing of energy vibrations. It has been proposed that the nurse can facilitate health patterning by fostering resonance of environmental energy and information (Leddy, 2003).

It is proposed here that universal essence is manifested in two energy fields. One field, "vital" energy, is associated with the informational aspect of universal essence. Vital energy ensures the cohesiveness and unity of the human. The other field, "metabolic" energy, is associated with the matter aspect of universal essence. Metabolic energy encompasses the potential processes that ensure the effective functioning of the human. Capacity, as it is conceptualized in this book, requires system integration, although the ways in which the fields engage in mutual processes are not articulated yet.

Capacity is composed of both vital and metabolic energy. It enables a "quantity" of material matter and the movement necessary for process. Capacity is an active strength, expressed in vigor and vitality. Peterson and Seligman (2004, p. 273) describe vitality as "a dynamic aspect of well-being marked by the subjective experience of energy and aliveness." Capacity can be decreased by factors such as conflict, stress, illness symptoms (e.g., pain and fatigue), and unbalanced nutrition. Capacity can be increased by contact with outdoor natural environments, relatedness, enjoyable physical activity, a nutritious diet, and noninvasive therapeutic modalities (e.g., meditation, yoga, and imagery) that facilitate calmness and harmony.

Capacity has a reciprocal relationship with the other strengths in the healthiness theory. Capacity "energizes" the other strengths, as it is rejuvenated by them.

Chapter Key Points

- Health can be perceived as a single process of ups and downs, in which disease and nondisease are viewed as complementary facets of health. Illness, like wellness, simply represents a pattern of life at a particular moment.

- The primary focus in this book is on promoting strengths and positive manifestations such as well-being, harmony, and growth. In this model, change is inevitable and provides an opportunity for growth and the development of potential toward increased complexity.

- The emphasis for nursing knowledge development and practice is on appreciation of changing pattern manifestations, facilitation of self-healing, and deliberate environmental manipulation to promote growth.

■ Health promotion focuses on positive health and the building of strengths, competencies, and resources. Human strengths are resources for health. By identifying, acknowledging, concentrating on, and increasing strengths and environmental resources, it is believed that individuals can be helped to improve human functioning and well-being.

■ One manifestation of health pattern is healthiness, which is defined as a measurable process characterized by mutual processes among perceived purpose, connections, and the power to achieve goals.

■ The healthiness theory includes the dimensions of meaningfulness, goals, connectedness, challenge, confidence, capacity, choice, capability to function, and control.

References

Abend, S. M. (2001). Expanding psychological possibilities. *Psychoanalytic Quarterly, 70*, 3–14.

Aspinwall, L. G., & Staudinger, U. M. (Eds.), (2003). A psychology of human strengths: Some central issues of an emerging field. *A psychology of human strengths. Fundamental questions and future directions for a positive psychology* (pp. 9–22). Washington, DC: American Psychological Association.

Bandura, A. (1997). *Self-efficacy: The exercise of control.* New York: Freeman.

Bauer, J. J., & McAdams, D. P. (2004). Growth goals, maturity, and well-being. *Developmental Psychology, 40*, 114–127.

Baumeister, R. F., & Vohs, K. D. (1998). In P. T. P. Wong & P. S. Fry (Eds.), *The human quest for meaning: A handbook of psychological research and clinical applications* (pp. 608–618). Mahwah, NJ: Lawrence Erlbaum.

Bavetta, S., & Del Seta, M. (2001). Constraints and the measurement of freedom of choice. *Theory and Decision, 50*, 213–238.

Blundo, R. (2001). Learning strengths-based practice: Challenging our personal and professional frames. *Families in society: The Journal of Contemporary Human Services, 82*, 296–304.

Caprara, G. V., & Cervone, D. (2003). A conception of personality for a psychology of human strengths: Personality as an agentic, self-regulating system. In L. G. Aspinwall & U. M. Staudinger (Eds.), *A psychology of human strengths. Fundamental questions and future directions for a positive psychology* (pp. 61–74). Washington, DC: American Psychological Association.

Carver, C. S., & Scheier, M. F. (2003). Three human strengths. In L. G. Aspinwall & U. M. Staudinger (Eds.), *A psychology of human strengths: Fundamental questions and future directions for a positive psychology* (pp. 87–102). Washington, DC: American Psychological Association.

Clark-Plaskie, M., & Lachman, M. E. (1999). The sense of control in mid-life. In S. L. Willis & J. D. Reid (Eds.), *Life in the middle: Psychological and social development in middle age* (pp. 182–208). San Diego, CA: Academic Press.

Davis, C. G., Nolen-Hoeksema, S., & Larson, J. (1998). Making sense of loss and benefiting from the experience: Two construals of meaning. *Journal of Personality and Social Psychology, 75*, 561–574.

Deci, E. L., & Ryan, R. M. (1985). *Intrinsic motivation and self-determination in human behavior.* New York: Plenum Press.

Drach-Zahavy, A., & Erez, M. (2002). Challenge versus threat effects on the goal-performance relationship. *Organizational Behavior and Human Decision Processes, 88,* 667–682.

Emmons, R. A. (2003). Personal goals, life meaning, and virtue: Wellsprings of a positive life. In C. L. M. Keyes & J. Haidt (Eds.), *Flourishing: Positive psychology and the life well-lived* (pp. 105–123). Washington, DC: American Psychological Association.

Frankl, V. E. (1978). *The unheard cry for meaning. Psychotherapy and humanism.* New York: Simon & Schuster.

Griffith, B. A., & Graham, C. C. (2004). Meeting needs and making meaning: The pursuit of goals. *Journal of Individual Psychology, 60,* 25–41.

Grob, A. (2000). Perceived control and subjective well-being across nations and across the life span. In E. Diener & E. M. Suh (Eds.), *Culture and subjective well-being* (pp. 319–339). Cambridge, MA: MIT Press.

Hagerty, B. M. K., Lynch-Sauer, J., Patusky, K. L., & Bouwsema, M. (1993). An emerging theory of human relatedness. *Image: Journal of Nursing Scholarship, 25,* 291–296.

Hagerty, B. M., & Patusky, K. L. (2003). Reconceptualizing the nurse-patient relationship. *Journal of Nursing Scholarship, 35,* 145–150.

Hanley, S. J., & Abell, S. C. (2002). Maslow and relatedness: Creating an interpersonal model of self-actualization. *Journal of Humanistic Psychology, 42,* 37–57.

Hanton, S., Mellalieu, S. D., & Hall, R. (2004). Self-confidence and anxiety interpretation: A qualitative investigation. *Psychology of Sport & Exercise, 5,* 477–495.

Held, B. S. (2004). The negative side of positive psychology. *Journal of Humanistic Psychology, 44,* 9–46.

Kear, M. (2000). Concept analysis of self-efficacy. Retrieved May 5, 2004, from http://www.graduateresearch.com/Kear.htm

Kenny, D. A. (1994). Using the social relations model to understand relationships. In R. Erber & R. Gilmour (Eds.), *Theoretical frameworks for personal relationships* (pp. 111–127). Hillsdale, NJ: Lawrence Erlbaum.

Keyes, C. L. M., & Lopez, S. J. (2002). Toward a science of mental health. In C. R. Snyder & S. J. Lopez (Eds.), *Handbook of positive psychology* (pp. 45–59). Oxford: Oxford University Press.

King, G. A. (2004). The meaning of life experiences: Application of a meta-model to rehabilitation sciences and services. *American Journal of Orthopsychiatry, 74,* 73–84.

Kobasa, S. C., Maddi, S. R., & Kahn, S. (1982). Hardiness and health: A perspective study. *Journal of Personality and Social Psychology, 42,* 168–177.

Lazarus, R. S., & Folkman, S. (1984). *Stress, appraisal, and coping.* New York: Springer.

Leddy, S. K. (1996). Development and psychometric testing of the Leddy Healthiness Scale. *Research in Nursing & Health, 19,* 431–440.

Leddy, S. K. (1997). Healthiness, fatigue, and symptom experiences in women with and without breast cancer. *Holistic Nursing Practice, 12,* 48–53.

Leddy, S. K. (2003). A nursing practice theory: Applying a unitary perspective of energy. *Visions: The Journal of Rogerian Scholarship, 11,* 21–28.

Locke, E. A. (2003). Setting goals for life and happiness. In C. R. Snyder & S. J. Lopez (Eds.), *Handbook of positive psychology* (pp. 299–312). Oxford: Oxford University Press.

Lowe, J. (2002). Balance and harmony through connectedness: The intentionality of Native American nurses. *Holistic Nursing Practice, 16,* 4–11.

Nakamura, J., & Csikszentmihalyi, M. (2003). The motivational sources of creativity as viewed from the paradigm of positive psychology. In L. G. Aspinwall & U. M. Staudinger (Eds.), *A psychology of human strengths. Fundamental questions and future directions for a positive psychology* (pp. 257–269). Washington, DC: American Psychological Association.

Park, C. L., & Folkman, S. (1998). Meaning in the context of stress and coping. *Review of General Psychology, 1,* 115–144.

Patusky, K. L. (2002). Relatedness theory as a framework for the treatment of fatigued women. *Archives of Psychiatric Nursing, XVI,* 224–231.

Pearlin, L. I., & Paoli, M. F. (2003). Personal control: Some conceptual turf and future directions. In S. H. Zarit, L. J. Pearlin, & K. W. Schaie (Eds.), *Personal control in social and life course contexts* (pp. 1–21). New York: Springer.

Peterson, C., & Seligman, M. E. P. (2004). *Character strengths and virtues: A handbook and classification* (pp. 273–289). Washington, DC: American Psychological Association.

Peterson, C., & Stunkard, A. J. (1989). Personal control and health promotion. *Social Science and Medicine, 28,* 819–828.

Reis, H. T. (2001). Relationship experiences and emotional well-being. In C. D. Ryff & B. H. Singer (Eds.), *Emotion, social relationships, and health* (pp. 57–86). Oxford: Oxford University Press.

Rodin, J. (1990). Control by any other name: Definitions, concepts, and processes. In J. Rodin, C. Schooler, & K. W. Schaie (Eds.), *Self-directedness: Cause and effects throughout the life course* (pp. 1–17). Hillsdale, NJ: Lawrence Erlbaum.

Ross, C. E., & Sastry, J. (1999). The sense of personal control: Social-structural causes and emotional consequences. In C. A. Aneshensel & J. C. Phelan (Eds.), *Handbook of the sociology of mental health* (pp. 369–394). New York: Kluwer Academic/Plenum.

Ryan, R. M., & Deci, E. L. (2000). Self-determination theory and the facilitation of intrinsic motivation, social development, and well-being. *American Psychologist, 55,* 68–78.

Ryan, R. M., & Solky, J. A. (1996). What is supportive about social support? In G. R. Pierce, B. R. Sarason, & I. G. Sarason (Eds.), *Handbook of social support and the family* (pp. 249–267). New York: The Plenum Press.

Ryff, C. D., & Singer, B. (1998). The role of purpose in life and personal growth in positive human health. In P. T. P. Wong & P. S. Fry (Eds.), *The human quest for meaning* (pp. 213–225). Mahwah, NJ: Lawrence Erlbaum.

Sastry, J. & Ross, C. E. (1998). Asian ethnicity and the sense of personal control. *Social Psychology Quarterly, 61,* 101–120.

Schmuck, P., & Sheldon, K. M. (2001). Life goals and well-being: To the frontiers of life goal research. In P. Schmuck & K. M. Sheldon (Eds.), *Life goals and well-being: Towards a positive psychology of human striving* (pp. 1–17). Seattle, WA: Hogrefe & Huber.

Schwarzer, R., & Knoll, N. (2003). Positive coping. Mastering demands and searching for meaning. In S. J. Lopez & C. R. Snyder (Eds.), *Positive psychological assessment. A handbook of models and measures* (pp. 393–409). Washington, DC: American Psychological Association.

Schwarzer, R., & Taubert, S. (2002). Tenacious goal pursuits and striving toward personal growth. In E. Frydenberg (Ed.), *Beyond coping: Meeting goals, visions, and challenges* (pp. 19–35). Oxford: Oxford University Press.

Seligman, M. E. P. (2002). Positive psychology, positive prevention, and positive therapy. In C. R. Snyder & S. J. Lopez (Eds.), *Handbook of positive psychology* (pp. 3–9). Oxford: Oxford University Press.

Sen, A. (1988). Freedom of choice. *European Economic Review, 32,* 269–294.

Skinner, E. A. (1996). A guide to constructs of control. *Journal of Personality and Social Psychology, 71,* 549–570.

Skinner, N., & Brewer, N. (2002). The dynamics of threat and challenge appraisals prior to stressful achievement events. *Journal of Personality and Social Psychology, 83,* 678–692.

Smith, M. S., Wallston, K. A., & Smith, C. A. (1995). The development and validation of the Perceived Health Competence Scale. *Health Education Research, 10,* 51–64.

Suzuki, S. (2002). Preference for freedom of choice. In S. P. Shohov (Ed.), *Advances in psychology research* (Vol 9, pp. 115–128). Huntington, NY: Nova Science.

Thompson, S. C. (2002). The role of personal control in adaptive functioning. In C. R. Snyder & S. J. Lopez (Eds.), *Handbook of positive psychology* (pp. 202–213). Oxford: Oxford University Press.

Tomaka, J., Blascovich, J., Kibler, J., & Ernst, J. M. (1997). Cognitive and physiological antecedents of threat and challenge appraisal. *Journal of Personality and Social Psychology, 73,* 63–72.

van der Bijl, J. J., & Shortridge-Baggett, L. M. (2001). The theory and measurement of the self-efficacy construct. *Scholarly Inquiry for Nursing Practice: An International Journal, 15,* 189–205.

Wong, P. T. P. (1998). Meaning-centered counseling. In P. T. P. Wong & P. S. Fry (Eds.), *The human quest for meaning: A handbook of psychological research and clinical applications* (pp. 395–435). Mahwah, NJ: Lawrence Erlbaum.

World Health Organization, Health and Welfare Canada, and the Canadian Public Health Association. (1986). *Ottawa charter for health promotion.* Copenhagen, Denmark: FADL.

THE MEANING OF HEALTH
Health Care Belief Systems

Abstract

Western biomedicine is assumed to be the world's standard health care system. However, this system only provides 10% to 30% of human health care. In this chapter, a number of popular (lay and community-based) and professional (Western biomedicine and traditional) health care belief systems are described. The intent is to help the student to appreciate the diversity of belief systems that provide a context for integrative health promotion.

Learning Outcomes

By the end of the chapter the student should be able to:

- Differentiate between popular and professional belief systems
- Discuss how mechanism, reductionism, and science have affected the development of values of the Western biomedical model
- Describe characteristics of several traditional medical belief systems

Today's rapidly changing environment creates important implications for health and health care delivery. Because of the conflicts inherent in many issues, the desirability and viability of potential approaches for resolution of an issue are strongly influenced by personal and cultural values.

Values are the criteria a person uses to evaluate the relative desirability, merit, usefulness, worth, or importance of objects, ideas, acts, feelings, or events (Hester, 1996). They are a standard for determining a preference between two or more alternatives, and are criteria for deciding what is desirable or desired. Values are also highly subjective. They are an underlying reason for a preference between choices, and are a motivating force for a particular choice of action. Discomfort results when choices and decisions are in conflict with a person's values.

Values are the result of multiple influences, which include the societal culture of which the person or group is a part. In order to better understand the values that underlie health and health care choices, beliefs within popular and professional medical care systems will be explored in this chapter. An understanding of these medical care systems provides one context for the integrative promotion of health in nursing practice.

Popular Health Care

LAY HEALTH CARE

Lay health care is what most people practice and receive at home, such as gargling with hot water and salt to relieve a sore throat. People get information about popular health care primarily from family or friends, but also learn from magazines, television, and other informal sources. Use of herbal preparations and food supplements, such as echinacea and zinc at the first signs of a cold, are examples of practices that are increasingly being popularized. In many cases, people are committed to popular practices that have the legitimacy of family tradition. Usually, evidence to support many popular practices is anecdotal rather than research-based. It is important for nurses to understand common popular beliefs and practices, and differentiate between those that are exclusively tradition-based and those beliefs and practices that have theoretical, empirical, and/or scientific support.

COMMUNITY-BASED HEALTH CARE

Community-based health care refers to the nonprofessionalized yet specialized health care practices of both rural and urban people (Berman & Larson, 1994). Community-based health care is derived from indigenous (endemic) health beliefs and incorporates such concepts as "folk," "native," and "tribal," that have often been treated stereotypically and assumed to be primitive, whimsical, exotic, and/or outmoded (Andrews, 1995). For example, in Latin American cultures, *mal de ojo* (related to the Mediterranean concept of "evil eye") is treated by rolling an egg over the person's (usually a child) body, then cracking it into a glass of water and placing it under the child's bed. When the egg and water solution is discarded the next day, so is the problem (Novey, 2000). Models of community-based health care are discussed in Chapter 5, *The Meaning of Health: Cultural Influences*.

The *American Heritage Dictionary* (Soukhanov, 1992, p. 919) describes *indigenous* as "originating and growing or living in an area or environment." An indigenous group may be bound by ethnicity, or may be made up of individuals from diverse ethnic groups and united by cultural role models and norms or religion. Most indigenous groups are distinct from what most would consider "mainstream society." Family may mean the extended family, a clan, a community, or an entire village. A great deal of importance is placed on social networks to maintain traditions, values, and beliefs, including health beliefs, that have endured over time and space. When one individual is sick, the entire community is viewed as having a problem (Berman & Larson, 1994). Health beliefs are often based on common sense and life experience. Similar to lay beliefs, information about community-based health care is commonly passed on orally and through informal and popular media sources.

Because the concepts of "medicine" and "religion" in community-based systems often are fused, no sickness can affect only one part of the body. Rather, it affects the whole network of existence, the natural world, and the spiritual world. Illness may be believed to be due either to not following the laws of nature or not maintaining harmony in one's life (Wing, 1998). Living in harmony with nature and maintaining balance in one's life are essential for health. Balance involves an equalization of opposites. The most frequent opposites that must be in balance are male and female, hot and cold, yin and yang, expulsion and retention, power or life force of one individual versus another, and good and evil. There is an implicit theme that a person with a naturally caused illness had a role in precipitating the illness by allowing him or herself to become stressed, not adhering to a taboo, or violating a law of nature. On the other hand, unnatural illness results from being an innocent victim of another's admiration or envy.

Another universal belief is that there is a biological energy that is present in every physical and mental event. This life energy has been called by many names including chi (qi) in China, prana in India, doshas in the Vedic tradition, and spirit in the Native American and Voodoo cultures. It is believed that if this energy is not kept moving, illness will occur due to imbalance and stagnation. Other aspects of motion are within the surrounding environment. "Wind, rain, flowing water, rustling trees, and animal life all contribute to the motion of the earth, necessary for peace and tranquility" (Wing, 1998, p. 148).

Professional Health Care

In contrast to lay and community-based health systems, professional health systems can be characterized by a(n):

- Tendency to be urban and complexly organized
- Theory of health and disease
- Educational curricula and schools to teach its concepts
- Delivery system involving practitioners who usually practice in hospitals, offices, or clinics
- Material support system to produce its medicines and therapeutic devices
- Legal and economic mandate to regulate its practice
- Set of cultural expectations about the role of the medical system
- Means to confer "professional" status on the approved providers

The values and beliefs that affect many professional health systems will be presented, after a brief discussion of the values that underpin the professional health system of biomedicine in the United States.

WESTERN BIOMEDICINE

Contemporary American Values

A number of American societal values have influenced the development of Western biomedical health beliefs, including the perceived desirability of morality, individualism, achievement, and progress.

Morality

Most of the original American pilgrims (settlers) were Puritans, a branch of Protestants within the Anglican church. Their beliefs were derived from the Judeo-Christian heritage of morality and belief in the inherent worth of the individual. The Puritans believed in an ordering of values, culminating in a supreme good. They were scrupulous in their adherence to a standard of right and wrong. Products of this religious past include belief in the sanctity of personal life, a sense of destiny, belief in the moral law that transcends the laws on the books, and a compulsive commitment to work.

The belief in the value of religion, values, and morality persists to this day. Some people argue that America is in a state of moral decay (e.g., rise in crime, illegitimacy, and high divorce rate) and that "as individuals and as a society, we need to return religion to its proper place. Religion, after all, provides us with moral bearings" (Bennett, 1995, p. 114). Although discussion of moral and bioethical issues (e.g., euthanasia, abortion, and rationing of resources) is still often based on an assumed collective standard of right and wrong, in contemporary society, there are now conflicting views of right and wrong (no absolute standards), and differences in valuing the legislation of morality versus individual belief and judgment.

Individualism

Historically, the hard life on the frontier encouraged self-reliance, which confirmed the individualism that was inherent in Puritanism. In contemporary society, self-motivation and willpower are considered to be essential to success. Individualism is now associated with autonomy, or self control, with an emphasis on both individual responsibility and rights. Personal freedom and liberty are associated with dignity.

However, an emphasis on individualism sets up a number of conflicts. Equality of relationships conflict with valuing of upward mobility in social status or standing. Self-reliance, or inner directedness, is in reaction to being directed by others (government). Therefore, a focus on independence, standing on one's own, and having a desire for privacy, compete with the need for community and association with others. In addition, there is concern that individualism threatens traditional community morality. Consensus and cooperation (instead of conformity) in order to succeed, and belongingness in the organization, are current reflections of the desire for community.

Achievement

With the industrial revolution and the development of business, achievement has come to be equated with success. Success is achieved through hard work, but also requires aggressiveness, competitiveness, courage and toughness in the pursuit of goals. It is believed that self-sacrifice will be rewarded with productivity. But, achievement may also come to be associated with the refusal to admit defeat. The emphasis on conquest over disease in American medicine may be viewed as an effort to achieve mastery over the "ultimate defeat": death.

Within this context, achievement requires an active agency in one's life. A person must work hard at being fit, strong, and healthy if he or she is to achieve success. As a consequence, the stereotype for physical attractiveness has become youth and vitality, which are viewed as functional advantages. For example, erect posture has become a metaphor for social stature. On the other hand, age has become associated with decline and handicap. Decreased mobility has become associated with dependence. Disease and dysfunction become a deviation, also leading to dependency.

Progress

Valuing the achievement of goals is naturally associated with a time orientation focused on the future rather than the past or present. Change, associated with optimism and faith in the future, can be viewed as growth, with newness seen as improvement and innovation. Education is valuable as a tool toward such growth. However, at its extreme, the possibility of progress without parameters becomes a quest for perfectibility. In addition, in American culture, the concept of progress has also become associated with materialism, as progress is equated with wealth. Another outcome of this orientation is "conspicuous consumption."

Biomedical Health Beliefs

Three major influences that have affected the development of values of the biomedical model of medicine are mechanism, reductionism, and science.

Mechanism

Western biomedicine developed as a profession during the industrial revolution, with an emphasis on mechanism and technology. A machine is comprised of separate interchangeable and replaceable components. Normative functioning (a standard based on group averages) is taken for granted as the desirable state of being, and any deviation from normal is labeled a disease with universal form, progress, and treatment. Since a machine is unable to modify itself, any change is the result of external influences (e.g., invasion of the individual by a microorganism). A machine is a passive recipient of being fixed. The machine metaphor applied to medicine leads to dehumanization of the "patient" with an emphasis on disease as a deviance from normal to be actively and quickly "cured" by the expert mechanic.

Reductionism

The machine metaphor is supported by reductionism, an analytical process that involves the division of a whole into parts to facilitate systematic and orderly thinking. Processes are broken into sequential steps, and complex systems are viewed in terms of distinct, separable, and often competitive components. For example, the body (matter) is seen as separate from the mind (spirit), with illness arising from one or the other. Individuals are viewed as separate from their environment and society. Specialization allows for depth of knowledge about isolated bits while hierarchy allows the division and organization of specialized laborers.

Science

The influence of science can be attributed to the desire for a rational system of truths from which accurate information about the world can be deduced with certainty and precision.

Science values rationality, logical thinking, and numerical measurement. Subjective feelings have little value. All "facts" have a specific cause which can be discovered through objective and verifiable observation. Effects can be attributed to a specific cause.

Other essential values of the Western biomedical system are (Dacher, 1995; Fulder, 1998; Larson-Presswalla, 1994):

- A healthy person is a symptom-free person; symptoms are defined as abnormalities that are recognized by professionals. They are not necessarily connected to the client's subjective experiences of illness.

- Phenomena must be observable or measurable to be considered real or acceptable.

- The aim is to repair biophysiologic abnormality and re-establish health, which is defined as the restoration of normal function. Health is a fixed, defined condition of the organism.

- The purpose of treatment is to cure, by killing or removing the "causative agent" (germs, tumors, faulty parts). The body can then restore balance to the system if intervention hasn't damaged it beyond the point where it can reestablish balance (Ranjan,1998).

"In its short history, modern medicine has proven to be so apparently effective, and so well adapted to the industrial worldview that it gave the impression that indigenous, ancient, or traditional medicine had no validity, and was nearly extinct" (Fulder, 1998, p. 147). However, Western biomedicine should be viewed as one of many professional belief systems and not a standard against which all other healing traditions should be evaluated (Thorne, 1993).

TRADITIONAL MEDICAL BELIEF SYSTEMS

Several labels are commonly used in the literature, often interchangeably, to describe non-conventional, non-Western biomedical health care systems. *Alternative* is currently interpreted as meaning in the place of mainstream medicine. *Complementary* is interpreted as meaning in addition to mainstream medicine. *Integrative* is interpreted as meaning in combination with mainstream medicine. In this book, the label *traditional* is used, to avoid defining all medical systems in relation to Western biomedicine. All of these labels refer to professional medical systems to diagnose and treat disease.

In the United States, many people assume that mainstream, Western biomedicine is the world's standard health care system and is accepted by most people most of the time. Actually, it has been estimated that "only 10% to 30% of human health care is delivered by the conventional, biomedically oriented health care system. The remaining 70% to 90% of health care includes everything from self-care according to folk principles to care rendered in an organized health care system based on an alternative tradition of practice" (Berman & Larson, 1994, pp. 67-68).

Changing needs and values in society, which include a rise in prevalence of chronic disease, an increase in public access to worldwide health information, reduced tolerance for paternalism, an increased sense of entitlement to a quality life, declining faith that scientific breakthroughs will have relevance for the personal treatment of disease, an increased interest in spiritualism, and concern about the adverse effects and escalating costs of conventional health care, are fueling the search for more traditional approaches (Jonas, 1998). Traditional health care systems "are safe and practitioners provide patients with understanding, meaning, and self-care methods for managing their condition. Empowerment, participation in the healing process, time, and personal attention are essential elements of all medicine. These elements are easily lost in the subspecialization, technology, and economics of modern medicine.... Conventional medicine can learn from [traditional health care systems] how to 'gentle' its approach by focusing on the patient's inherent capacity for self-healing" (Jonas, 1998, p. 1617).

Many traditional health care users are apparently not dissatisfied with conventional medicine, but find traditional alternatives to be more congruent with their own values, beliefs, and philosophical orientations toward health and life (Astin, 1998). "Use of at least 1 of 16 [traditional] therapies during the previous year increased from 33.8% in 1990 to 42.1% in 1997" (Eisenberg et al., 1998, p. 1569). According to Eisenberg and colleagues, the therapies that increased the most included herbal medicine, massage, megavitamins, self-help groups, folk remedies, energy healing, and homeopathy. Traditional therapies were used most frequently for chronic conditions such as back problems, anxiety, depression, and headaches. However, there is a danger that the "economic promise of growing markets may lead to a focus on developing profitable [traditional health care] products rather than on improving health care and may also lead away from addressing issues that have prompted the public to seek [traditional health care] practices" (Eskinazi, 1998, p. 1623).

Major Values of Traditional Health Systems

There are a number of values that differentiate traditional health systems from Western biomedicine. For example, the person and not his or her symptoms is treated and self-healing is most important. The client is actively involved in partnership with the provider, and the client is empowered to accept responsibility for part of the task of recovery and future health maintenance. Major values of traditional health systems, derived from the following sources, Burton Goldberg Group, 1995, pp. 14-15; Fulder, 1993, pp. 110-111; Fulder, 1998, pp. 148-155; Lyng, 1990; Wing, 1998, p. 151, are presented in Box 3-1.

Fulder (1998, pp. 155-156) has described the following characteristics of health within traditional health belief systems:

1. Living a nontoxic life, with emphasis on sound nutrition, a balanced lifestyle, adequate and appropriate exercise, rest, sleep, and emotional tranquillity.

2. Being sensitive to deep signs of function and dysfunction.

3. Understanding ones' own constitution and its patterns and needs.

4. Respecting the unknown, indeterminacy, the wild side of life, and change.

5. Knowing health as a journey, a process.

6. Knowing when to use what remedies or professional help.

7. Having a life-affirming attitude or the will to be well.

Box 3-1

Values of Traditional Health Systems

- Mind-body-heart-spirit and environment-society-individual are viewed as integrated and without boundaries.

- The individual, not his or her symptoms is treated. Each person's background, condition, and treatment path is different. Symptoms are a guide in the journey to a cure and an opportunity to learn about oneself. They are managed, not suppressed. Clients may be essentially symptom-free, or symptoms can precede the appearance of pathology.

- Self-healing is paramount. Resistance is improved by preventive measures, restoration of vital force, and trust in self-healing energy.

- The individual is empowered to accept responsibility for at least a part of the task of recovery and future health maintenance. Conscious attention can lead to informed choices.

- Health is a process and a journey without a beginning or ending.

- Health is considered "movement toward balance," which is not synonymous with homeostasis.

- Active involvement of the client in partnership with the provider. The practitioner is expected to share information and help the individual use the power of self-conscious will rather than to use power as a healer.

- Tends toward a state of harmony and balance between internal and external worlds such as seasons, environment, and social relations. Illness and wellness are defined contextually and the energetic dimension is often the best access point for the treatment of bodily dysfunction.

- Deals not only with disease but also with vulnerabilities. Disease does not result from a pathogen attack alone; it results from the interaction of the pathogen and a susceptible organism. Therefore, in order to decrease disease susceptibility and risk, the focus should be on increased resistance.

- There is a greater sense and respect for the unknown and a trust in empiricism (sensory experience as a source of knowledge) with a lack of urgency to construct explanatory models.

8. Having longevity.

9. Exhibiting vitalism and energy.

10. Having a subjective sense of well-being.

11. Developing a total accommodation to life and death.

No one major medical belief system has a monopoly over the right to practice medicine. A variety of traditional professional medical alternatives to the Western biomedical health care system currently exist. The traditional medical health belief systems of traditional Chinese medicine, Ayurvedic medicine, homeopathic medicine, anthroposophically extended medicine, naturopathic medicine, osteopathic medicine, chiropractic medicine, bioenergetic medicine, mind-body medicine, orthomolecular medicine, and environmental medicine will be reviewed briefly.

Traditional Chinese Medicine

The fundamental concepts of traditional Chinese medicine (TCM) are embedded in the philosophical and metaphysical worldviews of Taoism, Confucianism, and Buddhism. In the Eastern philosophies, all living processes are patterns of connected relationships and conditions, with health a result of the proper balance of conflicting influences, while the incidence of diseases might result from "transformations of the seasons and the 24 lunar sections in every year, day and night, morning and evening, noon and midnight, changes of weather, cold and hot, rain and wind; bright and dark, different regions, orientations and directions; [and] the varied changes of the body in the past and now" (Chongcheng & Qiuli, 2003, p. 310). Health is considered to be the ability of the organism to respond appropriately to a wide variety of challenges while maintaining equilibrium, integrity, and coherence" (Beinfield & Korngold, 1995, p. 45). Thus, purposes of TCM include relief of symptoms, increased physiological competence, enhanced recuperative power and immunity, decreased drug-reliance, and a contribution to a sense of greater health (Beinfield & Korngold, 1995). The first and most important principle of TCM is the prevention of illness through an appropriate lifestyle (Lao, 1999).

Major Concepts of TCM

According to TCM, there are five major concepts that interact to affect health. These are qi, yin/yang, energy phases, organ networks, and body climates.

Qi. "A human being is composed of qi (pronounced chee), moisture (body fluids), and blood (tissue) existing along a continuum that ranges from intangible to tangible. Shen, or mind, represents the nonmaterial expression of the individual; qi, the animating force that manifests as activity (moving, thinking, feeling, working) and warmth; moisture, the liquid medium that protects and lubricates tissue is tangibly more dense than qi but less so than blood; blood, the material out of which bones, nerves, skin, muscles, and organs are created, is yet more substantial; and essence (jing), the most dense substance, is the fundamental seed of reproduction and regeneration from which the physical body arises. Put simply, health exists if adequate qi, moisture, and blood are distributed equitably and smoothly" (Beinfield & Korngold, 1995, p. 45).

The most striking characteristic of Eastern medicine is its emphasis on diagnosing disturbances of qi, or vital energy, in health and disease. According to TCM theories, energy needs to flow, in balance, for the body to stay healthy, resistant to disease, and able to activate its own healing. Imbalances or blockages affect physiology and eventually pathologic changes (McGee et al., 1996).

Yin/yang. "Yin and yang are two stages of cyclical, opposing, but complementary, phenomena that exist in a state of dynamic equilibrium, with one constantly changing into the other. The concept of yin and yang harmony is a basic description of the interaction between the active and passive, stimulating and nurturing, masculine and feminine, and 'heavenly' and 'earthly' qualities that characterize living things" (Berman & Larson, 1994, p. 71). Every part of the human body has a predominantly yin or yang character. Yang corresponds to function and yin corresponds to structure. Yin and yang can be considered substitutes for inhibition and excitation (Chongcheng & Qiuli, 2003). All symptoms and signs can be interpreted as a loss of balance of yin and yang (Maciocia, 1989).

Energy phases. The five-phase theory explains relationships between the human body and the environment as well as relationships among internal organs. Each phase of energy is represented by the elemental natures of fire, earth, metal, water, and wood, which "define the various stages of transformation in the recurring natural cycles of seasonal change, growth and decay, shifting climatic conditions, sounds, flavours, emotions, and human physiology" (Reid, 1995, p. 49). Each phase of energy takes its name from the natural element that most closely resembles its function and character.

Organ networks. In addition, there are five functional systems (not physical organs) known as organ networks: liver, heart, spleen, lung, kidney. "Each organ network refers to a complete set of functions, physiological and psychological, rather than to a specific and discrete physical structure fixed in an anatomical location.... By treating the organs, emotional and mental processes can be modulated and enhanced" (Beinfield & Korngold, 1995, p. 48). Although some physiologic functions are similar to those in Western biomedicine, others are very different. For example, the heart is said to control mind activities as well as blood circulation.

Body climates. Finally, TCM identifies external, internal, and other factors that are pathogenic when they are excessive or the defensive qi of the body declines. The external body climates are described as cold, heat, wind, dampness, and dryness, and sometimes also fire. "The principle of complementarity applies: for cold, warm; for heat, cool; for congested qi, moisture; for blood, encourage movement; for depletion, nourish; for internal wind, subdue; for external wind, relieve surface congestion; and for phlegm, dissolve" (Beinfield & Korngold, 1995, p. 49). "The internal factors refer to the seven emotions: joy, anger, melancholy, worry, grief, fear, and fright... [while] the other factors include dietary irregularities, obsessive sexual activity, taxation fatigue, trauma, and parasites" (Lao, 1999, pp. 221-222).

"Diagnosis in TCM involves the classical procedures of observation, listening, questioning, and palpation, including feeling the quality of the pulses and the sensitivity of various body parts" (Beinfield & Korngold, 1995, p. 71). To reveal the severity, nature, and location of illness, "pulse diagnosis involves palpation along the radial artery at six positions and two depths" (p. 49), while tongue inspection involves observing the size, shape, and texture as well as the quality of fur. For further discussion of these techniques, see Chapter 7, Beyond Physical Assessment.

TCM Treatment Modalities

Treatment modalities most associated with TCM and used regularly by practitioners include acupuncture, moxibustion, acupressure, remedial massage, cupping, qigong, herbal medicine, and nutritional and dietary interventions.

Acupuncture. The therapeutic goal of acupuncture is to regulate or correct the flow of qi to restore health. By directly manipulating the network of energetic meridians, acupuncture increases the circulation of congested qi, moisture, and blood, relieving stagnation and obstruction of the organ networks associated with the channels. "Many of the therapeutic effects of acupuncture can be clearly related to the mechanism of chemical neurotransmitter release via peripheral nerve stimulation by puncturing the skin with a needle, heat, direct physical pressure (acupressure), fracture, suction, or impulses of electromagnetic energy to stimulate specific anatomic points, and, by so doing, enhances the self-regulatory, self-protective, and self-aware capacities of the organism" (Beinfield & Korngold, 1995, p. 50). Studies have shown evidence for the efficacy of acupuncture for osteoarthritis, chemotherapy-induced nausea, asthma, back pain, painful menstrual cycles, bladder instability, migraine headaches, chronic pain, and drug addiction.

Moxibustion. Moxibustion refers to the burning of the dried and powdered leaves of the artemesia vulgaris plant either on or in proximity to the skin. This leads to heating the body on the energetically active points in order to affect the movement of qi in the channel, locally or at a distance (Berman & Larson, 1994; Ergil, 2001).

Remedial massage. In remedial massage, vigorous pressing and rubbing hand motions (an-mo) tonify the system, while thrusting and rolling hand motions (tuina) soothe and sedate (Berman & Larson, 1994).

Cupping. Cupping "involves introducing a vacuum in a small glass or bamboo cup, and promptly applying it to the skin surface. This [suction] therapy brings blood and lymph to the skin surface under the cup, increasing local circulation" (Ergil, 2001, p. 325).

Qigong. Qi means "vital energy"; and gong means "training." Thus, qigong is "the art and science of using breath, movement, and meditation to cleanse, strengthen, and circulate vita; life energy and blood. Three basic principles of qigong exercises are relaxation and repose, association of breathing with attention, and the interaction of movement and rest" (Berman & Larson, 1994, pp. 72-73). Qigong exercise has been shown to affect strength, health, and longevity, and may reduce symptoms and improve appetite. (McGee et al., 1996). In human studies, qigong training (in the presence of a master instructor) has demonstrated the capacity to increase parasympathetic and decrease sympathetic activities, and produce analgesia. For example, qigong training was found to result in transient pain reduction and long-term anxiety reduction in a sample of 22 patients with late-stage complex regional pain syndrome (Wu et al., 1999, p. 45). In addition, qigong exercise has been shown to alter serum levels of epinephrine, dopamine, and serotonin. Some researchers report improvements in energy levels, bowel irregularity, body weight, leukopenia, and other side effects of chemotherapy in terminal cancer patients. Qigong training also appears to improve cardiac reserve in hypertensive, coronary heart disease (Wu et al., 1999). Qigong is discussed in depth in Chapter 13, *Re-establishing Energy Flow: Physical Activity and Exercise.*

Herbal medicine. "With herbs, active ingredients are enfolded within the whole plant, and this tends to buffer their side effects. Also, as herbs are often blended together to counteract undesired effects and enhance intended results, when they are used properly they rarely cause disagreeable consequences" (Beinfield & Korngold, 1995, p. 50). In TCM, medications are classified according to their energetic qualities and prescribed for their action on corresponding organ dysfunction, energy disorders, disturbed internal energy, blockage of the meridians, or seasonal physical demands. Herbs are discussed in depth in Chapter 12, *Relinquishing Bound Energy: Herbal Therapy and Aromatherapy*. A typical Chinese herbal formula usually includes the four components listed in Box 3-2.

Dietary interventions. Dietary interventions are individualized. "Foods, like herbs, are characterized according to their energetic qualities (e.g., tonifying, dispersing, heating, cooling, moistening, drying). Emphasis is given to eating in harmony with seasonal shifts and life activities" (Berman & Larson, 1994, p. 73). Nutrition is discussed in depth in Chapter 16.

Ayurvedic Medicine

Ayurveda, one of the oldest health care systems in the world, has its origins in the Sanskrit roots *ayu*, which means "longevity," and *ved*, which means "knowledge" (Mishra et al., 2001a). "In Vedic knowledge, the purpose of life is to know or realize the Creator (cosmic consciousness) and to express this divinity in one's daily life" (Lad, 1999, p. 200). Ayurveda provides an integrated approach to the prevention and treatment of illness through lifestyle interventions and a wide range of natural therapies.

The structural aspect of the body is made up of five elements, but the functional aspect of the body is governed by three metabolic principles, the *doshas*. The doshas are forces of energy, patterns, and movements, not substances and structures. Ether and air together constitute *vata* (the energy of movement); fire and water, *pitta* (the energy of digestion or metab-

Box 3-2

Components of Chinese Herbal Medicine

- The chief (principal) ingredient, which treats the principal pattern or disease.

- The deputy (associate) ingredient, which assists the chief ingredient in treating the major syndrome or serves as the main ingredient against a coexisting symptom.

- The assistant (adjuvant) ingredient, which enhances the effect of the chief ingredient, moderates or eliminates the toxicity of the chief or deputy ingredients, or can have the opposite function of the chief ingredient to produce supplementing effects.

- The envoy (guide) ingredient, which focuses the actions of the formula on a certain meridian or area of the body or harmonizes and integrates the actions of the other ingredients" (Lao, 1999, p. 225).

olism); and water and earth, *kapha* (the energy that forms the body's structure and holds the cells together). When balanced, vata creates energy and creativity, pitta creates perfect digestion and contentment, while kapha yields strength, stamina, immunity, and even temperament (Larson-Presswalla, 1994). In every person, the doshas that make up one's nature (prakriti) differ in emphases and combinations. To promote health, it is important to know one's prakriti, choose supportive influences, and avoid undermining influences (Titus, 1995).

According to Ayurveda, health is a state of balance between the body, mind, and consciousness. The body has its own intelligence to create balance, with therapeutic interventions helping in that process. Disharmony among the body and mental doshas constitutes disease. The essence of disease management is the restoration of harmonious dosha balance through "lifestyle interventions, spiritual nurturing, and treatment with herbo-mineral formulas based on one's mental and bodily constitution" (Mishra et al., 2001a, p. 36).

Disease and illness management in Ayurveda has four elements: 1) *shodan*, cleansing; 2) *shaman*, palliation; 3) *rasayan*, rejuvenation; and 4) *satwajaya*, mental nurturing and spiritual healing (Mishra et al., 2001b, p. 45). The primary Ayurvedic therapeutic methods are listed in Box 3-3.

Box 3-3

Primary Ayurvedic Therapeutic Methods

- *Pranayama.* The practice of alternative nostril breathing. It has an almost universal calming effect.

- *Abhyanga.* The practice of rubbing the skin with oil, usually sesame oil, to increase circulation and move lymph and toxins out of the body through the skin.

- *Rasayana.* Incorporates dosha-specific herbs and spoken mantras during meditation for the purpose of rejuvenation.

- *Yoga* (union, or joining in Sanskrit). Meditation through movement. Yoga has been demonstrated to improve blood pressure, metabolism, respiration, cardiac rhythms, skin resistance, alpha and theta brain waves, and body temperature.

- *Panchakarma.* A cleansing therapy. Patients are encouraged to sweat, eliminate fecal waste, and even vomit in an effort to cleanse the body of toxins (ama). Believed by some to prevent susceptibility to disease with change of season.

- *Herbal medicines.* Prescribed according to their effects on vayus (energy flow). Often given with warm milk, ghee (clarified butter), or nasyas (nasal rinse) (Lad, 1995, pp. 62-63; 1999).

In Ayurveda, all of life and nature are viewed as an interconnected expression of wholeness. Adjustment of diet and lifestyle in order to balance the doshic influences of the seasons is considered an important principle of Ayurvedic living (Titus, 1995). Specific lifestyle interventions are a major preventive and therapeutic approach in Ayurveda as well. Each person is prescribed an individualized dietary, eating, sleeping, and exercise program depending on his or her constitutional type (prakruti) and the underlying energy imbalance at the source of the illness.

Published studies have documented reductions in cardiovascular disease risk factors, including blood pressure, cholesterol, and reaction to stress, in individuals practicing Ayurvedic methods. Ayurvedic therapies have been shown to be potentially beneficial for the prevention and treatment of breast, lung, and colon cancers; mental health; infectious disease; health promotion; and aging (Berman & Larson, 1994). A considerable amount of data from both animal and human trials suggest the efficacy of Ayurvedic interventions in managing diabetes (Elder, 2004).

Homeopathic Medicine

The term homeopathy is derived from the Greek words *homeo* (similar) and *pathos* (suffering from disease). The first basic principles of homeopathy were formulated by the German physician Samuel Hahnemann in the late 1700s. Homeopathy considers illness to be primarily a disturbance of the vital force producing symptoms that are unique to each person (Jacobs & Moskowitz, 2001). What is needed is to treat the particular individual with the unique combination of substances that will relieve those symptoms.

The principle of similars, or "like cures like," proposes that a substance that can cause certain symptoms when given to a healthy person can cure those same symptoms in someone who is sick. The one remedy that most closely fits all of the symptoms of a given individual is called the similimum for that person. Homeopathic remedies are produced by a process called potentization, in which, by diluting them in a water-alcohol solution and then shaking, side effects can be diminished. When potentized to high dilutions, these remedies still produce a medicinal effect, with minimal side effects. By using the smallest possible doses and only repeating them if necessary, homeopaths allow remedies to complete their action without further interference. It is exceedingly unlikely that any untoward or dangerous side effects will occur, given the minuteness of the dose (Berman & Larson, 1994).

The effectiveness of homeopathic remedies has been demonstrated in many studies. For example, a study by Kuzeff (1998) found evidence for the ability of homeopathic prescribing to improve "sensation of well-being." Studies have suggested a positive effect of homeopathy on allergic rhinitis, fibrositis, rheumatoid arthritis, and influenza. A 1992 review of homeopathic clinical trials found that 15 of 22 well-designed studies showed positive results (Berman & Larson, 1994).

Seventeen schools in the United States and four in Canada offer homeopathic training. There are separate laws in each state governing who can practice homeopathy. Only medical doctors and osteopathic doctors can practice homeopathy in every state. There is no legal requirement for these practitioners to have any specific homeopathic qualifications. Many states also license naturopaths to practice homeopathy as well as physician's assistants and nurse practitioners. No diploma or certificate is recognized as a license to practice homeopathy in the United States (Bailey, 2002, p. 424).

Anthroposophically Extended Medicine

The foundations of anthroposophically extended medicine were laid down by the Austrian philosopher and spiritual scientist Rudolf Steiner (1861-1925). Steiner's anthroposophy (*anthropos* [human]; *sophia* [wisdom]) builds on naturopathy, homeopathy, and Western bioscientific medicine. The model includes the "sense-nerve system," which includes the mind and thinking process; the "rhythmic system," which includes the emotional or feeling processes; and the "metabolic-limb" system, which includes digestion, elimination, energetic metabolism, and the voluntary movement processes. This model provides "a scheme for understanding an illness as a deviation from the harmonious internal balance of the functions of the bodily self and the spiritual self" (Berman & Larson, 1994, p. 86). Medications seek to match the "archetypal forces" in plants, animals, and minerals with disease processes in humans.

Naturopathic Medicine

Naturopathic medicine integrates traditional natural therapeutics, including botanical medicine, clinical nutrition, homeopathy, acupuncture, traditional Eastern medicine, hydrotherapy, and naturopathic manipulative therapy, with modern scientific medical diagnostic science and standards of care. There are eight primary principles of naturopathic medicine (Berman & Larson, 1994, pp. 88-89):

1. Recognition of the inherent healing ability of the body.

2. Identification and treatment of the cause of diseases rather than mere elimination or suppression of symptoms.

3. Use of therapies that do no harm. Use the least invasive intervention.

4. Implementation of the physician's primary role as a teacher.

5. Establishment and maintenance of optimal health and balance.

6. Treatment of the whole person.

7. Prevention of disease through a healthy lifestyle and control of risk factors.

8. Therapeutic use of nutrition to promote health and to combat chronic and degenerative diseases.

Naturopaths emphasize identification and treatment of a disease source more than reducing the severity of symptoms. "In addition to physical and laboratory findings, important consideration is given to the [client's] mental, emotional, and spiritual attitude; lifestyle; diet; heredity; environment; and family and community life.... [Client] education and responsibility, lifestyle modification, preventive medicine, and wellness promotion are fundamental to naturopathic practice" (Pizzorno & Snyder, 2001, pp. 181-182). Other treatment modalities, in addition to the use of diet as therapy, include herbs, homeopathy, acupuncture, hydrotherapy, therapeutic use of touch, heat, cold, electricity and sound (physical medicine), endogenous and exogenous toxicity, counseling and lifestyle modification, and minor surgery (Pizzorno, 1996).

In general, licensing laws in all jurisdictions require completion of a naturopathic degree and diploma program at one of only five institutions in North America (Washington, Oregon, Arizona, Connecticut, and one in Canada). Laws governing naturopathic medicine require the successful completion of basic science and clinical board examinations (Smith & Logan, 2002).

Osteopathy

Osteopathy, a blend of holistic and conventional medical practices, was developed in the late 1800s by Andrew Taylor. It is based on treating illness through the manipulation of muscles and joints to restore the structure and balance of the musculoskeletal system. Asymmetry and pain are hallmark diagnoses, but osteopaths holistically consider the client's entire constitution, lifestyle, and psychology (Integrative Medicine Consult, 1998). Pharmacology and a symptom-oriented medical model are also integrated.

Osteopaths, whose educational degree is Doctor of Osteopathy (DO), are licensed as medical doctors in the United States. Important therapies include manipulative and re-educative approaches such as:

- *Gentle mobilization*. Moving a joint slowly through its range of motion, and then gradually increasing the motion to free the joint from restrictions.

- *Articulation*. A quick thrust (similar to chiropractic) when motion is severely restricted.

- *Functional and positional release methods*. Placing the client in a specific position to allow the body to relax and release muscle spasms that may have been caused by strain or injury.

- *Muscle energy technique*. Gently tensing and releasing specific muscles to produce relaxation.

- *Other soft tissue techniques*. Techniques to relax and release restrictions in the soft tissues of the body.

- *Cranial manipulation*. Very gentle and subtle cranial techniques used to treat conditions such as headaches, strokes, spinal cord injury, and tempromandibular joint syndrome dysfunction.

- *Relaxation*. Techniques to help reduce levels of excessive tension in muscles of people with joint and back problems.

- *Improved breathing methods*. Decrease the stress of back and neck muscles.

- *Postural correction*. To use the body in less stressful, more efficient and economical ways, reduce damage and tension affecting joints and soft tissues, and decrease fatigue.

- *Individualized nutritional guidance* (Integrative Medicine Consult, 1998, pp. 408-409).

Chiropractic

The three largest independent health professions in the Western world are allopathic medicine, dentistry, and then chiropractic medicine (Redwood, 1996). The chiropractor's scope of practice excludes surgery and pharmaceutical therapy, and centers on the manual adjustment or manipulation of the spine and nervous system to maintain or restore health.

Core chiropractic principles include (Redwood, 1996, p. 96):

1. Structure and function exist in intimate relation with one another.

2. Structural distortions can cause functional abnormalities.

3. Vertebral subluxation (misalignment) is a significant form of structural distortion and leads to a variety of functional abnormalities.

4. The nervous system plays a prominent role in the restoration and maintenance of proper bodily function.

5. Subluxation influences bodily function primarily through neurologic means.

6. Chiropractic adjustment is a specific and definitive method for the correction of vertebral subluxation.

Chiropractic treatment has been shown to be effective for controlling acute low back pain when used within the first month of symptoms and chronic, disabling lower back pain in cases where standard biomedical interventions have been exhausted. Chiropractic medicine has been shown to be more effective than the tricyclic antidepressant amitriptyline for long-term relief of pain from muscle tension headaches, while spinal manual therapy has been shown to be significantly more effective than a placebo treatment or treatment by a primary physician for persistent back and neck pain (Redwood, 1996). Studies are underway for migraine headaches, as is exploration of chiropracty's effects on visceral disorders.

Energy Medicine (Bioenergetic Medicine)

Bioenergetic medicine refers to therapies that "use an energy field—electrical, magnetic, sonic, acoustic, microwave, or infrared—to screen for or treat health conditions by detecting imbalances in the body's energy fields and then correcting them" (Integrative Medical Consult, 1998, p. 193). Bioenergetic medicine uses diagnostic screening devices to measure various electromagnetic frequencies in the body, including the electrocardiogram (EKG), electroencephalogram (EEG), electromyelogram (EMG), and magnetic resonance imaging (MRI).

It has been discovered that the electrical resistance of the skin decreases dramatically at the acupuncture points when compared with the surrounding skin. Each point appears to have a standard measurement for anyone who is in good health. This principle has been used in the development of assessment and treatment instruments. One instrument, the Dermatron, can be used for assessment of electrical resistance at acupuncture points. Another instrument, the MORA, raises or lowers aberrant electromagnetic waves and feeds the resultant normal waves back to the client through corresponding acupoints (Integrative Medical Consult, 1998).

Mind/Body Medicine

People have lost sight of the importance of the psychological, social, economic, and environmental influences on health and illness and of the extraordinary power of the mind to affect the body. Internal and external stimuli (e.g., memories, thoughts, emotions, body movements, sounds, smells, tastes, situations, and settings) can affect a variety of previously conditioned immune responses. Mind/body approaches focus on personal attitudes and lifestyle, the assumption of personal responsibility, and proactive self-motivation. The client/health practitioner relationship is considered a partnership, in which there is concern for "psychological development, individuation, personal transformation, and mastery, to the extent possible, over the activities of the mind and body" (Dacher, 1995, p. 191).

The principles of mind/body medicine (Benson, 1993; Burton Goldberg Group, 1995; Integrative Medical Consult, 1998) include:

- Each person is unique. No two people are alike, so even if they have the same disease, the paths to recovery may be different. Conversely, the same disease can be the result of different factors with different people.

- Chronic stress and lack of balance contribute to illness. Relaxation, positive methods of coping with stress, and restoration of balance lead to health.

- The client is an active partner in all stages of treatment, rather than a passive recipient of medical intervention.

- The healing process is viewed as a working partnership in which both parties respect the knowledge and intuition of the other.

- Illness may be only a manifestation of imbalance on the physical level, but the imbalance may also originate in other aspects of the self, such as the mental or emotional state.

- Part of healing involves the recognition and release of negative emotions. Having a sense of control, commitment, and connectedness—along with viewing change as a challenge rather than a threat—promotes the maintenance of good health even when under stress.

- Regulation of breathing plays an important role in mind/body medicine, because it is capable of bringing about a state of relaxation.

Orthomolecular Medicine

Orthomolecular medicine tries to create optimum nutritional balance in order to treat conditions such as depression, hypertension, schizophrenia, and cancer (Integrative Medical Consult, 1998). The types and amounts of the nutrients are determined by blood tests, urine analysis, and tests of nutrient levels based on biochemical individuality rather than recommended daily allowances (RDA) values. "Junk" foods, refined sugar, and food additives are eliminated, while promoting nutritious, whole foods, high in fiber and low in fat, supplemented by megavitamin therapy.

In support of orthomolecular medicine, it has been found that:

- Higher levels of beta-carotene (a precursor of vitamin A) are associated with lower rates of certain cancers.

- Intravenous magnesium sulfate (a mineral compound) is given in some hospitals to persons having a heart attack to speed recovery time.

- Chromium (a trace mineral) may be given to help regulate the body's response to sugar and insulin. It may help those with diabetes and hypoglycemia. It can also aid in lowering cholesterol.

- Essential fatty acids (unsaturated fats that the body cannot make for itself and must obtain from food sources), including omega-3 and omega-6, are now linked to a decrease in risk factors for heart disease and a lessening of symptoms of other diseases, including psoriasis and rheumatoid arthritis (Integrative Medical Consult, 1998, p. 401).

Environmental Medicine

Environmental medicine, with roots in the practice of allergy treatment by Theron Randolph in the 1940s, is based on the science of assessing the impact of environmental factors on health. It is the result of continuing study of the interfaces among chemicals, foods, and inhalants in the environment and the biological function of the individual. While the biomedical model holds that similar illnesses have the same cause in all clients and should be treated similarly, environmental medicine recognizes that an individual's illness can be caused by a broad range of substances, including foods and chemicals found in the home and workplace. Investigators are interested in things like "sick building syndrome;" the effects of chemicals like natural gas; industrial solvents; pesticides; car exhaust; chemicals in air, water, and food; and inhalant materials including pollens, molds, dust, dust mites, and danders (Berman & Larson, 1994).

The key to proper treatment is an accurate environmental history. Treatments, including immunotherapy, environmental controls, dietary management, and nutritional supplements, have been used to treat arthritis, asthma, chemical sensitivity, colitis, depression, eczema, eye allergy, fatigue, food allergy, hyperactivity, migraine, psychological complaints, and vascular disease.

Table 3-1 summarizes the cause of illness, treatment strategy, training, and other comments for six of the above traditional health belief systems.

Integrating Medical Belief Systems

Because each of the healing traditions has arisen in its own culture, each has its own strengths and weaknesses. However, Ballentine (1999, p. 6) proposes that "by integrating them, superimposing one upon another in layer after layer of complementary perspectives and techniques, we can arrive at an amalgam [composite] that is far more potent and thorough than any one of them taken alone." Ballentine believes that attitudes and emotional postures embedded in the mind and in the unconscious are hidden impediments to health because they shape the way in which subtle energy is organized, which in turn influences what happens in the physical body. By melding the philosophies and methods of the various traditions, it is proposed (Ballentine, 1999) that:

- The profound principles buried in each become clearer and stronger

- An intensity of effectiveness becomes possible

- Healing and reorganization accelerate and deepen

- Spurts of rapid transformation are made possible

These principles have been applied within the context of nursing practice in the remainder of this book. Each chapter contributes to a health promotion nursing practice matrix that draws upon theory and approaches from a variety of traditions. The practitioner is urged to develop competence in a wide variety of strategies, and to combine them in creative ways based on the individualized needs of clients.

Table
3-1

Professionalized Health Belief Systems

SYSTEM	CAUSE OF ILLNESS	TREATMENT STRATEGY
Acupuncture (TCM)	Imbalance of vital energies or qi (pronounced "chee").	Improve the flow of qi by strategically placing needles along any of the meridians that conduct energy between body surfaces and deep internal organs.
Anthroposophically extended medicine	Physical functioning is in discord with the patient's spiritual functioning.	Heal the soul and spirit, as well as the body.
Ayurveda	Disruption of the elements or doshas that form the patient's spiritual functioning.	Restore the doshas to their original equilibrium with lifestyle tactics.
Environmental medicine	Same as conventional medicine with one major exception: sensitivity to chemicals, foods, and inhaled substances can cause signs and symptoms not usually associated with allergies.	A thorough environmental history, physical examination, laboratory assessment, and hypersensitivity testing are used to uncover the cause of symptoms. Environmental controls and dietary management are basic to treatment. Immunotherapy may also be used to reduce sensitivity to antigens.
Homeopathy	A hereditary predisposition to an imbalance of the body's own vital energy.	Symptoms are treated with highly diluted preparations of naturally occurring animal, mineral, and plant substances capable of causing similar symptoms in a health patient.

continued

Table
3-1

Professionalized Health Belief Systems, continued

SYSTEM	PRACTITIONER'S TRAINING	COMMENT
Acupuncture (TCM)	More than 40 schools and colleges of acupuncture and Eastern medicine exist in the United States.* Conventional medicinal schools may teach the subject as well. Certification is offered by the Washington, DC-based National Commission for the Certification of Acupuncture and the American Academy of Medical Acupuncture, Los Angeles.	Most states regulate the practice in some way: 22 license or register acupuncturists; 12 limit the practice to MDs and DOs; two to MDs, DOs, and Doctors of Chiropractics; and eight allow the practice if supervised by a licensed physician.[1]
Anthroposophically extended medicine	MDs or DOs who have studied with others in the field. Board certification is available from the Physician's Association for Athroposophical Medicine but not required for practice.	Western scientific medical practices are blended with aspects of homeopathy and naturopathy.
Ayurveda	Centers providing Ayurvedic medicine frequently offer training programs. These vary in intensity. No standard qualifications exist.	A subtype of Ayurvedic medicine, known as Maharishi Ayurveda, includes transcendental meditation in its approach.
Environmental medicine	Practitioners are conventionally trained physicians—an estimated 3,000 of them practice worldwide, though the specialty is most common in the United States, Great Britain, and Canada.*	More than half of those belonging to the American Academy of Environmental Medicine are board-certified in one or more of 19 medical specialties.
Homeopathy	Formal training programs and home-learning courses are available, some through the Alexandria, VA-based Council on Homeopathic Education. No standard qualifications exist, though practitioners are licensed health care providers. However, Arizona, Connecticut, and Nevada maintain licensing boards for homeopathic physicians.	Homeopathy is commonly used in other parts of the world, particularly Asia, Europe, and Latin America.

continued

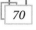

Table 3-1

Professionalized Health Belief Systems, continued

SYSTEM	CAUSE OF ILLNESS	TREATMENT STRATEGY
Naturopathy	Discord with nature.	Conventional diagnostic techniques are employed. Therapy is designed to spur the body's innate healing capacity. Nutritional and herbal tactics are fused with techniques such as acupuncture, homeopathy, hydrotherapy, and therapeutic massage.
Traditional Eastern medicine	Disruption of the vital energies.	Balance is maintained or restored with a variety of tactics, including acupuncture, dietary intervention, herbal remedies, and Qigong.

continued

Table 3-1

Professionalized Health Belief Systems, continued

SYSTEM	PRACTITIONER'S TRAINING	COMMENT
Naturopathy	Practitioners receive a Doctor of Naturopathy degree after 4 years of advanced study at a school of naturopathic medicine. Four currently exist in the United States: Bastyr College of Natural Health Sciences, Bothell, WA; National College of Naturopathic Medicine, Portland, OR;Southwest College of Naturopathic Medicine, Scottsdale, AZ; and University of Bridgeport College of Naturopathic Medicine, Bridgeport, CT.	Eight states have specific licensing laws pertaining to naturopaths.[1] A handful of others allow naturopathic physicians to practice. An increasingly common evaluation tool is a standardized national exam called the naturopathic physician licensing examination.
Traditional Eastern medicine	Acupuncture, as well as herbal medicine, Eastern massage, and pharmacology are among the courses taught at colleges of traditional Eastern medicine. Credentialing is the same as for acupunture.	Questions on herbal medicine are part of the state acupuncturist licensing exam in California and Nevada.* Practioners of Eastern medicine have the most authority in New Mexico, which allows them to operate much like MDs or DOs. In addition, other health care professionals in that state are not allowed to advertise or charge for acupuncture and other practices of Eastern medicine.

*National Institutes of Health. (1994). *Alternative medicine: Expanding medical horizons. A report to the National Institutes of Health on alternative medical systems and practices in the United States.* (NIH publication 94-066, pp. 67-112). Washington, DC: U.S. Government Printing Office.

[1]Collinge, W. (1997). *The American Holistic Health Association complete guide to alternative medicine.* (pp. 49-50). New York: Warner Books.

Table reprinted from Starr, C. (1997). Exploring the other health care systems. *Patient Care,* 140-141, with permission of Patient Care. Medical Economics.

Chapter Key Points

- Western biomedicine is one of many medical belief systems, providing 10% to 30% of worldwide health care.

- Mechanism, reductionism, and science are major influences that have affected the development of the values of the biomedical model.

- Traditional medical belief systems are complete diagnostic and treatment systems that provide many positive effects to promote health and treat disease.

- In traditional health systems, the individual, not his or her symptoms, is treated; and empowered self-healing is paramount.

References

Andrews, M. M. (1995). *Transcultural concepts in nursing care.* Philadelphia: Lippincott.

Astin, J. A. (1998). Why patients use alternative medicine: Results of a national study. *JAMA, 279,* 1548-1553.

Bailey, P. (2002). Homeopathy. In S. Shannon (Ed.). *The Handbook of Complementary and Alternative Therapies in Mental Health* (pp. 401-429). San Diego, CA: Academic Press.

Ballentine, R. (1999). *Radical healing.* New York: Harmony Books.

Beinfield, H., & Korngold, E. (1995). Chinese traditional medicine: An introductory overview. *Altern Ther Health Med, 1,* 44-52.

Bennett, W. J. (1995). Moral conduct is in decline. In J. Hurley (Ed.), *American values: Opposing viewpoints* (pp. 106-114). San Diego, CA: Greenhaven Press.

Benson, H. (1993). The relaxation response. In D. Goleman, & J. Gunn, *Mind-body medicine* (pp. 233-257). Yonkers, NY: Consumer Reports.

Berman, B. M., & Larson, D. B. (Eds.). (1994). *Alternative medicine: Expanding medical horizons.* Washington, DC: U.S. Government Printing Office.

Burton Goldberg Group (1995). *Alternative medicine: The definitive guide.* Fife, WA: Future Medicine.

Chongcheng, X., & Qiuli, Y. (2003). The model of traditional Chinese medicine., *23,* 308-311.

Collinge, W. (1997). *The American holistic health association complete guide to alternative medicine* (pp 49-50). New York: Warner Books.

Dacher, E. S. (1995). A systems theory approach to an expanded medical model: A challenge for biomedicine. *J Altern Complement Med, 1,*187-196.

Eisenberg, D. M., Davis, R. B., Ettner, S. L., Appel, S., Wilkey, S., Van Rompay, M., et al. (1998). Trends in alternative medicine use in the United States, 1990-1997: Results of a follow-up national survey. *JAMA, 280,* 1569-1575.

Elder, C. (2004). Ayurveda for diabetes mellitus: A review of the biomedical literature. *Altern Ther Health Med, 10,* 44-50.

Ergil, K. V. (1996). China's traditional medicine. In M. S. Micozzi (Ed.), *Fundamentals of complementary and alternative medicine* (pp. 185-223). New York: Churchill Livingstone.

Eskinazi, D. P. (1998). Factors that shape alternative medicine. *JAMA, 280,* 1621-1623.

Fulder, S. (1993). The impact of non-orthodox medicine on our concepts of health. In R. Lafaille, & S. Fulder (Eds.). *Towards a new science of health* (pp. 105-117). London: Routledge.

Fulder, S. (1998). The basic concepts of alternative medicine and their impact on our views of health. *J Altern Complement Med, 4,* 147-158.

Hester, J. P. (1996). *Encyclopedia of values and ethics.* Santa Barbara: ABC-CLIO.

Integrative Medicine Consult. (1998). *A primer: Integrative medicine.* Boston: Integrative Medicine Communications.

Jacobs, J., & Moskowitz, R. (2001). Homeopathy. In M. Micozzi (Ed.), *Fundamentals of Complementary and Alternative Medicine* (2nd ed., pp. 87-99). New York: Churchill Livingstone.

Jonas, W. B. (1998). Alternative medicine—Learning from the past, examining the present, advancing to the future. *JAMA, 280,* 1616-1617.

Kuzeff, R. M. (1998). Homeopathy, sensation of well-being and CD4 levels: A placebo-controlled, randomized trial. *Complement Ther Med, 6,* 4-9.

Lad, D. V. (1995). An introduction to Ayurveda. *Altern Ther Health Med, 1,* 57-63.

Lad, D. V. (1999). Ayurvedic medicine. In W. B. Jonas, & J. S. Levin (Eds.), *Essentials of complementary and alternative medicine* (pp. 200-215). Philadelphia: Lippincott Williams & Wilkins.

Lao, L. (1999). Traditional Chinese medicine. In W. B. Jonas, & J. S. Levin (Eds.), *Essentials of complementary and alternative medicine* (pp. 216-232). Philadelphia: Lippincott Williams & Wilkins.

Larson-Presswalla, J. (1994). Insights into eastern health care: Some transcultural nursing perspectives. *Journal of Transcultural Nursing, 5,* 21-24.

Lyng, S. (1990). *Holistic health and biomedical medicine.* New York: State University of New York.

Maciocia, G. (1989). *The foundations of Chinese medicine: A comprehensive text for acupuncturists and herbalists.* Edinburgh, UK: Churchill Livingstone.

McGee, C. T., Sancier, K., & Chow, E. P. Y. (1996). Qigong in traditional chinese medicine. In M. Micozzi (Ed.), *Fundamentals of complementary and alternative medicine* (pp. 225-230). New York: Churchill Livingstone.

Mishra, L., Singh, B. B., & Dagenais, S. (2001a). Ayurveda: A historical perspective and principles of the traditional healthcare system in India. *Altern Ther Health Med, 7,* 36-42.

Mishra, L., Singh, B. B., & Dagenais, S. (2001b). Healthcare and disease management in Ayurveda. *Altern Ther Health Med, 7,* 44-50.

National Institute of Health. (1994). *Alternative Medicine: Expanding Medical Horizons. A Report to the National Institutes of Health on Alternative Medical Systems and Practices in the United States.* (NIH publication 94-066, pp. 67-112). Washington, DC: U.S. Government Printing Office.

Novey, D. W. (2000). *Clinician's complete reference to complementary/alternative medicine.* St. Louis: Mosby.

Pizzorno, J. E. (1996). Naturopathic medicine. In M. Micozzi (Ed.), *Fundamentals of complementary and alternative medicine* (pp. 163-181). New York: Churchill Livingstone.

Pizzorno, J. E., & Snyder, P. (2001). Naturopathic medicine. In M. Micozzi, (Ed.), *Fundamentals of complementary and alternative medicine* (2nd ed., pp. 159-193). New York: Churchill Livingstone.

Ranjan. (1998). Magic or logic: Can alternative medicine be scientifically integrated into modern medical practice? *Adv Mind-Body Med, 14*, 43-73.

Redwood, D. (1996). Chiropractic. In M. S. Micozzi (Ed.), *Fundamentals of complementary and alternative medicine* (pp. 91-110). New York: Churchill Livingstone.

Reid, D. (1995). *The complete book of Chinese health and healing.* Boston: Shambhala.

Smith, M. J., & Logan, A. C. (2002). Naturopathy. In A. Perlman (Ed.). *Complementary and Alternative Medicine.* The medical clinics of North America (pp. 173-184). Philadelphia: W. B. Saunders.

Soukhanov, A. H. (Ed.). (1992). *The American heritage dictionary* (3rd ed.). Boston: Houghton Mifflin.

Starr, C. (1997, July 15). Exploring the other health care systems. *Patient Care*, 140-141.

Thorne, S. (1993). Health belief systems in perspective. *J Adv Nurs, 18*, 1931-1941.

Titus, G. W. (1995). Providing alternative health care: An ancient system for a modern age. *Advanced Practice Nursing Quarterly, 1*, 19-28.

Wing, D. M. (1998). A comparison of traditional folk healing concepts with contemporary healing concepts. *Journal of Community Health Nursing, 15*, 143-154.

Wu, W., Bandilla, E., Ciccone, D. S., Yang, J., Cheng, S. S., Carner, N., et al. (1999). Effects of Qigong on late-stage complex regional pain syndrome. *Altern Ther Health Med, 5*, 45-54.

THE MEANING OF HEALTH
Models and Theories

Abstract

Models and theories have been proposed to try to understand, explain, and promote health. An overview of health promotion as conceptualized within nursing models and theories by Roy, Neuman, King, Orem, Rogers, Parse, Newman, Watson, and Leddy is provided, followed by a discussion of the biophysiological theory of psychoneuroimmunology, and a discussion of energy healing theory. The chapter concludes with a description of alternative approaches to the selection of a model or theory to guide the promotion of health and healing in nursing practice.

Learning Outcomes

By the end of this chapter the student will be able to:

- Describe approaches to health promotion within selected nursing models and theories
- Discuss the theory of psychoneuroimmunology as it applies to the promotion of health
- Discuss energy theory as it applies to the promotion of health
- Identify personal preferences for a model or theories to guide practice

Nursing Conceptual Models and Theories

Until fairly recently, nursing practice was guided by social, biologic, and medical science theories. However, in addition to Nightingale's perspective of nursing formulated in the mid-1800s, from the 1950s to the present, nursing scholars have developed models of nursing that provide bases for the development of nursing theories and nursing knowledge.

A model, as an abstraction of reality, provides a way to visualize reality to simplify thinking. For example, an airplane model provides a representation of a real airplane. A conceptual model demonstrates one way that various concepts can be interrelated and guides the development of theories to predict or evaluate consequences of alternative actions. According to Fawcett (2000), each conceptual model provides a systematic structure and a rationale for scholarly and practical activities. A conceptual model "gives direction to the search for relevant questions about the phenomena of central interest to a discipline and suggests solutions to practical problems" (p. 16).

A conceptual model is made up of concepts and their interrelationships. Four concepts are generally considered central to the discipline of nursing: the person who receives nursing care (the patient or client); the environment (society); nursing (goals, roles, functions); and health. All existing conceptual models of nursing describe these four concepts. But the models vary in the amount of emphasis placed on each concept, as well as in the kinds of theories that might explain the interrelationships among the individual or family client, the environment, and nursing, to promote health.

According to Fawcett (2000, p. 18), a theory consists of "one or more relatively concrete and specific concepts that are derived from a conceptual model," and propositions that describe the concepts and specify relations between two or more of the concepts. Theories are less broad than conceptual models in level of abstraction and scope. The purposes of theory may be "describing what a phenomenon is, explaining why it occurs, or predicting how it occurs" (2000, p. 18). As a result, theories provide a specific structure for interpreting and/or modifying a situation or behavior. Theories are proposals about what might be rather than definitive fact. Multiple theories that are more or less supported by research findings usually co-exist in a discipline.

This section of the chapter focuses on health promotion implications of nursing models and theories: Roy's adaptation model, Neuman's system model, King's theory of goal attainment, Orem's self-care deficit theory, Rogers' science of unitary human beings, Parse's human becoming theory, Newman's theory of health as expanding consciousness, Watson's theory of human caring, and Leddy's human energy model.

ROY'S ADAPTATION MODEL

Roy's adaptation model focuses on the goal of enhancing the process and outcome through which humans use conscious awareness and choice to create human and environmental integration. Focal, contextual, and/or residual stimuli from the external or internal environment provoke a response by the human system. The human's ability to respond positively is represented by an integrated, compensatory, or compromised adaptation level, which reflect both challenges and strengths. Individuals cope through regulator and cognator subsystems, while groups use stabilizer and innovator subsystems to maintain integrated life processes to meet human needs. "Adaptive responses promote the integrity of the human system in terms of the goals of adaptation: survival, growth, reproduction, mastery, and person and environment transformations" (Roy & Andrews, 1999, p. 44). The behaviors that result can be observed in four categories or adaptive modes: physiologic-physical, self-concept-group identity, role function, and interdependence. The goal of nursing is to promote adaptation in each of the modes which contributes to health, "being and becoming an integrated and whole human being" (p. 54). Health promotion activities guided by this model would focus on the identification of environmental stimuli that require an adaptive response, and on strategies to promote adaptation within each of the adaptive modes.

In Roy's model, the individual, family, group, social organization, or community may be the unit of analysis and focus of nursing practice. In the initial assessment using Roy's adaptation model, behaviors of the human adaptive system and the current state of adaptation are noted first, and then the stimuli that contribute to those behaviors are explored. The analysis of the assessment data leads to the statement of focal, contextual, and residual stimuli for the individual or for the family as one entity. Nursing actions are focused on increasing, reducing, or maintaining the stimuli or strengthening adaptive processes in order to maintain or promote adaptation. In a study of the relationship among social support, parenting stress, coping style, and psychological distress in parents when caring for children with cancer with a sample of 246 mothers and 195 fathers, "hypotheses derived from the Roy adaptation model were supported for both mothers and fathers" (Yeh, 2003, p. 255). Table 4-1 summarizes selected concepts in Roy's model.

NEUMAN'S SYSTEMS MODEL

The focus of Neuman's systems model is maintenance of dynamic system stability (optimal wellness), which may be threatened by intrapersonal, interpersonal, or extrapersonal environmental stressors (tension producing stimuli). The client may be an individual, a family, a group, a community, or a social issue. The human is a composite of five harmoniously interacting variables-physiological, psychological, sociocultural, developmental, and spiritual. The human is protected by a flexible line of defense, and internal lines of resistance that are activated following invasion of the normal line of defense by environmental stressors. The normal range of response to the environment, the normal line of defense, is the usual "wellness/stability state" (Neuman, 2002, p. 14). When the flexible line of defense is no longer capable of protecting against an environmental stressor, the stressor breaks through the normal line of defense, resulting in system destabilization. Health "is equated with optimal system stability" (2002, p. 23), with wellness "a matter of degree, a point on a continuum running from the greatest degree of wellness to severe illness or death" (2002, p. 3). Nursing actions are aimed at retaining, attaining, and maintaining optimal client health or wellness, using the three preventions as interventions to keep the system stable.

Primary prevention is applicable before a person comes in contact with a stressor and focuses on protecting the client system's normal line of defense by strengthening the flexible line of defense. Secondary prevention is applicable after the stressor has penetrated the normal line of defense and includes activities to strengthen the flexible line of defense and resistance to the stressors, and reduce symptoms. Tertiary prevention accompanies reconstitution, moving in a circular manner toward primary prevention.

Table 4-1	**Roy's Adaptation Model**
Human System	"A whole with parts that function as a unit" (Roy & Andrews, 1999, p. 31).
Environment	The world within and around humans (Roy & Andrews, 1999, p. 51).
Health	"A state and a process of being and becoming an integrated and human being" (Roy & Andrews, 1999, p. 54). Integrity implies soundness or an unimpaired condition. Adaptation is a process of promoting integrity.
Goal of Nursing	To promote the health of individuals and society. To promote adaptation in each of the four modes, thereby contributing to health, quality of life, or dying with dignity.
Nursing Process	Assess adaptiveness of behaviors in the four modes and the stimuli influencing ineffective behaviors. State nursing diagnoses, determine goals and interventions, and evaluate as behavior changes.

In the Neuman systems model, health promotion is explicitly identified as "a component of the primary prevention-as-intervention modality" (Neuman & Fawcett, 2002, p. 29), but also works with both secondary and tertiary prevention to "prevent recidivism and to promote optimal wellness" (p. 29). The nursing process begins with the identification and evaluation of potential or actual stressors that pose a threat to the stability of the client system, as well as evaluation of lines of defense and resistance. Goals are negotiated and outcomes are evaluated with the client. "The major goal for nursing is to reduce stressor impact, whether actual or potential, and to increase client resistance" (p. 29) by augmenting existing strengths related to the flexible line of defense. "No explicit middle-range theories have yet been derived from the Neuman systems model" (Gigliotti, 2003, p. 201). Table 4-2 summarizes selected concepts in Neuman's model.

KING'S GENERAL SYSTEMS FRAMEWORK AND THEORY OF GOAL ATTAINMENT

The emphasis in King's general systems framework is on interactions between personal, interpersonal, and social systems which influence behavior. Each individual is a personal system, characterized by the concepts of self, body image, growth and development, perception, learning, time, and personal space. The interpersonal system (which includes family), com-

Table 4-2	*Neuman's Systems Model*
Client System	A composite of physiological, psychological, sociocultural, developmental, and spiritual variables in interaction with the internal and external environment.
Environment	All internal and external factors or influences surrounding the client system, including the created environment, a protective, perceptive coping shield developed unconsciously by the client.
Health	A continuum of wellness to illness, dynamic in nature. Optimal wellness, or stability, indicates that total system needs are being met.
Goal of Nursing	"To assist clients to retain, attain, or maintain optimal system stability" (Neuman, 1996, p. 69).
Nursing Process	Nursing diagnoses and goals. Primary, secondary, or tertiary revention as intervention.

posed of two or more interacting individuals, is characterized by the concepts of verbal and nonverbal communication, interaction, stress, role, and transaction. Social systems are groups that form in a community within a society and are characterized by the concepts of decision making, organization, power, authority, and status (King, 1995). The personal, interpersonal, and social systems are the "environments within which human beings grow, develop, and perform daily activities" (King, 1995, p. 18).

Health is "dynamic life experiences of a human being, which implies continuous adjustment to stressors in the internal and external environment through optimum use of one's resources to achieve maximum potential for daily living" (King, 1981, p. 5). Illness is "a deviation from normal" (1981, p. 5). "The goal of nursing is to help individuals and groups attain, maintain, and restore health" (King, 1971, p. 84).

The theory of goal attainment includes the concepts of self, perception, communication, interaction, transaction, growth and development, stress, time, personal space, and role from the Framework. King (1995, p. 27) describes a nursing situation as "the immediate environment, spatial and temporal reality, in which two individuals establish a relationship to cope with events in the situation." Transaction is the values element of the interaction, while communication is the informational element. Through an interaction-transaction process, "nurses interact with clients purposefully to mutually set goals and explore and agree on the means to attain the goals" (King, 1995, p. 28). The outcome is goal attainment. The theory

Table 4-3	*King's Theory of Goal Attainment*
Human Being	A personal system that interacts with interpersonal and social systems.
Environment	A context "within which human beings grow, develop, and perform daily activities" (King, 1995, p. 18).
Health	"Dynamic life experiences of a human being, which implies continuous adjustment to stressors in the internal and external environment through optimum use of one's resources to achieve maximum potential for daily living" (King, 1981, p. 5). Also, "an ability to function in social roles" (p. 143). Illness is a deviation from normal.
Goal of Nursing	"To help individuals and groups attain, maintain, and restore health" (King, 1971, p. 84).
Nursing Process	Assess perception, communication, and interaction of nurse and client. Agree on goals and means to attain goals. Make transactions and evaluate if goal was attained.

of goal attainment proposes that health promotion goals are more likely to be attained when there is mutual goal setting between nurse and client within the interaction-transaction process. Table 4-3 summarizes selected concepts in King's theory.

OREM'S SELF-CARE DEFICIT THEORY

Self-care is action by persons who have developed the capability to take care of themselves within their environment (self-care agency). "Self-care contributes to human structural integrity, human functioning, and human development" (Orem, 1995, p. 103). There are three reasons for doing actions that constitute self-care: universal, developmental, and health-deviation self-care requisites. The self-care actions to be performed that meet known self-care requisites are the therapeutic self-care demand. When self-care agency is not adequate to meet the therapeutic self-care demand, there is a self-care deficit. The goal of nursing is to help persons (through nursing systems) to meet therapeutic self-care demands when they are unable to provide for their own self-care requisites.

Orem (p. 129) suggests that universal self-care and developmental self-care, at the primary level of prevention, "is a requirement of each individual throughout life." Individuals might also have health promotion needs at the secondary and tertiary levels of prevention, such as

Table 4-4	**Orem's Self-Care Deficit Theory**
Patient	A person under the care of a nurse.
Health	"State characterized by soundness or wholeness of developed human structures and of bodily and mental functioning" (Orem, 1995, p. 101).
Environment	Physical, chemical, biological, and social contexts within which human beings exist.
Goal of Nursing	To help patients to meet their self-care needs.
Nursing Process	Actions to overcome or prevent the development of a self-care deficit or provide therapeutic self-care for a patient who is unable to do so.

"prevention of complicating diseases and adverse effects of specific diseases and prolonged disability," and "rehabilitation in the event of disfigurement and disability" (p. 131). Nursing systems and helping actions are performed for or with the client. Table 4-4 summarizes selected concepts in Orem's theory.

ROGERS' SCIENCE OF UNITARY HUMAN BEINGS

The essence of Rogers' model is the open, continuous, and mutual process of the unitary energy field that is the human being with the energy field that is the environment (principle of integrality). The unique pattern of energy fields evolves unpredictably in waves that change from lower frequency with longer patterns to higher frequency with shorter wave patterns (principle of resonancy), continually creating more diverse and complex field pattern (principle of helicy).

Health is an indication of field patterning, so an individual or his or her families' health potential can be promoted through deliberate nursing patterning of the environmental field. To promote health potential, the nurse would first appraise manifest behavior patterns of the client, including lifestyle parameters, rhythms and flow of energy, and manifestations of patterning. Then, empowering both nurse and client, accepting diversity as the norm, and viewing change as positive, the nurse would become attuned to patterning and use wave modalities for mutual deliberative patterning (e.g. light, color, music, and movement). Table 4-5 summarizes selected concepts in Rogers' model.

Table
4-5

Rogers' Science of Unitary Human Beings

Human Being	Unitary energy field with a unique pattern.
Environment	Energy field in mutual process with the human being.
Health	An "index of field patterning" (Malinski, 1986, p. 27). Health and illness are not separate states, good or bad, nor in a linear relationship.
Goal of Nursing	"To promote human health and well-being" (Rogers, 1988, p. 100).
Nursing Process	Mutual patterning to enhance health potential. "Health patterning is providing knowledgeable caring to assist clients in actualizing potentials for well being through knowing participation in change" (Malinski, 1986, p. 25).

PARSE'S HUMAN BECOMING THEORY

The emphasis in Parse's theory is on the meaning and values that influence a person's active choices of behavior. The person is defined as "an open being, more than and different from the sum of parts in mutual simultaneous interchange with the environment who chooses from options and bears responsibility for choices" (Parse, 1987, p. 160). Health is quality of life and a constantly changing process of becoming that incorporates values. Because it is not a state, health cannot be contrasted with disease. "The human becoming nurse's goal is to be truly present with people as they enhance their quality of life" (Parse, 1998, p. 69).

Parse (1987, p. 163) incorporates Rogers' principles with concepts from existential phenomenology into three principles. Meaning is structured multidimensionally as humans and the environment together create (cocreate) reality through "the language of valuing and imaging." In other words, the meaning of human beliefs and values is developed and demonstrated through words and movement. Rhythmicity of patterns of relating is cocreated through "living the paradoxical unity of revealing-concealing, enabling-limiting, and connecting-separating." In other words, human patterns in relating to others are derived from multiple choices and involve rhythmical processes of moving closer to and away from others. Contranscendence with possibilities is "powering unique ways of originating in the process of transforming." In other words, it involves the processes of distancing and moving closer in interrelationships that provide the force for change and creativity. Through presence, "a non-routinized, unconditional loving way of being" (Parse, 1996, p. 57), the nurse interacts with individuals and families to illuminate meaning, synchronize rhythms, and mobilize transcendence. Parse proposes that a discussion of lived experiences, in true presence between client

Table 4-6	*Parse's Human Becoming Theory*	
Person	An open being, more than and different from the sum of parts.
Environment	In mutual process with the person.
Health	The human being's way of living day-to-day, a personal commitment, a process originating with the person, a process of becoming. Emphasizes the meaning and values that influence a person's active choices of behavior.
Goal of Nursing	Nursing aims to affect the "quality of life as perceived by the person and the family" (Parse, 1987, p. 167).
Nursing Process	Focus is on the meaning constructed by the person. Uses true presence to explicate meaning, dwell with and synchronize rhythms, and move beyond in transforming.

and nurse (dialogical engagement), can shed light on the meaning of health for the client, and lead to moving beyond with changed health patterns. In three studies on feeling very tired, Bunkers (2003, p. 342) commented on the distinctiveness of each study and the "ebb and flow of rhythmical patterns of human-universe processes." Table 4-6 summarizes selected concepts in Parse's theory.

NEWMAN'S THEORY OF HEALTH AS EXPANDING CONSCIOUSNESS

The focus of Newman's theory is consciousness, which is defined as "the information of the system: the capacity of the system to interact with the environment" (Newman, 1994, p. 33). Newman's theory incorporates Rogers' concept of a unitary person as a center of constantly changing patterning of energy. The person does not possess consciousness, the person is consciousness. "The total pattern of person-environment can be viewed as a network of consciousness" (Newman, 1986, p. 33) that is expanding toward higher levels. Pattern has three dimensions: movement-space-time, rhythm, and diversity. The expansion of consciousness is health, which encompasses both disease and "nondisease." Disease is a manifestation of health. The goal of nursing "is not to make people well, or to prevent their getting sick, but to assist people to recognize the power that is within them to move to higher levels of consciousness" (Newman, 1994, p. xv). Nurses do not try to change the client's pattern, but recognize it "as information that depicts the whole and relate to it as it unfolds" (p. 13).

Using this theory for health promotion, the nurse would facilitate the process of evolving to higher levels of consciousness by "rhythmic connecting of the nurse with the client in an authentic way for the purpose of illuminating the pattern and discovering the new rules of a higher level of organization" (Newman, 1990, p. 40). Within a qualitative interview process,

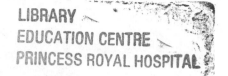

Table
4-7

Newman's Theory of Health as Expanding Consciousness

Human Being	"Unitary and continuous with the undivided wholeness of the universe" (Newman, 1994, p. 83).
Environment	"Undivided wholeness of the universe" (Newman, 1994, p. 83).
Health	"Manifest health, encompassing disease and nondisease, can be regarded as the explication of the underlying pattern of person-environment" (Newman, 1994, p. 11). "The patterns of interaction of person-environment constitute health.... Health is the expansion of consciousness" (1986, pp. 3, 18).
Goal of Nursing	"The pattern of the whole, health as the pattern of the evolving whole, with caring as a moral imperative" (Newman, 1994, p. xix). "Nursing is caring in the human health experience" p. 139).
Nursing Process	The process is practice driven and uses hermeneutic and dialectic approaches in partnership with the client.

participants tell their stories, while the nurse acts as an active listener. As person-environment patterns in the data emerge over time, they are diagrammed and interpreted. The intent is to foster recognition of the emerging pattern of the whole that is health. Although this theory was developed for use with individuals, it is also applicable to family health promotion. Table 4-7 summarizes selected concepts in Newman's theory.

WATSON'S HUMAN SCIENCE AND THEORY OF TRANSPERSONAL CARING

Watson's theory focuses primarily on the "centrality of human caring and on the caring-to-caring transpersonal relationship and its healing potential" (Watson, 1996, p. 141) for the nurse as a caregiver and the client who receives care. A transpersonal caring relationship is "a human-to-human connectedness" (Watson, 1989, p. 131) that is reflected in caring occasions or moments. Transpersonal caring is "actualized" and "grounded" through 10 carative factors (Watson, 1996, p. 156) as follows:

1. Forming a humanistic-altruistic system of values.

2. Enabling and sustaining faith-hope.

3. Being sensitive to self and others.

4. Developing a helping-trusting, caring relationship (seeking transpersonal connection).

5. Promoting and accepting the expression of positive and negative feelings and emotions.

Table 4-8	***Watson's Human Caring Theory***
Human	A "unity of mind/body/spirit/nature" (Watson, 1996, p. 147).
Environment	A "field of connectedness" at all levels (Watson, 1996, p. 147).
Health (Healing)	Manifested by harmony, wholeness, and comfort.
Goal of Nursing	"Nursing, as a profession, exists in order to sustain caring, healing, and health" (Watson, 1996, p. 146). "The ultimate goal can be stated as protection, enhancement, and preservation of human dignity and humanity" (p. 148). The emphasis is on helping other(s) to gain more self-knowledge, self-control, and self-healing potential.
Nursing Process	Reciprocal transpersonal relationship in caring moments guided by carative factors.

6. Engaging in creative, individualized, problem-solving caring processes.

7. Promoting transpersonal teaching-learning.

8. Attending to supportive, protective, and/or corrective mental, physical, societal, and spiritual environments.

9. Assisting with gratification of basic human needs while preserving human dignity and wholeness.

10. Allowing for, and being open to, existential-phenomenological and spiritual dimensions of caring and healing.

Watson (1996, p. 147) views the human as a "unity of mind/body/spirit/nature." There is "a field of connectedness between and among persons and environments at all levels, into infinity and into the universal or cosmic level of existence" (1996, p. 147). The purpose of nursing is to "expand human consciousness, transcend the moment, and potentiate healing and a sense of well-being—a sense of being reintegrated, more connected, more whole" (p. 160). The theory emphasizes healing potential for both the one who is caring and the one who is being cared for. Both the individual or family client and the nurse have human freedom, choice, and responsibility. Human caring is viewed as the moral ideal of nursing, with a strong emphasis on human dignity, caring-healing consciousness, and the potential for transformation of self. Table 4-8 summarizes selected concepts in Watson's theory factors.

Watson's latest writings (1996) discuss healing rather than health. By focusing on the carative factors within a transpersonal relationship, the nurse and client can promote healing and a sense of well-being through the use of caring competencies such as therapeutic presence, intuition, and active listening; caring modalities such as therapeutic touch, music, and guided imagery; and caring strategies such as ethics, aesthetics, and caring for the caregiver.

Over 50 doctoral dissertations and master's theses based on Watson's theory have been conducted. In a review of 40 published studies, Smith (2004) determined that one strength of published research is a recent focus on the relationship between caring and healing through evaluation of theory-guided practice models. One weakness is that many of the published studies have weak theoretical-empirical linkages. One middle-range theory (Swanson) and several theory-guided practice models have been developed (Smith, 2004).

LEDDY'S HUMAN ENERGY MODEL

Influenced by Rogers' science of unitary human beings, Leddy (2004) views the human being (person) as a unitary energy field that is open to and continuously interacting with an environmental energy field. Self-organization distinguishes the human energy field from the environmental field with which it is inseparably intermingled. "Self-organization is a synthesis of continuity and change, that provides identity while the human evolves toward a sense of integrity, meaning and purpose in living" (Leddy, 1998, p. 192). The human being also possesses awareness, which makes possible intention, the construction of self-identity and meaning, and the ability to influence change through choice.

The environment is viewed as dynamic, changing through continuous transformation of energy with matter and information. These transformations occur as a web of connectedness in relationships within the self and with the environment, including other humans and/or an "ultimate other." Change is partially unpredictable, but is also influenced by inherent order in the universe, history, pattern and choice.

Health is the pattern of the whole. This changing pattern of harmony/dissonance varies over time in quality and intensity. Knowledge-based consciousness in a goal directed relationship with an individual or family client is the basis for nursing, during which the nurse is a knowledgeable, concerned facilitator, and the individual or family client is responsible for choices that influence health and healing. The facilitation of harmonious health patterning is accomplished through health pattern appraisal and subsequent energetic interventions (see the Practice Theory of Energy later in this chapter). Table 4-9 summarizes selected concepts in Leddy's model.

The models and theories discussed previously in this chapter have been developed within nursing, with contributions from the biological and social sciences. Psychoneuroimmunology utilizes biophysiological concepts to address health and its promotion.

Psychoneuroimmunology

Can thought, emotion, and behavior directly enhance immune function and thereby prevent the onset or alter the course of diseases involving immunity (Hafen et al., 1996)? These questions are addressed by psychoneuroimmunology (PNI), the study of the "mechanisms of

Table 4-9	*Leddy's Human Energy Model*
Human Being	A unitary, self-organized energy matter and information field.
Environment	A dynamic, ordered, connected web in continuous transformation of energy, matter, and information with the human being.
Health	The pattern of the whole. This pattern is rhythmic, varying in quality and intensity over time. Health is characterized by a changing pattern of harmony and dissonance.
Goal of Nursing	Knowledge-based awareness in a goal-directed relationship with the client is the basis for nursing. A nurse-client relationship is a commitment characterized by intentionality, authenticity, trust, respect, and genuine sense of connection. The nurse is a knowledgeable, concerned facilitator. The client is responsible for choices that influence health and healing.
Nursing Process	The facilitation of harmonious health patterning is accomplished through health pattern appraisal and subsequent energetic interventions.

bidirectional communication between the neuroendocrine and immune systems" (Zeller et al., 1996, p. 657).

Consistent with the disease perspective, medical science considers the body to be a system composed of separate and interacting subsystems. For some time, it has been recognized that the nervous and endocrine subsystems interact to coordinate coping and adaptation efforts of the entire system when stressors affect the body. However, since the 1980s, increasing evidence supports the expansion of this coordinating framework to include the immune system. The emphasis is on the variety of ways in which information from subjective experience, emotions, memory, and cognition is shared throughout the total system to facilitate resistance and healing.

Zeller, McCain, and Swanson (1996) describe four pathways for neuroendocrine-immune communication, as depicted in Figure 4-1.

■ *Path* A. Direct autonomic (sympathetic, parasympathetic) neural innervation via neurotransmitters (catecholamines, opioid peptides, dopamine) and neuropeptide messengers (vasoactive intestinal polypeptide [VIP], B-endorphin, corticotropin [ACTH] on the surface of immune system tissues including lymphocytes).

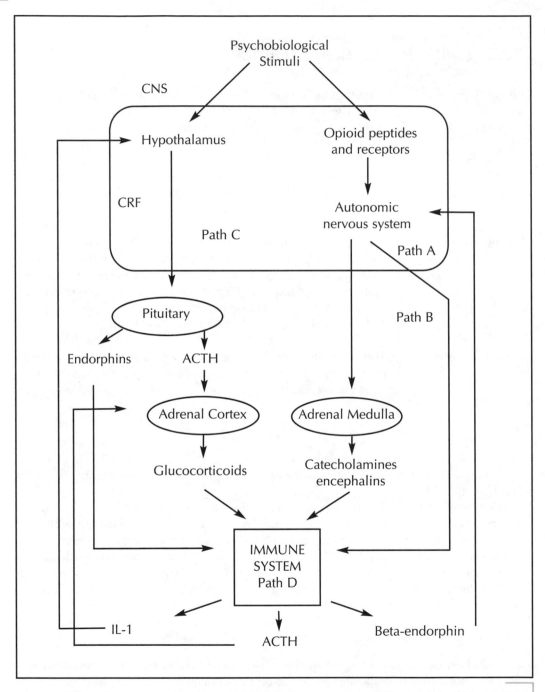

Figure 4-1. Psychoneuroimmunology interaction pathways. (reprinted from Zeller, J. M., McCain, N. L., & Swanson, B. (1996). Psychoimmunology: An emerging framework for nursing research. *J Adv Nurs, 23*, 658. Used with permission of Blackwell Scientific Ltd.).

- *Path B.* Sympathetic-adrenomedullary system activation results in release of catecholamines and encephalins, which circulate by way of the blood to immune system tissues.

- *Path C.* Hypothalamic-pituitary-adrenocortical activation result in corticotropin (ACTH), endorphins, and glucocorticoids that have immunopotentiating and immunosuppressive effects.

- *Path D.* Immune-derived products (cytokines), such as interleukin-1 (IL-1), communicate directly and indirectly with the brain.

The immune system not only recognizes foreign substances and arranges for their destruction and removal, but also functions as a diffuse sense organ distributed throughout the body (Maier & Watkins, 1998). As a result, "social and physical conditions, emotional states, neuropeptide interactions, and immune surveillance capabilities are inseparable aspects of a seamless organismic response" (Pert et al., 1998, p. 35). While "acute stress associated with activation of the sympathetic nervous system (fight or flight) often causes increases in NK cell activity, chronic, inescapable, or unpredictable stress that yields a sense of helplessness and habitual repression of strong emotions results in chronically high levels of endogenous opioid peptides, which in turn are responsible for immune deficits that reduce resistance to infections and neoplastic disease" (pp. 34-35).

Both brief and longer-term stressors are associated with declines in functional aspects of immunity, and both the duration and intensity of stressors are related to the breath and magnitude of immune changes (Kiecolt-Glaser, McGuire, Robles, & Glaser, 2002). However, the ability to unwind after stressful encounters influences the total burden. In general, the narrower the scope of a behavioral intervention and the shorter its time course, the smaller and less enduring the impact.

Altering subjective feelings of well-being through various interventions such as relaxation training, hypnosis, exercise, classical conditioning, self-disclosure, cognitive-behavioral interventions, and support groups may enhance immune function (Kiecolt-Glaser & Glaser, 1992; Micozzi, 2001). In addition, a series of therapeutic touch treatments was associated with immune changes in both practitioners and recipients (Quinn & Strelkauskas, 1993). However, it may not be possible to enhance immune function above normal levels.

An association between personal relationships and immune function has been supported by a number of studies. "Distress and poorer personal relationships appear to be associated with the down-regulation of immunity" (Kiecolt-Glaser & Glaser, 1992, p. 574), while "social support may mitigate the harmful effects of stressful life events" (Houldin et al., 1991, p. 14). However, although the preliminary evidence is promising, "it is not clear to what extent positive immunological changes translate into any concrete… alterations in the incidence, severity, or duration of infectious or malignant disease" (Kiecolt-Glaser & Glaser, 1992, p. 569). In addition, minimal research has investigated relationships between enhanced immunity and the promotion of health.

Booth and Ashbridge (1993, p. 19) suggest that "metaphorically, we might profitably consider the immune system less as a soldier and more as a gardener." Evidence from psychoneuroimmunology studies could provide a bridge between the disease and person perspectives of health. There is now increasing scientific support for nursing interventions that enhance subjective feelings of well-being as a way to enhance the environment within which health can "grow" and "flourish." Some of these approaches are discussed in Chapters 12 through 16.

The concept of energy is integral to several nursing models (e.g., Rogers and Leddy). The next section will provide an overview of energy healing theory derived from Eastern healing traditions.

Energy Healing Theory

According to Slater (1997, p. 52), energetic healing occurs through the medium of energy, "a metaphoric term used to mean healing that occurs at the quantum and electromagnetic levels of a person, plant, or animal." All matter is energy. "Matter and energy are now known to be interchangeable and interconvertible" (Gerber, 1988, p. 58). Energy varies in quantity and quality (vibration), has polarity (yin and yang), and is arranged in specific patterns.

Energy can be viewed as a phenomenon, an actuality or thing with an inherent ability to change, or as part of a process resulting in change. "In the idea of energy as part of a process, the universe is portrayed as mechanistic; things are viewed as particulate, and change comes about from efficient causes. In this view, energy is gained, lost, transferred, or transmitted, and change is a consequence of cause and effect. In the idea of energy as a phenomenon the universe is portrayed as dynamic; all things are viewed as forming an intricate whole, and change emerges from the whole. In this view energy isn't exchanged, transmitted, lost, or gained; instead, it is transforming or manifesting itself eternally and in unique ways" (Todaro-Franceschi, 1999, p. 30).

According to Kaptchuk (2001), energy is known by different names in different health belief systems.

- Homeopathy connects with the "spiritual vital force"

- Chiropractic calls it "innate" or "universal intelligence"

- Psychic healing manipulates "auric," "psi," or psionic powers

- Acupuncture utilizes "qi"

- Ayurveda is in touch with "prana"

- Naturopaths invoke the "vis medicatrix naturae"

Energy healing, also known as the laying on of hands, or biofield therapeutics, occurs in the human energy field surrounding, supporting, and interpenetrating the human body. Energy healing is a systematic, purposeful intervention which uses focused intention, hand contact, and "aligning with the universal energy field" (Starn, 1998, pp. 209-210). A field is described as "a domain of influence, presumed to exist in physical reality, that cannot be observed directly but that is inferred through its effects" (Dossey, 2000, p. 112). For example, a magnetic field around a bar magnet cannot actually be seen, but it is known that a field exists because of the pattern demonstrated by iron filings.

ANATOMY OF THE BIOFIELD

Gerber (1988) and Kunz and Peper (1982) provide an extensive description of the anatomy of human energy fields as follows:

- "The human organism is a series of interacting multidimensional [interpenetrating, interactive] energy fields" (Gerber, 1988, p. 91).

- "The energetic network... is organized and nourished by 'subtle' energetic systems which coordinate the life-force with the body" (Gerber, 1988, p. 43).

- "The physical body is actually a complex network of interwoven energy fields... the cellular matrix of the physical body can be seen as a complex energetic interference pattern" (Gerber, 1988, p. 60).

- The physical system (nerve, muscle, flesh, and bones) is "only one of several systems which are in dynamic equilibrium.... All of these systems are physically superimposed upon one another in the very same space" (Gerber, 1988, p. 119). "Bodies of higher energetic frequencies are interconnected and in dynamic equilibrium with the physical body" (Gerber, 1988, p. 120). The difference between physical matter and etheric matter is only a difference of frequency" (Gerber, 1988, p. 120).

- "The higher the frequency of matter, the less dense, or more subtle the matter" (Gerber, 1988, p. 69).

- The etheric body (vital field), an energetic form that underlies and energizes all aspects of the physical body, extends 1 to 6 inches from the body or 2 inches on the average (Kunz & Peper, 1982).

- "The astral [or emotional] body... is a subtle substance of even higher energetic frequencies than etheric matter" (Kunz & Peper, 1982, p. 136), and extends about 18 to 48 inches beyond the body. "Through thoughts and intention, the individual emotional field can be stretched to considerable distances, such as 10 to 15 feet.... Relaxation tends to expand the field while anxiety tends to constrict the field" (pp. 398, 400). Figure 4-2 is a depiction of the human energy fields.

The mental, causal, and astral subtle energetic bodies exist beyond the etheric, in what might be referred to as a nonphysical or nonspace, nontime level of existence. "The mental body is concerned with the creation and transmission of concrete thoughts and ideas to the brain." The next highest level of subtle energetic substance from the mental body is the causal body (intuitional field), which "is involved with the area of abstract ideas and concepts.... Causal consciousness deals with the essence of a subject while the mental level studies the subject's details" (Gerber, 1988, pp. 154-55). The astral body (emotional field), through the astral chakras, provides "a subtle-energy connection whereby a person's emotional state can disturb or enhance health.... The astral body also functions as a vehicle of consciousness which can exist separately, yet connected to, the physical body" (Gerber, 1988, pp. 137, 139).

The chi dynamic force of energy is constantly circulating within the body in 12 well-defined channels, or physical ducts called meridians, which exist as a series of points following line-like patterns. Energy always flows from high to low potential (Gerber, 1988). "The meridian system forms an interface between the etheric and the physical body. The meridian system is the first physical link established between the etheric body and the developing physical body.... Illness is caused by energetic imbalance within the meridians supplying the nutritive chi energies to the organs of the body" (Gerber, 1988, pp. 126-127).

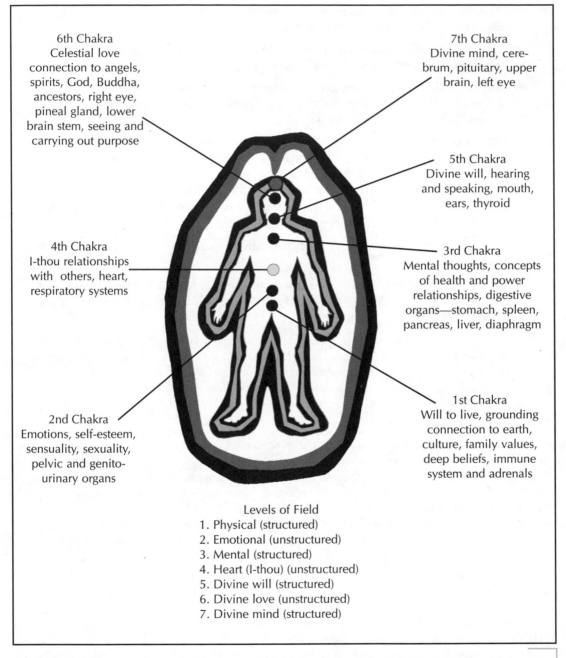

6th Chakra
Celestial love
connection to angels,
spirits, God, Buddha,
ancestors, right eye,
pineal gland, lower
brain stem, seeing and
carrying out purpose

7th Chakra
Divine mind, cere-
brum, pituitary, upper
brain, left eye

5th Chakra
Divine will, hearing
and speaking, mouth,
ears, thyroid

4th Chakra
I-thou relationships
with others, heart,
respiratory systems

3rd Chakra
Mental thoughts, concepts
of health and power
relationships, digestive
organs—stomach, spleen,
pancreas, liver, diaphragm

2nd Chakra
Emotions, self-esteem,
sensuality, sexuality,
pelvic and genito-
urinary organs

1st Chakra
Will to live, grounding
connection to earth,
culture, family values,
deep beliefs, immune
system and adrenals

Levels of Field
1. Physical (structured)
2. Emotional (unstructured)
3. Mental (structured)
4. Heart (I-thou) (unstructured)
5. Divine will (structured)
6. Divine love (unstructured)
7. Divine mind (structured)

Figure 4-2. The human energy field (reprinted with permission from Stern, J. K. (1998). The path to becoming and energy healer. *Nurse Practitioner Forum*, 9, 211. W. B. Saunders).

Special energy centers known as *chakras* exist within the etheric body. Chakras (Sanskrit meaning "wheels"), "resemble whirling vortices of subtle energies, that 'take in' higher energies and transmute them to a utilizable form within the human structure" (Gerber, 1988, p. 128). There are at least seven major chakras associated with the physical body, in a vertical line ascending from the base of the spine to the head. These are the root chakra (I) near the coccyx, the sacral chakra (II) located either just below the umbilicus or near the spleen, the solar plexus chakra (III) in the upper middle abdomen below the tip of the sternum, the heart chakra (IV) in the midsternal region directly over the heart and the thymus, the throat chakra (V) directly over the thyroid gland and larynx, the brow chakra (VI) in the region of the mid-forehead slightly above the bridge of the nose, and the crown chakra (VII) located on the top of the head. Each is associated with a major nerve plexus and a major endocrine gland (Gerber, 1988).

Because chakras separate vibrations into various frequencies (not the same as frequencies of visible light and audible sound), a specific color, tone, function, organ, and nervous structure is associated with each chakra. "Chakras seem to have [the more] moment-to-moment responsibility of receiving, processing, transforming, and transmitting energy, information, and emotions that may be stored in the aura" (Slater, 1995, pp. 215, 218, 221). "The specific frequency of a particular chakra may modulate a particular emotion, need, drive, and/or organ" (Slater, 1997, p. 54).

Connecting the chakras to each other and to portions of the physical-cellular structure are up to 72,000 fine subtle-energetic channels, known as nadis, that are interwoven with the physical nervous system (Gerber, 1988). "Nadis, or channels of electromagnetic energy, subdivide finally to the cellular level, supporting the concept that healing can affect the cellular level of the physical body" (Starn, 1998, pp. 211-212). It is assumed that "there is a special alignment between the major chakras, glands, and nerve plexuses that is necessary for optimal human functioning" (Gerber, 1988, p. 131).

Mechanism of Action of Energetic Healing

There are two alternative beliefs about causation in energetic healing (Berman & Larson, 1994). One belief is that the "healing force" comes from a source other than the practitioner, such as God, the cosmos, or another supernatural entity. For example, reiki, qigong, and prayer, are based on channeling of a spiritual energy that has innate intelligence or logic and knows where and to what extent it is required. A second belief is that a human biofield—directed, modified, or amplified in some fashion by the practitioner—is the operative mechanism. For example, music, color therapy, and therapeutic touch pattern the vibrations of the environmental energy field for healing purposes. However, as the biofield is metaphysical (outside the four observable dimensions of space and time), these causal beliefs are currently untestable.

A Practice Theory of Energy Intervention

The practice theory of energy intervention is one of three theories that have been derived from Leddy's human energy model. This theory is based on the assumption that the universe is composed of an essence that has a dual nature: particle and wave. Universal essence has three aspects that are not differentiated in reality: matter is the potential for structure and identity, information is the potential for coordination and pattern, and energy is the potential for process, movement, and change. Universal essence creates fields of mutually transformable manifestations such as electromagnetism, light, sound, heat, and gravitation. These fields are open and in mutual process between living beings and the environment. Through magnetic emissions from a healer's hands, vibrational coupling between similar wave frequencies can be induced, resulting in resonance (increased wave amplitude and intensity) and entrainment (harmony of oscillation). Conscious focusing of intention is also suggested as a mechanism to increase frequency (and therefore intensity), complexity, and harmony of energy (Leddy, 2003).

The theory proposes that nursing interventions to facilitate energy flow, and resonant and harmonious pattern of both client and nurse are accomplished through energetic patterning of human-environmental fields. The six proposed domains of energetic patterning are:

1. *Connecting.* Promotes harmony of energetic patterning.

2. *Coursing.* Re-establishes free movement of energy.

3. *Conveying.* Fosters redirection of energy away from excess to depleted areas.

4. *Converting.* Transforms and augments energy resources.

5. *Conserving.* Reduces energy depletion.

6. *Clearing.* Releases energy tied to old patterns.

A number of types of interventions are consistent with this theory, including those found in Section IV of this book. Table 4-10 presents examples of noninvasive therapies that are appropriate for each of the domains of energetic patterning.

Using Models/Theories to Guide Practice

Nursing theory "provides the language, concepts, and worldview to reflect on nursing care" (Frisch, 2001, p. 4). In selecting a model or theory to guide practice, the nurse should first be aware of his or her philosophical or worldview beliefs. According to Fawcett (2000), different worldviews lead to different conceptualizations of human beings, the environment, health and nursing, and the nature of the relations between them. After the identification of a worldview perspective that is consistent with philosophical beliefs, several different approaches might be used to select model(s) or theories for practice.

In the coherence approach there is a commitment to one specific model based on beliefs about the nature of metaparadigm concepts or beliefs about how knowledge should be developed. For example, a nurse who truly believes in the person perspective might select Rogers' model and an energy theory to guide nursing care. Commitment to one model, in this case Rogers' model, is the guideline. Several theories may be consistent with the chosen model.

In the integrative approach, theories and strategies from diverse sources, models and orientations are interwoven. The nurse integrates these to develop a personal approach. For example, Mantle (2001) suggests that each nurse develops a unique and constantly evolving model of nursing. The integrative approach has some philosophical similarities with the pragmatic or eclectic approach in which those knowledge claims and theories that are considered

Table 4-10

Selected Noninvasive Therapies for Each Domain of Energetic Patterning

CLEARING

Music/color therapy
Acupressure
Postural movement
Aromatherapy

COURSING

Massage
Yoga
Polarity therapy
Exercise

CONVEYING

Acupressure
Reflexology

CONVERTING

Nutrition
Herbal therapy
Music/color therapy
Exercise

CONSERVING

Relaxation/meditation
Biofeedback
Sleep and rest
Breathing
Herbal therapy

CONNECTING

Guided imagery
Reiki
Therapeutic touch
Aromatherapy
Music/color therapy

to be most capable or useful in solving nursing problems are selected. In the reflective approach, new theories and empirical approaches are adopted based on congruence with reflections by the nurse and with the client. The view of situation or meanings of the problem drive the choice.

It should be clear that there is no one "best" model or theory, just as there is no "correct" model or theory for use by every nurse in every situation. Models and theories are alternative viewpoints, each with potential strengths and weaknesses. It is suggested that students first select the perspective (disease or person) that seems the more consistent with their beliefs about the nature of the person, environment, health, and nursing. Then, the dominant models/theories within that perspective should be explored. Ideally, one or more model or theory will seem consistent (coherence approach) with the student's beliefs, or potentially useful (pragmatic or eclectic approach) to guide practice. Some students may try to combine elements (integrative approach) of different models or theories (within the same worldview perspective of course) to develop their own personal model. Some students may feel that it is necessary to develop their own theory or model to reflect their beliefs. Regardless of how the particular model or theory is selected, it then becomes a framework that guides assessment, planning, and facilitation of health and healing with the client.

Chapter Key Points

- Models and theories within the disease and person perspectives provide alternative frameworks to guide health promotion and healing nursing practice and science.

- Nursing models and theories are needed to focus on enhancing the awareness, meaning, and potential of families' health and healing patterns and experiences.

- Roy, Neuman, King, Orem, Rogers, Parse, Newman, Watson, and Leddy have developed models/theories that provide structures for understanding how nursing can promote the health of individuals or families within the environment.

- Most nursing and non-nursing models and theories emphasize the individual in the context of family and focus on the diagnosis and treatment of health concerns (or deviations from norms) with the overall goal being the restoration of balance (Hartrick, 1998).

- Given that the disease and person perspectives are distinct, one of the two perspectives will seem more consistent with the nurse's beliefs or useful to guide practice.

- Once a choice of perspective has been made, a model or theory that seems most consistent with the individual's beliefs, or useful to guide practice is selected.

- In-depth study of the selected model or theory will be needed before it will be useful as a framework to guide practice.

References

Berman, B. M., & Larson, D. B. (Eds.). (1994). *Alternative medicine: Expanding medical horizons.* Washington, DC: US Government Printing Office.

Booth, R. J., & Ashbridge, K. R. (1993). A fresh look at the relationship between the psyche and immune system. Theolological coherence and harmony of purpose. *Advances: The Journal of Mind-Body Health, 9*(2), 4-28.

Bunkers, S. S. (2003). Comparison of three Parse method studies on feeling very tired. *Nursing Science Quarterly, 16,* 340-344.

Dossey, L. (2000). Creativity: On intelligence, insight, and the cosmic soup. *Altern Ther Health Med, 6,* 12-17, 108-117.

Fawcett, J. (2000). *Analysis and evaluation of contemporary nursing knowledge: Nursing models and theories.* Philadelphia: Davis.

Frisch, N. C. (2001, May 31). Nursing as a context for alternative/complementary modalities. Online *Journal of Issues in Nursing, 6*(2), manuscript 2. Retrieved March 19, 2002, from http://www.nursing-world.org/ojin/topic15/tpc15_2.htm

Gerber, R. (1988). *Vibrational medicine.* Santa Fe, NM: Bear & Company.

Gigliotti, E. (2003). The Neuman systems model institute: Testing middle-range theories. *Nursing Science Quarterly, 16,* 201-206.

Hafen, B. Q., Karren, K. J., Frandsen, K. J., & Smith, N. L. (1996). *Mind body health.* Boston: Allyn and Bacon.

Hartrick, G. (1998). Developing health promoting practices: A transformative process. *Nurs Outlook, 46,* 219-225.

Houldin, A. D., Lev, E., Prystowsky, M. B., Redei, E., & Lowery, B. J. (1991). Psychoneuroimmunology: A review of the literature. *Holistic Nursing Practice, 5*(4), 10-21.

Kaptchuk, T. J. (2001). History of vitalism. In M. S. Micozzi (Ed.), *Fundamentals of complementary and alternative medicine* (2nd ed., pp. 43-56). New York: Churchill Livingstone.

Kiecolt-Glaser, J. K., & Glaser, R. (1992). Psychoneuroimmunology: Can psychological interventions modulate immunity? *J Consult Clin Psychol, 60,* 569-575.

Kiecolt-Glaser, J. K., McGuire, L., Robles, T. F., & Glaser, R. (2002). Psychoneuroimmunology: Psychological influences on immune function and health. *Journal of Consulting and Clinical Psychology, 70,* 537-547.

King, I. M. (1971). *Toward a theory for nursing.* New York: John Wiley.

King, I. M. (1981). *A theory for nursing: Systems, concepts, process.* New York: John Wiley & Sons.

King, I. M. (1995). A systems framework for nursing. In M. A. Frey, & C. L. Sieloff (Eds.), *Advancing King's framework and theory of nursing* (pp. 14-22). Thousand Oaks, CA: Sage.

Kunz, D., & Peper, E. (1982, December). Fields and their clinical implications. *American Theosophist, 70,* 395-401.

Leddy, S. K. (1998). *Leddy and Pepper's conceptual bases of professional nursing* (4th ed.). Philadelphia: Lippincott.

Leddy, S. K. (2003). A unitary energy-based nursing practice theory: Theory and application. *Visions: The Journal of Rogerian Science, 11,* 21-28.

Leddy, S. K. (2004). Human energy: A conceptual model of unitary nursing science. *Visions: The Journal of Rogerian Science, 12,* 14-27.

Maier, S. F., & Watkins, L. R. (1998). Cytokines for psychologists: Implications for bidirectional immune-to-brain communication for understanding behavior, mood, and cognition. *Psychol Rev, 105,* 83-107.

Malinski, V. M. (1986). Nursing practice within the science of unitary human beings. In V. M. Malinski (Ed.), *Explorations on Martha Rogers' science of unitary human beings* (pp 25-32). Norwalk, CT: Appleton-Century-Crofts.

Mantle, F. (2001). Complementary therapies and nursing models. *Complementary Therapies in Nursing and Midwifery, 7,* 142-145.

Micozzi, M. S. (Ed.). (2001). *Fundamentals of complementary and alternative medicine* (2nd ed.). New York: Churchill Livingstone.

Neuman, B. (1996). The Neuman systems model in research and practice. *Nursing Science Quarterly, 9,* 67-70.

Neuman, B. (2002). The Neuman systems model. In B. Neuman, & J. Fawcett, *The Neuman systems model* (4th ed., pp. 3-33). Upper Saddle River, NJ: Prentice Hall.

Neuman, B. & Fawcett, J. (2002). *The Neuman systems model* (4th ed., pp. 3-33). Upper Saddle River, NJ: Prentice Hall.

Newman, M. A. (1986). *Health as expanding consciousness.* St. Louis: Mosby.

Newman, M. A. (1990). Newman's theory of health as praxis. *Nursing Science Quarterly, 3,* 37-41.

Newman, M. A. (1994). *Health as expanding consciousness* (2nd ed.). St Louis: Mosby.

Orem, D. E. (1995). *Nursing: concepts of practice* (5th ed.). St. Louis: Mosby.

Parse, R. R. (1987). *Nursing science: Major paradigms, theories, and critiques.* Philadelphia: Saunders.

Parse, R. R. (1996). The human becoming theory: Challenges in practice and research. *Nursing Science Quarterly, 9,* 55-60.

Parse, R. R. (1998). *The human becoming school of thought.* Thousand Oaks, CA: Sage.

Pert, C. B., Dreher, H. E., & Ruff, M. R. (1998). The psychosomatic network: Foundations of mind-body medicine. *Altern Ther Health Med, 4*(4), 30-41.

Quinn, J. F., & Strelkauskas, A. J. (1993). Psychoimmunologic effects of therapeutic touch on practitioners and recently bereaved recipients: A pilot study. *Advances in Nursing Science, 14*(4), 13-26.

Rogers, M. E. (1988). Nursing science and art: A prospective. *Nursing Science Quarterly, 1,* 99-102.

Roy, S. C., & Andrews, H. A. (1999). *The Roy adaptation model* (2nd ed.). Stamford: Appleton & Lange.

Rubik, B. (1997). Information, energy, and the unpredictable whole. *Advances: The Journal of Mind-Body Health, 13,* 67-70.

Slater, V. E. (1995). Toward an understanding of energetic healing. Part I: Energetic structures. *Journal of Holistic Nursing, 13,* 209-224.

Slater, V. E. (1997). Energetic healing. In B. M. Dossey, *Core curriculum for holistic nursing* (pp. 52-58). Gaithersburg, MD: Aspen.

Smith, M. (2004). Review of research related to Watson's theory of caring. *Nursing Science Quarterly, 17,* 13-25.

Starn, J. R. (1998). The path to becoming an energy healer. *Nurse Practitioner Forum, 9,* 209-216.

Todaro-Franceschi, V. (1999). *The enigma of energy: Where science and religion converge.* New York: Crossroad Publishing.

Watson, J. (1989). Watson's philosophy and theory of human caring in nursing. In J. P. Riehl-Sisca (Ed.), *Conceptual models for nursing practice* (pp. 219-235). East Norwalk, CT: Appleton & Lange.

Watson, J. (1996). Watson's theory of transpersonal caring. In P. H. Walker, & B. Neuman (Eds.), *Blueprint for use of nursing models: Education, research, practice, and administration* (pp. 141-162). New York: National League for Nursing.

Yeh, C. (2003). Psychological distress: Testing hypotheses based on Roy's adaptation model. *Nursing Science Quarterly, 16,* 255-263.

Zeller, J. M., McCain, N. L., & Swanson, B. (1996). Psychoneuroimmunology: An emerging framework for nursing research. *J Adv Nurs, 23,* 657-664.

THE MEANING OF HEALTH

Cultural Influences

Abstract

Cultural forces are powerful determinants of health-related behaviors in any group or sub-population. The beliefs, ideologies, knowledge, institutions, religion, governance, and nearly all activities (including efforts to achieve health-related behavior change) are affected by cultural influences. Thus, the nurse's cultural awareness and sensitivity must be reflected in the planning, design, and implementation of health promotion activities.

The chapter begins with a consideration of the differences between culture, ethnicity, and race, and continues with a discussion of racial and ethnic disparities in health status. Next, the influence of health and illness beliefs and the influence on health promotion of indigenous cultural beliefs of Asian Americans (Vietnamese Americans), Appalachians, Hispanics (Mexican Americans), African Americans, and Native Americans are considered. After a discussion of the effects of medicocentrism, and models or theories, the chapter concludes with approaches to understanding cultural and ethnic differences and commonalities for culturally competent health promotion care.

Learning Outcomes

By the end of the chapter the student will be able to:

- Differentiate between ethnicity, culture, and race

- Describe characteristics of lay/folk theories of health and illness

- Discuss indigenous cultural beliefs of Asian Americans (Vietnamese Americans), Appalachians, Hispanics (Mexican Americans), African Americans, and Native Americans

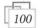

- Describe the implications of medicocentrism
- Describe factors to be considered in planning multicultural health promotion programs

Differentiating Ethnicity, Culture, and Race

Ethnicity "relates to the sense of identity an individual has based on common ancestry and national, religious, tribal, linguistic, or cultural origins.... Ethnicity, then, helps shape the way in which we think, relate, feel, and behave within and outside our reference group and defines the patterns of behavior that provide an individual with a sense of belonging and continuity with his or her ethnic group over time" (Huff & Kline, 1999, p. 8). The primary characteristics of ethnic identification include:

- Common geographic origin, language, and religion
- A sense of community transmitted over generations by families
- An internal sense of distinctiveness
- A comfortable sense of security, belonging, and understanding

In contrast, race distinguishes groups of people exclusively on the basis of genetically transmitted physical characteristics.

Although ethnic identity tends to persist through time, culture changes when individuals and groups modify their beliefs and practices to survive and adapt. Cultural differences exist among groups with the same ethnic or racial background (Huff & Kline, 1999). Culture is defined as "a learned and shared system of symbolic meanings that shape social reality and personal experiences" (Drew, 1997, p. 82), "above all a system of meanings and symbols" (Corin, 1995, p. 273). Culture determines health values and behavior, beliefs about the etiology of disease and illness, and the interpretation of these phenomena (Toumishey, 1993). Cultural beliefs provide several functions (Drew, 1997, p. 83):

- Enables the recognition of health status
- Attaches significance to a health problem
- Ascribes meaning to health and illness events
- Contributes to explanatory models of causation and expected healing outcomes
- Identifies acceptable behaviors related to seeking help

Racial and Ethnic Disparities in Health Status

According to Tarlov (1999), health status is influenced by five major categories, including genes and associated biology (including race); health behaviors such as nutrition, use of tobacco, alcohol or drugs, and physical activity; medical care and public health services; the ecology of all living things; and social and societal characteristics (including ethnicity and culture). These factors are interactive in complex and dynamic ways. An approximation of the relative influence of the categories on health status is portrayed in Figure 5-1.

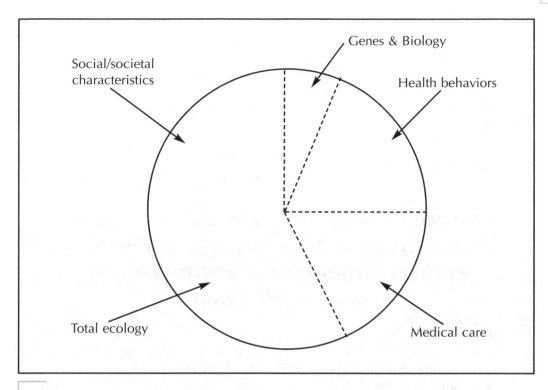

Figure 5-1. Determinants of population health. Relative influence of the five major determinant categories of population health: rough approximations (reprinted with permission from Tarlov, A. R. (1999). Public policy frameworks for improving population health. *Annals of the New York Academy of Sciences, 896,* 281-93).

Race and ethnicity are associated with persistent health status disparities among U. S. populations. Underlying causes for health status disparities include poverty, lack of access to high-quality health services, environmental hazards in homes and neighborhoods, and lack of effective prevention programs designed for specific community needs (USDHHS, 2001). Socioeconomic position and race (ethnicity) are variables that can affect health care include affordability and access, transportation, education, knowledge, literacy, health beliefs, attitudes and preferences, provider bias, and competing demands including work and childcare (Fiscella et al., 2000). Many of these variables, especially macro influences such as socio-economic inequalities and disadvantage, require broad societal involvement. In 1996, the poverty rate among African Americans was 28.4% and among Hispanics was 29.4%, in contrast to 11.2% among whites and 14.5% among Asian Americans (Flaskerud & Winslow, 1998). Improved access to appropriate and effective health care services is a variable that can be influenced by nurses through activities such as identification of need, advocacy within the health care system, and community empowerment efforts (Yali & Revenson, 2004). In fact, "public health approaches, in general, may provide a better model of health care than individually based models as practitioners strive to reach more people, particularly those in under-

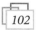

served groups (Yali & Revenson, 2004, p. 148). Nurses need to be social advocates who work with advocacy groups, policymakers, and community-based organizations, and use their expertise to change policy on the local and national levels.

The U.S. Department of Health and Human Services' (USDHHS) *Initiative to Eliminate Racial and Ethnic Disparities in Health* has identified several areas for concentrated focus that affect the health of multiple racial and ethnic minority groups at all life stages. Four areas are highlighted in Box 5-1.

Box 5-1

Selected Racial and Ethnic Disparities in Infant Mortality, Cancer Screening and Management, Cardiovascular Disease, and Diabetes

1. Infant mortality rates:
   - The average rate for whites in 1996 was 6.0 per 1,000 live births, compared with an average rate of 14.2 for African Americans, 9.0 for Native Americans overall, and 7.6 for Hispanics overall.
   - In 1996, 84% of white pregnant women, compared with 71% of African American and Hispanic pregnant women, received early prenatal care.
   - Sudden Infant Death Syndrome deaths, which account for about 10% of all infant deaths in the first year of life, are three to four times as high among Native Americans as among whites.
   - Reductions will require changes in behaviors such as smoking, substance abuse, poor nutrition, and conditions such as stress, domestic violence, lack of prenatal care, medical problems, and chronic illness. Babies should be placed on their backs to sleep to prevent SIDS.

2. Cancer screening and management:
   - For men and women combined, African Americans have a cancer death rate about 35% higher than for whites (171.6 vs. 127.0 per 100,000).
   - The death rate for cancer for African American men is about 50% higher than it is for white men (226.8 vs. 151.8 per 100,000).
   - Vietnamese women in the United States have a cervical cancer incidence rate more than five times greater than white women (47.3 vs. 8.7 per 100,000). Hispanic women's rates of cervical cancer are also elevated.
   - The mortality rate from breast cancer is higher for African American women than for white women.

continued

Box 5-1 CONTINUED

- ■ Hispanic, Native American, and Asian American women also have low rates of screening and treatment, limited access to health facilities and physicians, and barriers related to language, culture, and negative provider attitudes.

- ■ Lifestyle change might prevent many cancers. Tobacco use is responsible for nearly 33% of all cancer deaths, and diet and nutrition may by related to 30 to 40% of deaths. Reducing sun exposure could prevent many of the 900,000 yearly diagnosed skin cancers. Regular mammography and appropriate follow-up might reduce deaths from breast cancer by 30% for women over 50. Pap test screening and follow-up could virtually eliminate cervical cancer, and colorectal cancer screening is now recommended.

3. Cardiovascular disease (the leading cause of death for all ethnic groups):

- ■ Compared with rates for whites, coronary heart disease mortality was 40% lower for Asian Americans, but 40% higher for African Americans in 1995.

- ■ Racial and ethnic minorities have higher rates of hypertension, tend to develop hypertension at an earlier age, and are less likely to be treated.

- ■ Among adult women, the age-adjusted prevalence of being overweight continues to be higher for African American women (53%) and Mexican American women (52%) than for White women (34%).

- ■ Only 50% of Native Americans, 44% of Asian Americans, and 38% of Mexican Americans have had their cholesterol checked within the past 2 years.

- ■ The major modifiable risk factors are high blood pressure, high blood cholesterol, cigarette smoking, excessive body weight, and physical inactivity.

4. Diabetes:

- ■ Compared with whites, the prevalence of diabetes in African Americans is about 70% higher and in Hispanics is nearly double. The prevalence rate of diabetes among Native Americans is more than twice that for the total population.

- ■ Rates for diabetes-related complications such as end-stage renal disease and amputations are higher among African Americans and Native Americans compared to the total population.

continued

Box 5-1 Continued

■ African Americans are more likely to be hospitalized for signs of poor diabetic control such as septicemia, debridement, and amputations, even though careful control of blood glucose levels can prevent these complications.

Source: USDHHS. Initiative to eliminate racial and ethnic disparities in health. Retrieved September 3, 2001, from http://www.omhrc.gov/rah

A major national commitment is necessary if the underlying causes of higher levels of disease and disability in ethnic and racial minority communities are to be identified and addressed. Based on a commitment made by President Clinton in February 1998 to eliminate disparities in selected areas of health status while continuing to improve the overall health of the American people, *Healthy People 2010* was published in 2000. *Healthy People 2010* outlines national health objectives and provides specific targets and evaluation strategies under the coordination of the United States Department of Health and Human Services (see Chapter 1, *Health, Health Promotion, and Healing*).

Research into underlying causes and approaches to elimination of health disparities is needed. Flaskerud and Winslow (1998) have proposed a conceptual framework for research and practice with vulnerable populations, that is, "social groups who have an increased relative risk or susceptibility to adverse health outcomes" (p. 69). Socioeconomic conditions have been labeled human capital (such as income, jobs, education, and housing), social connectedness or integration, and social status; environmental resources have been operationalized as access to health care and quality of care; and relative risk factors include lifestyle, behavior and choices, use of screening procedures, immunization programs and health promotion services, and exposure to or participation in stressful events including abuse, violence and crime. There may be a relationship between increased risk factors, increased morbidity, and premature mortality.

Flaskerud and Winslow (1998) propose a variety of primary, secondary, and tertiary prevention community nursing intervention strategies, including:

■ Population-based education efforts

■ Immunization programs

■ Safety programs to prevent risk behaviors

■ Screening for early detection of health problems

■ Support groups for caregivers of persons with chronic disease

■ Public policy efforts to change societal and environmental resources

Additional intervention strategies will be discussed at the end of this chapter.

Health/Illness Beliefs

An individual or group's definitions of health and illness are culturally determined. The experience of illness is related to an individual's perception and is not necessarily the same as a biomedical interpretation of disease (Toumishey, 1993). When lay or popular beliefs about health and illness are closely aligned with Western biomedicine (see Chapter 3, *The Meaning of Health: Health Care Belief Systems*), for example, cancer as an abnormal growth, there is high potential for a good exchange of ideas between practitioners and clients with regard to mutually acceptable treatment options. However, when there is an incompatibility between lay or popular beliefs and biomedical beliefs, for example, high blood pressure caused by too much blood, there may be client resistance to Western biomedical assessment and treatment recommendations.

Folk illnesses are based on very different theories of explanation than disease in Western biomedicine. In addition to a cluster of signs and symptoms, folk illnesses, which are commonly recognized or associated with specific cultural groups, also have symbolic meaning to the individual and the culture from which the folk illness arises. Helman (1994) outlines four categories of causality of lay/folk theories of illness:

1. *Biological causality.* Illness may result from malfunctions of the body as a result of factors such as diet or behavior over which the person has some control. This category also recognizes that hereditary, social, economic, and personality factors may play a role in illness causality and response. Here it is important to identify the individual's locus of control to determine whether he or she will take responsibility for health or regard health as lying outside of the self.

2. *Natural causality.* Includes both animate and inanimate factors thought to cause illness. For example, illness might be attributed to bacteria and viruses (e.g., flu, tuberculosis), parasitic infections (pinworms), and injuries caused by animals, birds, or fish. Other factors include environmental irritants such as smog, pollens, and poisons; natural disasters such as earthquakes, floods, and fires; and climatic conditions such as extremes of heat, cold, wind, rain, or snow.

3. *Social causality.* Concerned with interpersonal conflicts that include physical injuries inflicted by people on others (such as personal assaults resulting from gang violence, war, or other similar causes). Stresses resulting from conflicts with family, friends, or the work environment also are part of social causality. In more traditional non-Western cultures, illness is often ascribed to sorcery or witchcraft in which certain people have the power to cast spells, create potions, or carry out rituals that can result in illness or death for individuals against whom the sorcerer or witch has a personal vendetta.

4. *Supernatural causality.* Includes ancestral and other spirits and gods who can directly intercede in human life and cause personal difficulties, illness, and death. Illnesses inflicted from the supernatural world include spirit possessions, spirit aggression, and soul loss as retribution for behavioral lapses (e.g., sinful behavior such as getting drunk, offending a particular ancestor's spirit, or breaking a particular social taboo). When supernatural causes of illness are suspected by the client and/or the family or community, neither traditional home remedies nor a Western medical practitioner is considered useful in treating and curing the illness. Such situations call for repentance, prayer, and intercession of a shaman, priest, or other spiritual advisor or healer.

Many clinical encounters can be viewed as an interaction between the culture of the client and the culture of biomedicine or nursing. Both cultures are likely to have divergent perceptions, knowledge, attitudes, behaviors, and communication styles relative to the illness or health issue as a result of their explanatory models of health, disease, causality, and treatment. An individual's model is generally a composite of his or her "ethnocultural beliefs and values; personal beliefs, values, and behaviors; and understanding of biomedical concepts" (Huff, 1999, p. 25). The meanings people attach to various symptoms and illnesses are key factors in considering the implications for healing.

In contrast to the biomedical beliefs of most professional providers, the concept of illness (a subjective feeling of being unhealthy), rather than disease (a medical label for a recognizable clinical syndrome), is central to the average person's subjective response to not being well. Beliefs are the basic guidelines for perceiving, interpreting, organizing, and understanding meaningful experiences. Illness beliefs include the meaning and significance of the experience for the individual and "form the cognitive basis of the reasoning processes used by individuals to link plausible predictions about how to alter or control threats to health" (Drew, 1997, pp. 84-85).

Hufford (1995) suggests that too much emphasis on narrowly defined medical goals over the existential concerns of sick people is responsible for many of the concerns being expressed with conventional biomedicine. It is important for nurses to begin to understand clients' health, illness, and healing beliefs and behaviors from their own perspectives. Although health practitioners bring their personal cultural beliefs to each interaction with their clients, it is not acceptable to impose on clients "certain cherished and 'habitual' interventions" (Toumishey, 1993, p. 117). Provider ethnocentrism, even when unintended, communicates to the client disregard for perceptions, knowledge, and cultural health beliefs and practices (Drew, 1997). Most cases of lay illness have multiple causalities and may require several different approaches to diagnosis, treatment, and cure, potentially including home remedies, care by a nonprofessional healer, treatment by a biomedical physician, and/or intercession by a shaman.

Influence of Indigenous Cultural Beliefs

"America is a multicultural society.... There is an effort to maintain a respect for differences while recognizing that differences conspire against equity" (Huff & Kline, 1999, p. 504). The relationship of culture to health beliefs and practices is highly complex, dynamic, and interactive, involving family, community, and/or supernatural agents in cause, effect, placation, and treatment rituals to prevent, control, or cure illness (Huff, 1999). This section will review similarities of indigenous beliefs of Asian Americans (Vietnamese Americans), Appalachians, Native Americans, African Americans, and Hispanics (Mexican Americans) that can influence their health promotion care.

ASIAN AMERICAN INDIGENOUS HEALTH BELIEFS

Asian and Pacific Islander Americans are the fastest growing ethnic minorities in the United States (Huff & Kline, 1999). The term Asian American encompasses at least 23 subgroups, including Asian Indian, Cambodian, Chinese, Filipino, Hmong, Japanese, Korean, Laotian, Thai, Vietnamese, and "other Asian," with 32 linguistic groups. Although Asian groups share some similarities based on religious background and the influence of Chinese culture throughout Asia, health and disease patterns among Asian Americans differ by generations and immigration dates (Huff & Kline, 1999).

Indigenous beliefs can have a major impact on health. "A shift in the balance of natural forces can result in illness.... [A belief] among Vietnamese, Khmer, and Hmong is that illness is caused by eating spoiled food or eating an excess of 'hot' or 'cold' foods... energizing (hot) or calming (cold).... Spiritual beings can also cause illness. Malicious spirits can enter the body as a result of a violation of a taboo or spells of black magic. Benign spirits, believed to reside in the trees, can punish an offensive person who fails to show proper respect.... There are also guardian spirits" (Frye, 1995, p. 271).

Health is generally viewed as a state of harmony with nature or freedom from symptoms or illness. The concept of balance is related to health promotion, and the concept of imbalance is related to disease This balance, or equilibrium, applies to temperature in foods, climate, body elements, emotions, relationships, work and relaxation patterns, food intake, and spiritual life (Huff & Kline, 1999).

Confucian ideology, Buddhism, and Taoism are prominent in Asian cultures. These religions focus on upholding a public façade and sanctions against public admission of problems. For example, mental illness is regarded as shameful and as a punishment for misdeeds (Huff & Kline, 1999). Buddhism teaches that suffering should be accepted with calm resignation and expectation of future improvement in another lifetime (Frye, 1995). Therefore, some Asian cultures value stoicism and restraint of public display of emotion. People of some Asian cultures believe that suffering is a part of life, which may postpone seeking treatment for symptoms until they become unbearable.

Traditionally, elderly persons have held critical helper roles. "Monks, healers, and traditional birth attendants have provided stability and have been the bearers and gatekeepers of culture and tradition" (Frye, 1995, p. 273). Buddhism advocates merit-making actions such as feeding the monks or being kind to children and elders as ways to balance the scales for sinful transgressions in this life or past lives. This balance is further promoted through generosity and nonconfrontational behavior in interpersonal relationships (Frye, 1995).

An essential characteristic of Asian families is kinship solidarity, the view that "the individual is subservient to the kinship-based group or family.... Most Asian family patterns are characterized by filial piety, male authority, and respect for elders.... The contentment and happiness of their children is paramount to the notion of Chinese families of 'normal family functioning'" (Huff & Kline, 1999, pp. 349-350). In threatening situations, family solidarity is paramount (Frye, 1995).

A number of factors have contributed to the decline of the traditional multigenerational household, including loss of family, breaking of family units into manageable sizes for sponsorship, smaller housing units available in America, and challenges to the traditional family authority over adolescents. Marital roles also have changed. Many Khmer and Vietnamese refugee women have obtained informal or formal employment, often finding jobs more easily than their husbands. This factor has created a shift in power and challenged traditional gender roles. In addition, refugee families have frequently settled in cities, which are quite different from their rural backgrounds. They have often responded to the violence of the urban environment with passivity and withdrawal (Frye, 1995).

Language and literacy barriers are major factors in alienation from the American culture. Within the health care setting, one barrier is the use of bilingual children as translators for their elders. This practice, although expedient at times, exposes adult problems to the children. This practice does not support the traditional strong sense of hierarchy and authority. Of concern, in addition to the language barrier, is the illiteracy of much of the older Southeast Asian refugee population (Frye, 1995).

Vietnamese American Health Beliefs (Researched by Eden Zabat)

The Vietnamese are one of the largest Southeast Asian groups resettling in the United States (D'Avanzo, 1992; Frye, 1995). Vietnamese health beliefs are deeply rooted in Eastern philosophy. Eastern-influenced health assumptions assert that humans are a microcosm of nature and knowledge is subjective and relative (Beinfield & Korngold, 1995). The principal assumption is that there is order in the processes of heaven and earth with harmony and regularity in the order (Calhoun, 1985). Central beliefs of the Vietnamese are harmony with nature, and the integrative wholeness of the person. Health is "one facet of life in the universe, functioning as part of a unified, comprehensive scheme" (Calhoun, 1985, p. 63) and "rooted in a sense of balance and harmony within a person" (Healy, 1997, p. 40). The nature of health is harmony with nature.

Illness is related to a disharmony with nature. Illness is believed to be caused by traditional, supernatural (animism), and metaphysical (Am [yin] and Duong [yang] theory) factors. Animists believe in the existence of spirits, with both animate and inanimate things possessing a soul. While in an induced trance, shamans use rituals and negotiation with spirits to intercede for an ill person.

Excess or insufficiency of either *am* (cold, female) or *duong* (hot, male) can lead to illness through eating rotten foods, "bad wind," or excess ingestion of hot or cold food elements (Frye, 1995). "Foods are divided into two groups: hot—spices, coffee, beef, wild game; and cold—tea, most fruits, chicken, duck, seafood" (Nguyen, 1985, p. 411). Health care practices center on balancing the hot and cold elements. For example, Chinese herbs are seen as cold, while Western medicine is considered hot (Calhoun, 1985). Antibiotics are hot, and should always be taken with vitamin C, which is seen as cooling (Craig, 2000).

Other common indigenous health belief practices related to illness and disease that Vietnamese Americans use concurrently with professionalized health care include (Giger & Davidhizar, 1995; Louie, 1995; Nguyen, 1985):

- *Cao gio* ("coin rubbing"). Use of hot balm oil over the neck, back, chest, and arms to bring the "bad wind" to the surface.
- *Bat gio* ("skin pinching"). Commonly used for a headache.
- *Gia* ("cup suctioning"). Used for "bad wind."
- *Xong*. Herbal steam inhalation for colds or "bad wind."
- *Ingestion of gelatin-like tiger bones*. Brings strength.
- *Ingestion of hot foods*. Cures a "cold" illness.
- *Chinese herbs*. Balance am and duong.

Access and barriers to health care for Asian Americans are similar to those for other ethnic groups and focus on socioeconomic factors such as availability of health insurance, access and location of health care facilities, transportation, poverty, and unemployment.

APPALACHIAN HEALTH BELIEFS (RESEARCHED BY SANDRA ROZENDAL SCHULTZE, BSN, MS)

The term Appalachians refers to individuals who were either born in or live in a large area known as the Appalachian Mountain region of the United States (Purnell & Counts, 1998). The region crosses 13 different states. Although the population of the Appalachian Mountain region is diverse, most Appalachians are "largely white, primarily of Scottish-Irish or British descent, and predominantly fundamentalist Protestant. For the most part, the Appalachian region is classified as a rural, nonfarming area" (Small, 1995, p. 263), dominated by mining, timber, and textile industries. However, not all Appalachians live in the mountains; some have migrated to urban settings in the region.

Given the rural environment within which many Appalachians live, harmony with the environment is important. Burkhardt (1994) conducted a qualitative study in which she interviewed 12 Appalachian women about their spirituality. The women frequently spoke of connecting with the earth. They stated that they derived strength from nature, were knowledgeable regarding various plants and animals, and had a sense of the weather. Burkhardt noted that "there was a general sense that the environment was a source of strength and health" (p. 15).

Fundamentalist religion is an important aspect of the Appalachian culture, although for the most part, religious convictions are not associated with organized churches (Small, 1995). This is due in part to the mountainous terrain, which makes travel difficult. Instead, people develop informal social networks to support their faith. For the Appalachians, good health is seen as a gift from God (Purnell & Counts, 1998). They believe that God's will must prevail (Small, 1995), a present-oriented view that has been labeled by some writers as fatalistic.

Appalachians have an inherent distrust of health care providers, who are considered "outsiders." They are hesitant to discuss personal matters, including health-related issues, with outsiders (Sortet & Banks, 1997). When they do have contact with Western health care providers, they want to "sit a spell" and talk, allowing the health care provider an opportunity to gain acceptance (Reed et al., 1995).

A variety of nonprofessional healers may deliver care. Appalachian folk healers, including the "granny midwife," usually are older women. Many grannies take great pride in knowing that they delivered all of the children in a particular region (Helton, 1996). Because they are well known and trusted by those in need of health care, most herbal and folk practitioners are highly respected for their treatment (Purnell & Counts, 1998). Because of the social, geographical, or cultural isolation, folk healers are often the primary health care providers.

To restore harmony, folk practitioners may use a variety of items from nature, including herbal medicines, poultices, or teas. For example, to control bleeding, a spider web may be placed across the wound, and if a person has a burn, a poultice of egg whites and castor oil can be used. To treat arthritis, a tea is made by boiling the roots of ginseng. This tea is then either drunk or rubbed on the arthritic joint. As is the case with any cultural group, professional health care providers (outsiders) need to gain the support of indigenous providers (insiders) and work within the indigenous traditions and beliefs in order to influence health.

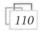

HISPANIC HEALTH BELIEFS

The term Hispanic originated as an official government label by the Office of Budget and Management in 1978, creating an ethnic category that included populations bound by a common ancestral language and cultural characteristics such as persons of Mexican, Puerto Rican, Central American, South American, or some other Spanish origin (Suarez & Ramirez, 1999). "The majority (61%) of the 22 million Hispanics in the United States are of Mexican origin" (Suarez & Ramirez, 1999, p. 116), three-quarters of whom live in Texas or California. The other two major Hispanic groups consist of 2.7 million Puerto Ricans and 1.0 million Cuban Americans, 65% of whom live in Florida. "By the next decade, the number of Hispanics will exceed that of African Americans to become the second largest racial/ethnic group in the country" (Suarez & Ramirez, 1999, p. 116).

Within the Hispanic culture, there is a strong identification with one's family and strong feelings of support from nuclear and extended family members. "Embedded in the structure of *la familia* is the authority and protection of the father, the sacrificing nature of the mother's role, and the *respeto* (respect) that children must give to family members.... For Hispanics, decisions about the use of medical care or preventive care or treatment are family based" (Suarez & Ramirez, 1999, pp. 120-121). The collective needs and achievements of the family take precedence over those of the individual members. Group togetherness and the physical presence of family and friends are valued. Help and advice are usually sought from within the family system first, and important decisions are made as a group.

Mexican American Health Beliefs

Within the Mexican American culture, children are highly desired and valued. Mexican American women are primarily responsible for maintaining the health of the family but may be uncomfortable touching their own bodies. A female provider can help to address modesty during health care examinations. However, fatalism, the belief that an individual has little control over personal health outcomes, is common. There is a "hint of fatalism (*asi es la vida,* or 'such is life'), accompanied by spiritual faith" (Applewhite, 1995, p. 250). The individual perceives little personal ability or responsibility for success or failure in matters of health and illness (Burk et al., 1995; Suarez & Ramirez, 1999). The belief that health is a matter of chance and controlled by forces in nature, may hinder the compliance of Mexican Americans with a health care regimen.

Value is placed on achieving harmony in interpersonal relationships. *Simpatia* (being nice) is the Hispanic tendency to avoid conflict in social and personal encounters. Respeto (respect) toward individuals is acknowledged and reciprocated and is based on age, sex, and social positions of authority. Respeto dictates appropriate deferential behavior toward others on the basis of age, sex, social position, economic status, and position of authority. Deferential behavior is demonstrated by using formal, rather than informal, Spanish language and by listening attentively to clients and providing information in a courteous manner. It incorporates diplomacy and tactfulness and discourages confrontation (Suarez & Ramirez, 1999).

Personalismo emphasizes that the client's relationship is with the individual provider rather than the institution. Therefore, the nurse should greet the client by name and inquire about his or her general well-being or family before getting to the actual business of the visit. There is a valuing of physical touch, so a handshake is an appropriate greeting (Burk et al., 1995).

Curanderismo, or Mexican American folk healing, is a coherent, comprehensive system of healing primarily derived from a synthesis of Mayan and Aztec teachings with the Mexican heritage of Spanish Catholicism. The underlying concept is the spiritual focus of the healing (Krippner, 1995). The *curandero*, or folkhealer, views illness from a religious and social context. However, although curanderismo is a traditional healing system, it exists within the modern world. Biomedical beliefs, treatments, and practices are very much a part of curanderismo, and are supported by curanderos (Trotter, 1996).

Curanderismo has a community-based theoretical structure based on a duality of "natural" and "supernatural." There are three primary areas of concentration, called levels (niveles) by the healers: the material level (nivel material), the spiritual level (nivel espiritual), and the mental level (nivel mental). Physical (material) treatments are those that do not require supernatural intervention to assure a successful outcome. *Parteras* (midwives), *hueseros* (bone setters), *yerberos* (herbalists), and *sobadores* (people who treat sprains and tense muscles) accomplish cures without any need for supernatural knowledge or practices, while the supernatural aspect of the material level is involved in cures for common folk illnesses such as *mal de ojo*, *susto*, *empacho*, and *caida de mollera* (Trotter, 2001).

- *Mal de oyo* (evil eye). A person can make another sick by looking at him or her, but it usually is not thought to have been done on purpose. The one who gets ill is weak (usually an infant), fussy, and refuses to eat and sleep. Treatment is symbolic, by protecting with amulets or having the face covered in the presence of strangers.

- *Susto*. Fright, sudden shock. Herb tea and ritual cleansings (barrideas) are used to restore the harmony of body and soul (Giger & Davidhizar, 1995).

- *Empacho*. Thought to be caused by something getting stuck in the intestines causing blockage. Symptoms are diarrhea, constipation, indigestion, vomiting, and bloating. The most common treatment is massage along with herbal teas; the former is for dislodging the blockage and the later is for washing it out.

- *Caida de mollera* (fallen fontanelle). Diarrhea, excessive crying, fever, loss of appetite, and irritability. Treatment includes raising the fontanelle by pushing up on the palate.

Most practitioners of curanderismo are women who are typically "called" to their profession by spiritual entities. They apprentice themselves to a friend or relative until they are considered ready to practice. Most are part-time practitioners who do not charge a fee but are given a small offering or gift.

"Supernatural manipulations involve prayers and incantations in conjunction with such objects as candies, ribbons, water, fire, crucifixes, tree branches, herbs, oils, eggs, and live animals... Supernaturally induced illnesses are most commonly said to be initiated by either *espiritos malos* (evil spirits) or by *brujos* (individuals practicing antisocial magic)" (Trotter, 2001, p. 413). The spiritual level is comparable to the channeling found in New Age groups and in shaman healing rituals around the world. In addition, the mental level might be described as "the ability to transmit, channel, and focus mental vibrations in a way that would affect the [client's] mental or physical condition directly" (Trotter, 2001, p. 414).

Healers work by virtue of "a gift of healing" (*el don*) (Trotter, 2001, p. 413). The three levels are discrete areas of knowledge and behavior, each necessitating a separate gift for healing. They involve different types of training, and different methods of dealing with both the natural and the supernatural world. Treatment of natural illnesses is generally carried out by physician specialists. Herbal treatments are supervised by the *herbolaria*, *medica*, and *herbalista* while the *senora* prescribes home remedies. "The first person to be consulted at the time of illness is a key family member who is respected for her knowledge of folk medicine.... The *jerbero* is a folk healer who specializes in using herbs and spices for preventive and curative purposes.... The more serious physical and mental or emotional illnesses are brought to the curandero" (Giger & Davidhizar, 1995, p. 219). Illnesses with a supernatural source can be repaired only by the supernatural manipulations of curanderos.

The priorities and roles of society are to support the patient's recovery because the entire community is concerned and affected when a member becomes ill. The goal of the curanderismo model is to assist the recovery of the patient, restoring balance within a social framework that preserves the traditions of the family and the Mexican American subculture. Suffering and illness are not seen as a punishment from God but as an inevitable part of life, a challenge, and part of God's plan to instruct human beings and lead them to salvation (Krippner, 1999).

Another element of the belief in balance is the humoral model for classifying activity, food, drugs, and illness, in which good health is maintained by maintaining a balance of hot and cold. This model emphasizes balance in relationships and behavior. A balance of emotional "humors" and the avoidance of an excess of "hot" or "cold" foods (i.e., foods that stimulate the body versus foods that have a calming effect) is important as well. "Symbolically, cold is related to things that menace the individual, whereas hot is related to warmth and reassurance" (Giger & Davidhizar, 1995, p. 217).

Hispanics have much lower rates of cardiovascular disease and cancer than whites, but have higher death rates due to diabetes, the seventh leading cause of death in the country. Lack of health insurance is the major barrier to preventive care for the Hispanic population, which limits participation in dental care, cancer screening, and prenatal care (Suarez & Ramirez, 1999). The coexistence of curanderismo with biomedicine in Hispanic communities requires both cultural sensitivity and the ability to provide care that acknowledges the beliefs of the contrasting systems.

African American Health Beliefs

African American values are a combination of African heritage and the American experience. Some 80% of Africans, especially the economically deprived, still use traditional healing methods grounded on belief rather than knowledge, which have been sustained over the years because they are acceptable, available, and affordable (Hopp & Herring, 1999).

One important value includes the extended family, the belief that all the aunts and uncles are responsible parents of all their nieces and nephews, the belief in collectivism as opposed to individualism, and respect for age. Women, especially, are affected by "a legacy of struggle against racism, classism, and sexism that is inextricably linked with a parallel struggle for independence, self-reliance, and self-definition.... The goal of struggle is to live a meaningful life reflective of the uniqueness of African American culture" (Banks-Wallace, 2000, p. 35).

In the traditional African philosophy, knowledge obtained through Western formal education is a power that is reserved only for males who will inherit the land. Women's humanity is affirmed not only by their ability to have children, but also by their ability to have male children. Young girls are discouraged from becoming high achievers because of concern over their difficulty in finding husbands (Airhihenbuwa, 1995).

Traditional African values stress a lifestyle of "acquiescence" rather than challenge of nature. It is believed that a state of balance exists within the individual and between the individual and the environment. Good health is considered harmony with nature; illness and bad health, on the other hand, are viewed as disharmony with nature that may be caused by a variety of factors. In addition, there is an emphasis on oral tradition, in which people learn by listening. "Learning by seeing is important to the extent that what is seen is congruent with what is heard" (Airhihenbuwa, 1995, p. 9).

Illnesses deemed to be due to natural causes often result from stress; cold; impurities in the water, air, or food; improper eating habits or diet; weakness; or lack of moderation in daily activities. In contrast, illnesses or mishaps deemed to be due to unnatural causes may be blamed on the evil influences of the devil, witchcraft, demons, or bad spirits. Worry, according to traditional beliefs of many African Americans, is the main component in the course of unnatural illness. Unnatural illnesses can be terrifying because they usually do not respond to self-treatment or remedies administered by friends, relatives, or practitioners (Hopp & Herring, 1999).

"The remedies for treating calamities caused by evil influences include food, medicine, antidotes, healing, and prayer proposed to God by a medium with unusual powers" (Hopp & Herring, 1999, p. 208). Other traditional cures and treatments include:

- External aids such as magic and visible protection in the form of prayer, cards, and charms.

- Eating garlic for hypertension.

- Drinking teas made from herbs for colds.

- Applying tallow to the chest and covering it with a cloth for colds.

- Pouring kerosene into cuts as a disinfectant.

- Wearing garlic around the neck to keep from catching disease.

- Using vinegar, Epsom salts, pain-relief cream, and copper wire or bracelets for arthritis.

- Drinking horehound tea or buttermilk for diabetes, and tea made of rabbit tobacco and pine top for asthma.

Experience is strongly valued by African American women, and "separates knowledge from wisdom" (Banks-Wallace, 2000, p. 37). Opportunities to share experience, through dialogue and sharing stories, can build or nurture connections and establish the credibility of a health promotion intervention. Replenishment as an aspect of spiritual development is integrally associated with health in this group as well as in Native American tribes.

NATIVE AMERICAN (INDIAN) HEALTH BELIEFS

The term Native American is problematic because it implies a uniform culture and healing system. "The indigenous people of North America identify themselves by nation (commonly called tribe), band or community, clan, and family" (Cohen, 1998, p. 45). Although there are more than 500 distinct federally recognized tribes, there are many similarities and cultural bonds among them (Lowe & Struthers, 2001). Commonly, "health means restoring the body, mind, and spirit to balance and wholeness: the balance of life energy in the body; the balance of ethical, reasonable, and just behavior; balanced relations within family and community; and harmonious relationships with nature.... A healthy person has a sense of purpose... is committed to walking a path of beauty, balance, and harmony... and is grateful, respectful, and generous" (Cohen, 1998, pp. 45, 47).

Unlike Western biomedicine, Native American healing tends to consider disease in terms of morality, balance, and the action of spiritual power rather than specific, measurable causes. As a result, "native healers believe that among adults, some diseases are the [client's] responsibility and the natural consequence of his or her behavior; to treat these conditions may be to interfere with important life lessons" (Cohen, 1998, p. 47). The health of the land is integral to human health.

"Native American medicine is based upon a spiritual rather than a materialistic or Cartesian world view. The art of traditional healing places an emphasis on: (a) the spirit world, (b) supernatural forces, and (c) religion" (Struthers, Eschiti, & Patchell, 2004, p.142). The term "medicine" in Native American cultures has come to mean "supernatural power." Wholeness and interrelatedness are basic principles, and illness is associated with imbalance. Healing ability can be acquired in several ways that include inherited from ancestors, transmitted from another healer, and/or developed through training and initiation. Healers can be chosen by their own vision, or by their community (Struthers et al., 2004).

The causes of disease are internal and external. Internal causes include:

- Negative thoughts about oneself, including shame, despair, worry, and depression.

- Negative thoughts about others, including blame, jealousy, and anger.

- "Disturbances in flow of life energy and healing power within the individual or to/from the environment" (Cohen, 1998, p. 48).

External causes include:

- Pathogenic forces, objects (including microbes), people (sorcerers), and/or spirits.

- Environmental poisons, pollution, and contaminants, including alcoholic drinks and unhealthy food.

- Traumatic events that are physical, emotional, and/or spiritual.

- Breach of taboo, including unbalanced living and inconsiderate behavior; not demonstrating proper respect toward an animal, person, place, object, event, or spirit; improper performance of ritual or care of ritual objects (Cohen, 1998).

In describing characteristics of the Navajo tribe during illness, Bell (1994) notes that families gather together for consultation during a prolonged visit, often answering questions affirmatively in the presence of a primary care practitioner because of a desire to please. Direct eye contact is considered to be unacceptably rude and intrusive. Silence is highly respected, since speech connotes power and wisdom as well as communication. "Conflict and competitiveness are not valued, as they are not in keeping with a peaceful heart" (p. 238).

Lowe and Struthers (2001, p. 280) have identified seven dimensions forming a conceptual framework of "intertwined, related, and overlapping components" of nursing in Native American culture. This framework, which clearly demonstrates the uniqueness of the Native American culture, can provide a structure for nursing practice, education, and research with Native Americans.

Western biomedicine relies heavily on the precision of particular diagnostic techniques. However, within Native American cultures, diagnostic ability depends more on the intuition, sensitivity, and spiritual power of the healer—"the ability of the healer to see the patient with the inner eye of spirit, to sense disturbances of energy with the hands and heart, and to commune with higher sources of knowledge" (Cohen, 1998, p. 50). Some principles of Native American healing include (Mehl-Madrona, 1999, pp. 37-39):

- Healing takes time and time is healing. One should not begin the task of treating a sick person unless he or she has sufficient time to "give" to the client. The act of giving time to another person is healing in itself. Intent and power from the healer are passed on to the recipient.

- Healing takes place within the context of a relationship.

- Achieving an "energy of activation" is necessary, exerting maximum effort over a short period of time. As a result, one client at a time may be treated until the job is done.

- The distractions of modern life inactivate catalysts of change. Peace and quiet are needed for self-exploration and development of an awareness of emotional states.

- Modern culture systematically teaches us to ignore emotions and to maintain a low level of emotional awareness.

- Physiological change often requires a break in usual daily rhythms. Rest and quiet are needed to promote cellular repair.

- Ceremony such as a vision quest or purification ceremony is important as a means to receive help from the spiritual dimension.

"Methods of diagnosis, methodology, and treatment vary greatly from tribe to tribe and healer to healer. Specific skills are utilized to correct imbalance."

- Divination or prediction to foretell or forecast events or situations, e.g., a seer can foretell the future. This may include dreaming of events to come.

- Natural elements such as water, fire, smoke, stones, or crystals may be used as a projective field to help to see the reason and/or course of an imbalance.

- Prayer

- Chanting

- Use of music, singing, drums, and rattles

- Smudging with medicinal plants such as sage, cedar, and sweet grass

- Laying on of hands

- Talking or counseling

- Medicinal plants or botanical medicines that are made into teas, salves, ointments, purgatives, and other substances

- Ceremony

- Sweat lodge

- Shake tent

- Yuwipi

- Dancing

- Dreaming

- Use of tobacco, either as an offering or smoked

- Storytelling (Struthers, Eschiti, & Patchell, 2004, p. 146)

Therapeutic methods include prayer, music, ritual purification, herbalism, massage, ceremony, and the personal innovations of individual healers (Cohen, 1998).

Medicocentrism (Medical Ethnocentrism)

Medicocentrism is the bias produced by viewing health through the lens of medicine as it is currently found in modern society. Mastery over nature, future time orientation, doing, and individualism are stable, core American values (See Chapter 3, *The Meaning of Health: Health Care Belief Systems*). Stein (1990) discusses specific American medical decision making and treatment values that are associated with the core American values including:

- *Fantasized omnipotence*. Manifested by a compulsion to change others. In addition, theories provide an inexhaustible reserve of explanations and interventions in cases for which the rest of medicine has nothing to offer, assuring that there are never sicknesses about which medicine simply cannot say or do anything (Hufford, 1996).

- *Dichotomy between active and passive*. Passively listening, waiting, comforting, nondirective counseling, "going along with nature," or doing nothing are anathema. Actively intervening, aggressively treating, controlling, curing, and fixing the client increase self-esteem for the clinician and preserve the illusion of distance between clinician and client.

- *Health as an ideal*. Health is manifested by the absence or resolution of the presenting problem. Disease is a deviation.

- *Visualization*. Seeing what the pathology is and where is it located spatially is valued. Technology follows and endlessly elaborates on this visual mode of knowing. Subjective data are less valuable than objective data.

- *Control*. Medicine tends to move toward administrative control, based on technical knowledge, over all activities relevant to health.

- *Male language.* "'Hard science,' 'real medicine,' 'aggressive intervention,' the 'cure' and 'conquest' of 'real disease' are all idealized idioms of masculinity" (Stein, 1990, p. 51).

- *Functionality.* Dysfunction, and its associated dependency are dreaded. Consequently, what works is valued.

Additional, more specific values include "certainty, completeness, lack of ambiguity, power (omnipotence), knowledge (omniscience in the form of 'facts'), [and] goodness (omnibenevolence). So long as a [clinician] is able to exercise and fulfill these values, he or she feels competent, successful, good, validated, and vindicated as a [clinician]" (Stein, 1990, p. 50). However, medicocentrism negatively affects the establishment of an authentic therapeutic relationship between culturally diverse clients and their clinicians. As a result, clients feeling that their beliefs are not understood nor valued, may not seek biomedical or nursing assistance, or may not adhere to recommended regimens. At the least, medicocentrism leads to lack of mutual trust and collaboration between client and provider.

Culturally Competent Health Promotion Care

Leininger (1999, p. 9) blends concepts from anthropology and nursing to define transcultural nursing "as a legitimate and formal area of study, research, and practice, focused on culturally based care beliefs, values, and practices to help cultures or subcultures maintain or regain their health (well-being) and face disabilities or death in culturally congruent and beneficial caring ways." Culturally congruent care means to provide appropriate "care that is meaningful and fits with cultural beliefs and lifeways" (Leininger, 1999, p. 9). Smith (1998, p. 8) defines cultural competence as "a continuous developmental process of pursuing cultural awareness, knowledge, skill, encounters, sensitivity, and linkages among services and people."

Mensah (1993) defines terms somewhat differently in differentiating three types of culturally based care:

1. *Transcultural care.* Based on a comparative study and analysis of different cultures with respect to their caring behavior, health and illness values, beliefs and patterns of behavior. The focus is on the care-giver.

2. *Cross-cultural care.* Based on the assumption that the client and the professional helpers are of different cultural backgrounds. The focus is on the care.

3. *Multicultural care.* Health care which is both culturally appropriate and culturally sensitive; the focus is on the total health system.

The next section will present an overview of Leininger's theory of culture care diversity and universality, and Purnell's model for cultural competence. Both initiate a process for cultural competence through assessment of cultural differences in various categories of culture.

MODELS/THEORIES FOR CULTURALLY COMPETENT CARE

A prominent cross cultural nursing theory is Leininger's theory of culture care diversity and universality. She states that "the social structure and worldview of Western and non-Western cultures are strong influences on care practices leading to health or well-being" (Leininger, 1991, p. 57). Selected major elements of the theory of culture care diversity and universality, which have mutual influence in affecting culture congruent nursing care, are:

1. Culture and social structure dimensions:

   - Technological factors

   - Religious and philosophical factors

   - Kinship and social factors

   - Cultural values and lifeways

   - Political and legal factors

   - Economic factors

   - Educational factors

2. Care systems:

   - *Generic lay care system.* A folk, indigenous, or naturalistic lay care system.

   - *Professional health care system.* Care or cure services offered by personnel who have been prepared through professional programs of study.

3. Three major modalities guide nursing judgments, decisions, or actions so as to provide cultural congruent care:

   - *Cultural care preservation and/or maintenance.* "Assistive, supportive, facilitative, or enabling professional actions and decisions that help people of a particular culture to retain and/or preserve relevant care values so they can maintain their well-being, recover from illness, or face handicaps and/or death" (Leininger, 1991, p. 48).

   - *Cultural care accommodation and/or negotiation.* "Assistive, supportive, facilitative, or enabling creative professional actions and decisions that help people of a designated culture to adapt to, or to negotiate with, others for a beneficial or satisfying health outcome with professional care providers" (Leininger, 1991, p. 48).

   - *Cultural care repatterning or restructuring.* "Assistive, supportive, facilitative, or enabling professional actions and decisions that help a clients reorder, change, or greatly modify their lifeways for a new, different, and beneficial health care pattern" (Leininger, 1991, p. 49). Leininger's theory of culture care diversity and universality posits that "emic culture care knowledge from Western and non-Western cultures shows greater diversity than similarities or commonalties in cultural values, usage, and meanings" (Leininger, 1991, p. 57). The implication is that culture care knowledge specific to each culture is needed to guide nursing care.

In contrast to Leininger's theory, which is specific to nursing, Purnell (2000) developed a model for cultural competence to be used by all health disciplines in all practice settings. The core of the model is comprised of twelve cultural domains each of which relates to and is affected by all other domains:

- *Overview/heritage.* Concepts related to the country of origin; current residence; economics; politics; educational status; and occupation.

- *Communication.* Concepts related to the dominant language and its contextual use; nonverbal communication; past, present, or future temporality; and clock versus social time.

- *Family roles and organization.* Concepts related to head of the household and gender roles; family roles; child-rearing practices and roles of the aged; and social status.

- *Workforce issues.* Concepts related to autonomy; acculturation; assimilation; and health care practices from the country of origin.

- *Biocultural ecology.* Variations in ethnic and racial origins; and differences in the way drugs are metabolized by the body.

- *High-risk behaviors.* Includes the use of tobacco, alcohol, and recreational drugs; lack of physical activity; increased calorie consumption; and engaging in risky sexual practices.

- *Nutrition.* Includes having adequate food; the meaning of food; food choices, rituals, and taboos; and how food and food substances are used for health promotion and wellness and during illness.

- *Pregnancy and childbearing practices.* Includes fertility practices; birth control methods; and practices related to pregnancy, birthing, and postpartum.

- *Death rituals.* Includes behaviors to prepare for death and burial practices; and bereavement behaviors.

- *Spirituality.* Includes religious practices and the use of prayer; behaviors that give meaning to life; and individual sources of strength.

- *Health care practices.* Includes acute or preventive focus of health care; traditional, magicoreligious, and biomedical beliefs; individual responsibility for health; self-medicating practices; and barriers to health care.

- *Health care practitioner concepts.* Includes status, use, and perceptions of providers; and gender of the health care provider.

According to Purnell (2000, p. 43), "cultural competence is the adaptation of care in a manner that is congruent with the culture of the client." The model provides a structure for identifying cultural elements to assess, plan, and intervene in a culturally competent manner.

Duffy (2001) directly challenges the current emphasis in providing culturally competent care by adapting care from the dominant culture of the health care provider to the culture of the client. Duffy (2001, p. 487) disagrees with the highlighting of unique, exotic, or unusual differences between groups, contending that by developing a composite portrait, the group is homogenized and stereotyped, and, in addition, "globalization contributes to differences within cultures that may equal or exceed differences between cultures." This last assertion, which challenges Leininger's theory of culture care diversity and universality, can be evaluated through ongoing research.

Duffy (2001) contends that the emphasis on understanding stereotypes of another culture fosters feelings of cultural superiority, with care subsequently focused on changing the individual rather than society. She states that the emphasis should be on the "shared human attributes that create a common global culture" (p. 491), with emphasis on risk-taking, critical self-reflection, and shared power interactions co-creating cultural inclusion.

Andrews and Boyle (1999, p. 15) also contend that "transcultural nursing has done too little to encourage nurses to be actively involved in setting political, economic and social policy agendas." It is necessary to go beyond awareness of one's own and other cultures. Positive experiences and a genuine valuing of the contributions of other cultures are needed in order to alleviate and eventually eradicate prejudice, bigotry, discrimination, and ethnic or cultural violence.

Nurses need knowledge and skills for multicultural assessment and intervention of clients, organizations, government, and/or community agencies including abilities to:

1. recognize cultural diversity;

2. understand the role that culture and ethnicity/race play in the sociopsychological and economic development of ethnic and culturally diverse populations;

3. understand that socioeconomic and political factors significantly impact the psychosocial, political, and economic development of ethnic and culturally diverse groups;

4. help clients to understand/maintain/resolve their own sociocultural identification, and understand the interaction of culture, gender, and sexual orientation on behavior and needs.

UNDERSTANDING CULTURAL AND ETHNIC DIFFERENCES

Huff and Kline (1999) suggest ways in which understanding and appreciating cultural and ethnic differences can be used by the nurse to facilitate the success of health promotion efforts. Guidelines for working with diverse populations can be found in Box 5-2.

■ Be aware of the many ways of perceiving, understanding, and approaching health and disease processes across cultural and ethnic groups. Cultural differences can and do present major barriers to effective health care intervention, as competing values, beliefs, norms, and health practices may be in conflict with the traditional Western biomedical model.

■ Understand how the concepts of culture, ethnicity, acculturation, and ethnocentrism may affect the ability to assess, plan, implement, and evaluate health promotion development programs. Be careful in the assessment, intervention, and evaluation planning processes not to overlook, misinterpret, stereotype, or otherwise mishandle encounters with those who might be viewed as different.

■ Assess the degree to which the culture of the target group has been modified through contact with other cultures (acculturation) when working in a multicultural setting because there is a natural tendency on the part of many culturally diverse individuals to resist acculturation. Be aware that ethnicity often is used to stereotype diversity in human populations and frequently can lead to misunderstanding and/or distrust in all sorts of human interactions.

■ Be careful not to become caught in personal ethnocentrism, because culturally diverse target groups may view the nurse as foreign; ignorant of illness or disease causality; or uneducated to proper social customs, forms of address, and nonverbal behaviors deemed appropriate by the groups for dealing directly or indirectly with their health problems

Box 5-2

Guidelines for Working with Ethnically, Linguistically, and Culturally Diverse Populations

1. Incorporate an understanding of the client's ethnic and cultural background.
2. Be aware of how their own culture/background/experiences, attitudes, values, and biases influence psychological processes.
3. Help clients increase their awareness of their own cultural values and norms.
4. Help a client determine whether a problem stems from racism or bias in others.
5. Respect the roles of family members and community structures, hierarchies, values, and beliefs within the client's culture.
6. Respect clients' religious and/or spiritual beliefs and values, including attributions and taboos.
7. Interact in the language requested by the client.
8. Consider the impact of adverse social, environmental, and political factors in assessing problems and designing interventions.
9. Work to eliminate biases, prejudices, and discriminatory practices.
10. Document culturally and sociopolitically relevant factors in the records.

Source: American Psychological Association. APA guidelines for providers of psychological services to ethnic, lingistic, and culturally diverse populations. Accessed 1/4/05 at http://www.apa.org/pi/oema/guide.html.

or concerns. Seek to become more culturally competent and sensitive. The process is ongoing. Be willing to step out of your own current frames of reference and take the risk of discovering personal biases and stereotypes and opening up to new and perhaps quite divergent points of view about the world.

■ Be acutely aware that in an interaction between two or more individuals representing divergent cultural orientations, the rules governing the communication process may be different and the opportunity for miscommunication is significant. Remember that the typical Western biomedical model for health care communication seeks to quickly establish facts. This approach may be seen as cold, too direct, or otherwise in conflict with more traditional beliefs, values, and ways of communicating and of seeking and receiving health care.

■ Be aware that the health concepts held by many cultural groups may result in people choosing not to seek Western biomedical treatment procedures because they do not view the illness or disease as coming from within themselves (in Western cultures, the locus of control tends to be more internally oriented). Recognize that individuals from other cultures might not follow through with health-promoting or treatment recommendations because they perceive the medical or nursing encounter as a negative or perhaps even hostile experience.

■ Recognize that the more disparate the differences are between the biomedical model and the lay/popular explanatory models, the greater the potential for resistance to Western health development programs. If the more traditional person does seek Western biomedical treatment, then that person might not be able to provide or describe his or her symptoms in precise terms. Folk illnesses are generally learned syndromes that individuals from particular cultural groups claim to have and from which their culture defines the etiology, behaviors, diagnostic procedures, prevention methods, and traditional healing or curing practices.

■ Remember that most cases of lay illness have multiple causalities and may require several different approaches to diagnosis, treatment, and cure including folk and Western biomedical interventions. Folk illnesses, which are perceived to arise from a variety of causes, often require the services of a folk healer who may be a local curandero, shaman, native healer, spiritualist, root doctor, or other specialized healer.

UNDERSTANDING CULTURAL AND ETHNIC COMMONALTIES

In the spirit of Duffy's (2001) recommendation to focus on commonalties across cultural and ethnic groups, Box 5-3 proposes common strategies for understanding cultural and ethnic groups.

Box 5-3

Common Strategies for Cultural and Ethnic Understanding

■ Examine your own perceptions, stereotypes, and prejudices and be willing to suspend judgments (where they exist) in favor of learning who these people really are rather than who or what you might think they are. This is a critical first step in developing cultural competence and sensitivity.

continued

Box 5-3 CONTINUED

- All care requires co-participation of nurse and clients working together. Plans and decisions should be made with clients.

- Engage in active listening (rather than talking) and be alert to non-verbal cues.

- Autonomy is not the central value in many cultures. Appreciate the relative valuing of independence and cooperation.

- Appreciate that family and family support is one of the most important core values. Be aware how devastating separation from family members can be to a culture that values the nuclear and extended family.

- Be aware of the dynamics within the family. Recognize that one adult might be the spokesperson for the family, but try to elicit all opinions.

- Understand that a trusting relationship must be established before concerns are shared with the nurse.

- Recognize that belief in folk illnesses still is a strong cultural characteristic among many population groups with strong traditional roots.

- Recognize that traditional folk healers often are the first health practitioners consulted because they are culturally acceptable, willing to make house calls, and far less expensive than the Western health care system.

- Do not overlook traditional or cultural beliefs of spiritual or supernatural forces and balance with nature.

- Be aware that avoiding conflict and achieving harmony in interpersonal relationships may be a strong cultural value.

- Be aware that many traditional family patterns are characterized by filial piety, male authority, and respect for elders and that this pattern sometimes determines decision-making practices relating to health care. Knowledge is "shown" in a context of respect rather than through direct asking.

- Address illiteracy by using picture stories, videos, sociodrama, and story-telling with appropriate cultural imagery.

- Understand that health beliefs and practices will vary between urban and rural areas and between cultures of origin.

- Recognize that socioeconomic status has a greater impact on health status than does ethnicity.

- Recognize that lifestyle risk factors are more important predictors of diseases than is ethnicity (e.g. intravenous drug use and HIV infection) (Hopp & Herring, 1999, p. 218).

- Appreciate that there is a healthy suspicion in many communities about programs and services coming from outside the community.

Source: Adapted from Huff, R. M., & Kline, M. V. (1999). *Promoting health in multicultural populations: A handbook for practitioners* (pp. 383-394). Thousand Oaks, CA: Sage.

At the system level, "it is clear that the sociopolitical contexts of poverty, racism, immigration, and culture have had a significant bearing on access to health care, utilization of services, and health status" (Chin, 2000, p. 28). In addition to the acknowledged need for language access, cultural competence in health care requires attention to quick, convenient, and readily obtainable services (access to care), appropriate utilization of services, and quality of care. Unfortunately, language, cultural, and financial barriers can result in delayed entry into care, under utilization of services, and/or over utilization of the emergency room (Chin, 2000).

Clearly, it is appropriate for the nurse to take the time in an initial needs assessment to explore the explanatory models of the cultural or ethnic group with which he or she will be working, but also recognize "the influence of the global community, other groups, and individuals on the individual expression of culture" (Duffy, 2001, p. 490). Cultural interactions should emphasize shared power and mutual communication, learning, and changing. The individual, not the professional, is the expert. Health promotion activities can best be fostered by focusing on universal commonalities and individual distinctiveness.

Chapter Key Points

- Ethnic and cultural beliefs play a significant role in the development of a person's health beliefs.

- Indigenous health beliefs of Asian Americans (Vietnamese Americans), Appalachians, Native Americans, African Americans, and Hispanics (Mexican Americans) must be incorporated into multicultural health promotion care.

- Multicultural care is needed to reduce medicocentrism (medical ethnocentrism), and culturally based misunderstandings between nurses and their clients.

- Multifaceted assessment is critical to the development of multicultural health promotion interventions.

- Both cultural and ethnic differences and commonalties must be considered in planning for culturally competent health promotion.

References

Airhihenbuwa, C. O. (1995). *Health and culture: Beyond the Western paradigm.* Thousand Oaks, CA: Sage.

American Psychological Association. APA gruidelines for providers of psychological services to ethnic, lingistic, and culturally diverse populations. Accessed 1/4/05 at http://www.apa.org/pi/oema/guide.html.

Andrews, M. M., & Boyle, J. S. (1999). *Transcultural concepts in nursing care* (3rd ed.). Philadelphia: Lippincott.

Applewhite, S. L. (1995). Curanderismo: Demystifying the health beliefs and practices of elderly Mexican Americans. *Health & Social Work, 20,* 247-253.

Banks-Wallace, J. (2000). Womanist ways of knowing: Theoretical considerations for research with African American women. *Advances in Nursing Science, 22,* 33-45.

Beinfield, H., & Korngold, E. (1995). Chinese traditional medicine: An introductory overview. *Altern Ther Health Med, 1,* 44-52.

Bell, R. (1994). Prominence of women in Navajo healing beliefs and values. *Nursing & Health Care, 15,* 232-240.

Burk, M. E., Wieser, P. C., & Keegan, L. (1995). Cultural beliefs and health behaviors of pregnant Mexican-American women: Implications for primary care. *Advances in Nursing Science, 17,* 37-52.

Burkhardt, M. A. (1994). Becoming and connecting: Elements of spirituality for women. *Holistic Nursing Practice, 8*(4), 12-21.

Calhoun, M. A. (1985). The Vietnamese woman: Health/illness attitudes and behaviors. *Health Care for Women International, 6,* 61-72.

Chin, J. L. (2000). Culturally competent health care. *Public Health Rep, 115,* 25-33.

Cohen, K. B. (1998). Native American medicine. *Altern Ther Health Med, 4,* 45-57.

Corin, E. (1995). The cultural frame: Context and meaning in the construction of health. In B. C. Amick, S. Levine, A. R. Tarlov, & D. C. Walsh (Eds.), *Society and health* (pp. 272-303). Oxford, England: Oxford University Press.

D'Avanzo, C. E. (1992). Barriers to health care for vietnamese refugees. *J Prof Nur, 8*(4), 245-253.

Drew, J. C. (1997). The ethnocultural context of healing. In P. B. Kritek, (Ed.), *Reflections on healing. A central nursing construct.* New York: National League for Nursing.

Duffy, M. E. (2001). A critique of cultural education in nursing. *J Adv Nurs, 36,* 487-495.

Fiscella, K., Franks, P., Gold, M. R., & Clancy, C. M. (2000). Inequality in quality: Addressing socioeconomic, racial, and ethnic disparities in health care. *JAMA, 283,* 2579-2583.

Flaskerud, J. H., & Winslow, B. J. (1998). Conceptualizing vulnerable populations health-related research. *Nurs Res, 47,* 69-78.

Frye, B. (1995). Use of cultural themes in promoting health among southeast Asian refugees. *American Journal of Health, 9*(4), 269-280.

Giger, J. N., & Davidhizar, R. E. (1995). *Transcultural nursing: Assessment and intervention* (2nd ed.). St Louis: Mosby.

Healy, E. A. (1997). Health locus-of-control beliefs in vietnamese clients with latent tuberculosis. *Nursing Connections, 10*(2), 39-46.

Helman, C. G. (1994). *Culture, health and illness* (3rd ed.). Oxford, England: Butterworth-Heinemann.

Helton, L. R. (1996). Folk medicine and health beliefs: An Appalachian perspective. *Journal of Cultural Diversity, 3,* 123-128.

Hopp, J. W., & Herring, P. (1999). Promoting health among Black American populations: An overview. In R. M. Huff, & M. V. Kline, *Promoting health in multicultural populations: A handbook for practitioners* (pp. 201-221). Thousand Oaks, CA: Sage.

Huff, R. M. (1999). Cross-cultural concepts of health and disease. In R. M. Huff, & M. V. Kline, *Promoting health in multicultural populations: A handbook for practitioners* (pp. 23-39). Thousand Oaks, CA: Sage.

Huff, R. M., & Kline, M. V. (1999). Promoting health in multicultural populations: A *handbook for practitioners*. Thousand Oaks, CA: Sage.

Hufford, D. J. (1995). Cultural and social perspectives on alternative medicine: Background and assumptions. *Altern Ther Health Med, 1*, 53-61.

Hufford, D. J. (1996). Culturally grounded review of research assumptions. *Altern Ther Health Med, 2*, 47-53.

Kline, M. V., & Huff, R. M. (1999). Tips for the practitioner. In R. M. Huff, & M. Kline, *Promoting health in multicultural populations: A handbook for practitioners* (pp. 103-111). Thousand Oaks, CA: Sage.

Krippner, S. (1995). A cross-cultural comparison of four healing models. *Altern Ther Health Med, 1*, 21-29.

Leininger, M. M. (1991). *Culture care diversity and universality: A theory of nursing* (pp. 103-112). New York: National League for Nursing.

Leininger, M. M. (1999). What is transcultural nursing and culturally competent care? *Journal of Transcultural Nursing, 10*, 9.

Louie, K. B. (1995). Cultural considerations: Asian-Americans and pacific islanders. *Imprint, 42*, 41-44, 46.

Lowe, J., & Struthers, R. (2001). A conceptual framework of nursing in Native American culture. *Journal of Nursing Scholarship, 33*(3), 279-283.

Mehl-Madrona, L. E. (1999). Native American medicine in the treatment of chronic illness: Developing an integrated program and evaluating its effectiveness. *Altern Ther Health Med, 5*, 36-44.

Mensah, L. (1993). Transcultural, cross-cultural and multicultural health perspectives in focus. In R. Masi, L. Mensah, & K. A. McLeod (Eds.), *Health and culture: Exploring the relationships* (Vol. 1, pp. 33-41). Oakville, Canada: Mosaic Press.

Nguyen, M. D. (1985). Culture shock: A review of Vietnamese culture and its concepts of health and disease. *West J Med, 142*, 409-412.

Purnell, L. (2000). A description of the Purnell model for cultural competence. *Journal of Transcultural Nursing, 11*, 40-46.

Purnell, L. D., & Counts, M. (1998). Appalachians. In L. D. Purnell & B. J. Paulanka (Eds.), *Transcultural health care: A culturally complete approach*. Philadelphia: Davis.

Reed, B. W., Wineman, J., & Bechtel, G. A. (1995). Using a health risk appraisal to determine an Appalachian community's health care needs. *Journal of Cultural Diversity, 2*, 131-135.

Small, C. C. (1995). Appalachians. In: J. N. Giger & R. E. Davidhizer (Eds.), *Transcultural nursing: Assessment and intervention* (2nd ed.). St. Louis, MO: Mosby.

Smith, C. A. (1995). The lived experience of staying healthy in rural African American families. *Nursing Science Quarterly, 8*, 17-21.

Smith, L. S. (1998). Concept analysis: Cultural competence. *Journal of Cultural Diversity, 5*, 4-10.

Sortet, J. P., & Banks, S. R. (1997). Health beliefs of rural Appalachian women and the practice of breast self-examination. *Cancer Nurs, 20*, 231-235.

Stein, H. F. (1990). *American medicine as culture*. Boulder: Westview Press.

Struthers, R., Escheti, V. S., & Patchell, B. (2004). Traditional indigenous healing: Part I. *Complementary Therapies in Nursing and Midwifery, 10*, 141-149.

Suarez, L., & Ramirez, A. G. (1999). Hispanic/Latino health and disease: An overview. In R. M. Huff, & M. V. Kline (Eds.), *Promoting health in multicultural populations: A handbook for practitioners* (pp. 115-136). Thousand Oaks, CA: Sage.

Tarlov, A. R. (1999). Public policy frameworks for improving population health. *Annals of the New York Academy of Sciences, 896,* 281-293.

Toumishey, H. (1993). Multicultural health care: An introductory course. In R. Masi, L. Mensah, & K. A. McLeod (Eds.), *Health and culture: Exploring the relationships* (Vol. 1, pp. 113-138). Oakville, Canada: Mosaic Press.

Trotter, R. T. (1996). Curanderismo. In M. S. Micozzi (Ed.), *Fundamentals of complementary and alternative medicine* (pp. 259-277). New York: Churchill Livingstone.

Trotter, R. T. (2001). Curanderismo. In M. S. Micozzi (Ed.), *Fundamentals of complementary and alternative medicine* (2nd ed., pp. 411-428). New York: Churchill Livingstone.

U.S. Department of Health and Human Services. (n.d.). *The initiative to eliminate racial and ethnic disparities in health.* Retrieved September 3, 2001, from http://www.omhre.gov/rah

Yali, A. M., & Revenson, T. A. (2004). How changes in population demographics will impact health psychology: Incorporating a broader notion of cultural competence into the field. *Health Psychology, 23,* 147-155.

ETHICAL AND LEGAL INFLUENCES ON HEALTH PROMOTION

Abstract

Normative ethics, which addresses questions of value and action based on abstract principles, is the primary standard for ethical decision making in biomedicine and nursing. This chapter will discuss preferential valuing among the normative ethical principles of autonomy, nonmalefi- cence, beneficence, and justice, but will also discuss a model with the broader values of integrated humanity, ecological integrity, naturalism, relationalism, and spiritualism as a basis for profes- sional ethics in integrative health promotion. This content is followed by issues of power and empowerment, a review of licensing issues, negligence, electronic transmittal of health informa- tion, and implications of food and drug regulation, with special consideration for health promo- tion and healing. The chapter concludes with a brief discussion of the nurse's role in promoting health policy.

Learning Outcomes

By the end of this chapter the student will be able to:

- Differentiate between values, ethics, and morals
- Discuss ethical issues related to power and empowerment
- Discuss the differences between the ethical frameworks of utilitarianism, liberalism, contextualism, and deontology
- Differentiate ethical universalism from relational narrative

- Discuss the implications for integrative health promotion of the ethical principles of autonomy, nonmaleficence, beneficence, and justice

- Discuss licensure implications of incorporating noninvasive therapeutic modalities into integrative nursing care

- Describe ways to prevent claims of negligence

- Discuss the implications of "standard of care"

- Discuss the nurse's role in promoting health policy

Ethical Influences

Values are ideals or concepts that give meaning to an individual's life. They are most commonly derived from societal norms, religion, and family orientation and serve as the framework for making decisions and taking certain actions in everyday life. Values are very important in both moral behavior and ethical decisions. Morals are personal standards for right and wrong behavior that an individual learns and internalizes. Moral behavior is often manifested as behavior in accordance with a group's norms, customs, or traditions. Ethics are societal standards of what is right or wrong, and what ought to be. Ethics, which are usually presented as systems of valued behaviors and beliefs, serve the purpose of governing conduct to ensure the protection of individual or group rights.

Most of the ethical issues that affect nurses who incorporate health promotion and healing into their practice have been addressed with normative ethics. Normative ethics include questions about what ethical principles and values should be adopted, what reasons count as ethical reasons, what actions should be performed, and why some principles or values should be chosen over others (Kuhse, 1997). Traditionally, normative ethics have been considered reflective, involving sound reasoning, impartial, and universal.

Categories of Ethical Frameworks

Within normative ethics, there are several different frameworks for judging ethical or moral behavior. To provide a context for ethical decision making, each individual must decide which "ethical worldview" provides what seems to him or her to be the most acceptable framework for judgements. Some individuals will be most comfortable applying one perspective in all situations, while other individuals will modify their perspective depending on the particular situation.

Utilitarianism

Utilitarianism posits that behavior that leads to the greatest good, or lessens the greatest amount of bad for the greatest number, is moral. Utilitarian frameworks focus on the end (greatest good) and on the responsibility of the individual to the good of the community (Rothschild, 2000). Several clarifications or questions are indicated below:

- It is not required that all share equally in happiness or "the good" or that an attempt be made to serve all.

- By providing the greatest good, or greatest utility, to the greatest number, the ends justify the means.

- How does one decide what is the "greatest good?"

- How does one choose in conflicts between what is good for the individual and the group?

LIBERALISM

Liberalism focuses on individual rights and freedom from coercion. Several clarifications or questions are indicated below:

- Calls for the greatest good for the greatest number.

- All persons should have an equal right to free choice without coercion.

- Freely chosen behaviors should not impede any other person's ability to equally pursue free choice.

- What are the limits of freedom? (e.g., private liberty vs. public cost)

CONTEXTUALISM

Contextualism relates and binds ethics to time and place. Several clarifications or questions are indicated below:

- "In contextualism, there is a moral, bounded, or cultural relativism where ethical standards are dictated by the society and those in power, judged by the customs, rules, and norms of the society, and grounded in the history of the community" (Rothschild, 2000, p. 31).

- What is ethical or moral is seen as being the result of negotiations among those in power.

- Nothing is absolute.

DEONTOLOGY

Deontology proposes that absolute ethical standards hold universally and categorically. Several clarifications or questions are indicated below:

- Moral rightness or wrongness is considered separately from the consequences.

- What do you do when basic guiding principles conflict?

- Under what circumstances are exceptions to the rules applicable?

Conventional Normative Ethical Principles

Principle-based ethics is a systematic method of resolving ethical problems that involves reflection on general principles such as beneficence (producing benefit), justice (fairness), autonomy (independence), veracity (truth telling), fidelity (faithfulness to obligations, duties or observances), and avoidance of killing. In applying these principles to a specific situation, one must first identify which principles are involved and then weigh and balance the competing claims that each principle obligates us to honor. Furthermore, none of the principles is assumed to have priority over the other. "Principles also allow a distancing from the more subjective, contextual aspects of a particular situation and thereby help us to avoid bias and self-interest" (Haddad, 1998, p. 37). "Ethically, a 'right' is a morally justified claim that others should respect, and by extension, it entails a responsibility on the part of others either not to interfere with that claim or to provide assistance" (Schwarz, 2000, p. 64).

In contrast with Haddad (1998), who indicates that none of the ethical principles has assumed priority, Nash (1999, p. 92) states that "in descending order of priority," the four principles of biomedical ethics are:

- Autonomy
- Nonmaleficence
- Beneficence
- Justice

Hall (1996, p. 108) states that "the value of doing good [beneficience] is the highest value for nurses." None of these authors provides justification for their statements. However, it appears that if the nurse's beliefs are consistent with ethical universalism, an accepted hierarchy of biomedical ethical principles would facilitate clinical decision making, especially when competing ethical principles are involved. Respect for the autonomy of the client would always be the first consideration, followed by the avoidance of harm, action to "help," and, finally, fairness. In contrast, it is interesting that much of the discussion of medical ethics in the popular press seems to put fairness first as, for example, in policies for distribution of resources.

AUTONOMY

Autonomy requires that a person act in a manner that respects the rights of others to freely determine their own choices and destiny. "A competent [client] has absolute veto power over our best intentions. The [client] is in charge—ethically, legally, and morally—whether we like it or not" (Nash, 1999, p. 92). Autonomy presumes that the client is competent. Telling the truth, client confidentiality, privacy, informed consent, and allocation of resources are all part of autonomy. The first part of provision one of the Code of Ethics for Nurses (ANA, 2001) states that "the nurse, in all professional relationships, practices with compassion and respect for the inherent dignity, worth and uniqueness of every individual…"

The ethical obligation of respect for persons, or autonomy, is the basis for well-established expectations of shared nurse-client decision making and informed consent. The belief that in certain circumstances it is acceptable to disregard a person's views in favor of promoting his or her health is deeply ingrained in the biomedical model view of health care. This benevolent restriction of another person's freedom is called paternalism (from the Latin for father) or maternalism (from the Latin for mother). The assumption is that others need to be protected, because they do not know what is best for them (Bournes, 2000). However, "paternalism is seldom justified, despite our acts of mercy, kindness, and charity. Positive acts to prevent illness and promote health are ethical" (Nash, 1999, p. 93).

A high value is placed on individual independence in American culture, but it should be remembered that in many cultures autonomy is not the central value. Empathy and accommodation to the beliefs of a client or family are preferable to an overzealous insistence on handling all clients in one way. On the other hand, deception is not permissible, and nurses cannot avoid responsibility for willing participation in group decisions and actions, and physicians cannot assume authority over others in ethical matters. "A team can develop a self-righteous opinion of the good it is doing and thus give its decisions self-justification, thereby infantilizing the [client]" (Pellegrino, 1998, p. 1522).

Informed Consent

Informed consent arises from the ethical principle of respect for autonomy. The essence of informed consent should be the capacity of the client to understand and make a rational decision. However, unfortunately "the language of consent connotes compliance not collaboration or agreement" (Green, 1999, p. 108), which is contrary to the principle of autonomy. Informed consent should be a voluntary, uncoerced decision based on adequate information and deliberation by a sufficiently competent person. In addition, consent should be viewed as a process with ongoing discussion and negotiation to confirm the continued agreement of the client (Norton, 1995).

Often, the approach to informed consent is to satisfy an administrative requirement or to protect oneself from liability, rather than as a meaningful component of enhanced client involvement in the decision making process (Braddock et al., 1999). What is desired is a meaningful dialogue about healing methods and outcomes instead of a one-way dutiful disclosure of alternatives, risks, and benefits. According to Braddock and colleagues (1999), this expanded view is termed informed decision making. Green (1999), in turn, proposes a collaborative planning model that changes the understanding of professional liability from tort concepts that are based on standards of care to a contract model that is based on the doctrine of assumption of risk. He suggests that the scope of professional services should be formalized, and mutually agreed upon, in an early interview.

In order to enhance client involvement in the decision-making process, the following elements of informed decision making are proposed (Braddock et al., 1999):

- *Discussion of the client's role in decision-making.* Many clients are not aware that they can and should participate in decision making.

- *Discussion of the clinical issue or nature of the decision.* A clear statement of what is at issue helps to clarify what is being decided.

- *Discussion of the alternatives.* A decision is always a choice among certain options, including doing nothing at all.

- *Discussion of the pros (potential benefits) and cons (risks) of the alternatives.* Discussion of the pros of one option and the cons of another.

- *Discussion of the uncertainties associated with the decision.*

- *Assessment of the client's understanding.* Fostering understanding is really the central goal of informed decision making.

■ *Exploration of client preference.* It should be clear to the client that it is appropriate to disagree or ask for more time.

NONMALEFICENCE

Nonmaleficence requires that one avoid doing harm to others. It is a duty that applies generally, even in the absence of a professional obligation. Not harming clients unnecessarily in the process of providing care is a well-recognized ethical principle. For example, thorough history taking is critical in order to prevent potentially harmful interactions between conventional biomedicine and therapeutic noninvasive modalities. The principle of nonmaleficence (do no harm) is above beneficence, that is the principle to help (Nash, 1999). Nonmaleficence protects the incompetent client. However, "good intentions alone don't morally justify an act" (Schwarz, 2000, p. 61). The principles of nonmaleficence and beneficence are combined in provision three of the Code of Ethics for Nurses (ANA, 2001), "The nurse promotes, advocates for, and strives to protect the health, safety, and rights of the patient," and provision five, "The nurse owes the same duties to self as to others, including the responsibility to preserve integrity and safety, to maintain competence, and to continue personal and professional growth."

Is it ethical to hold the client personally responsible for behavior that may increase health risk? In consideration of the ethical principle of causing no harm, Guttman and Ressler (2001) suggest that a person can only be held responsible if s(he) is self-aware, free not to engage in potentially hazardous behavior, the behavior deemed risky is deliberate or carried out for personal gratification, and the undesirable health outcome can only be caused by the particular behavior(s) in question. There is concern that inappropriate attribution of culpability, particularly for highly vulnerable groups, may result in added suffering and fatalism or feelings of guilt.

Nurses who practice integrative health promotion have an ethical obligation to apply the principle of nonmaleficence. But, how can the nurse do no harm and also promote informed consent of clients "given the limited availability of scientific data regarding the safety, efficacy, optimal dosage, and side-effects or interactions of some therapies" (Clark, 2000, p. 448)? Of specific concern is the risk for potential adverse interactions involving prescription medications and herbal or high-dose vitamin supplements. Nurses must seek appropriate education to develop the relevant knowledge and skills to avoid client injury.

BENEFICENCE

Beneficence means taking action to "help" a client. Nurses have a duty to act positively and contribute to the well-being of their clients. Accountability extends to lack of care and the nurse may be asked to justify why certain care, including noninvasive therapies, was not performed. For example, massage is an essential component of nursing which is an effective intervention for pain, insomnia, and anxiety (Norton, 1995), but many nurses do not provide this therapy, relying exclusively on medically prescribed drugs. The principle of beneficence refers to a professional obligation to act "for the good" or to benefit others (Milton, 2000).

JUSTICE

A central concern of justice in health care relates to fairness. For example, the health care delivery system has been severely criticized for uneven access to health care due to a variety of societal conditions. Nurses need to be involved in addressing the issues that affect just distribution of health care. Another concern related to justice is that clients have fair access to noninvasive therapeutic modalities that are known to be safe, effective, and appropriate as well as to conventional biomedical therapies (Sugarman & Burk, 1998). The second part of provision one of the Code of Ethics for Nurses (ANA, 2001) states "...unrestricted by considerations of social or economic status, personal attributes, or the nature of health problems."

A global perspective is necessary in considering quality of life and justice issues such as living in poverty, surviving as victims of war, genocide, or environmental disasters, dealing with issues of racism and sexism, or "living in situations where there is a lack of humanitarian effort (responses to the struggles of humanity)" (Bunkers, 2001, p. 297). Johnstone (1998, p. 43) stresses "the need to advance a genuinely nursing perspective on...the otherwise neglected broader social justice issues associated with promoting the well-being and significant moral interests of marginalized groups."

Critiques of Conventional Ethics

THE CARE CRITIQUE

During the past 20 years, a number of philosophers have criticized and tried to find alternatives to traditional normative ethics. For example, in work that has significant implications for nursing, Gilligan (1982) suggested that there is a difference between women's and men's moral perspectives. She asserted that her research showed that many men have a language of impartiality, which fits comfortably with traditional ethical systems. In contrast, many women have a relational language, where the emphasis is on individualized caring that is contextualized within a relationship. Gilligan (1987) describes the difference between a care and the traditional justice approach as follows: "From a justice perspective, the self as moral agent stands as the figure against a ground of social relationships, judging the conflicting claims of self and others against a standard of equality or equal respect.... From a care perspective, the relationship becomes the figure, defining self and others. Within the context of relationship, the self as a moral agent perceives and responds to the perception of need. This shift in moral perspective is manifest by a change in the moral question from What is just? to How to respond?" (p. 23). An ethical approach based on care criticizes the abstraction and the universal application of principles of conventional normative ethics, arguing for the importance of the individual context for each particular situation.

SELECTED ETHICAL NURSING CONCERNS

Discussions of nursing ethics have typically tended to emphasize ethical decision making in clinical situations, with nurses and other health care providers paternalistically viewed as the primary decision makers. Each of the steps in the process for resolving ethical dilemmas tends to be described through the value priority lens of the nurse (Milton, 2000). Ironically, at the same time, "nurses views on ethical issues have been either invalidated, trivialized, or ignored altogether" (Johnstone, 1998, p. 43). Fry and Duffy (2001) identified 32 end-of-life treatment decisions, patient care issues, and human rights issues registered nurses are believed to encounter frequently in practice. These ethical issues are summarized in Box 6-1.

Box 6-1

Ethical Issues Frequently Encountered in Clinical Practice

1. End-of-treatment decisions:
   - Prolonging the dying process with inappropriate measures
   - Treatment or nontreatment despite client or family wishes
   - Use or removal of support including nutrition and hydration
   - To resuscitate or not to resuscitate
   - Treatment or nontreatment of a very disabled infant, child, or adult
   - Not considering the quality of client's life
   - Acting against one's own personal or religious views
   - Acting against client's personal or religious views
   - Determining when death occurs
   - Organ transplantation or organ or tissue procurement
   - Over- or underuse of pain management
   - Ordering too many or too few procedures, tests, etc.
   - Participation or refusal to participate in euthanasia or assisted suicide

2. Patient care issues:
   - Staffing patterns that limit client access to nursing care
   - Child, spousal, elderly, or client abuse or neglect
   - Allocation of human, financial, or equipment resources
   - Implementing managed care policies that threaten quality of care
   - Breaches of client confidentiality or privacy
   - An irresponsible, unethical, incompetent, or impaired colleague
   - Ignoring client or family autonomy
   - An uninformed or misinformed client or family about treatment, prognosis or medical alternatives
   - Rights of minors versus parental rights

continued

BOX 6-1 CONTINUED

- Discriminatory treatment of clients
- Unsafe equipment or environmental hazards
- Conflict in nurse, doctor, or other professional relationship
- Reporting unethical or illegal practice of a health professional or agency
- Implementing managed care policies threatening availability of care

3. Human rights issues:
- Use or nonuse of physical or chemical restraints
- Issues involving advance directives
- Protecting patient rights and human dignity
- Informed consent to treatment
- Providing care with possible risk to RNs' health (e.g., TB, HIV, violence)

Source: Adapted from Fry, S. T., & Duffy, M. E. (2001). The development and psychometric evaluation of the Ethical Issues Scale. *Journal of Nursing Scholarship, 33,* 273–277.

Nurses face multiple and frequently conflicting imperatives "as organizational members and subordinates to physician's orders.... The realities of business values permeating health care, work settings operating within severe economic constraints, and redistribution of nursing manpower away from direct practice are not explicitly addressed in the current ANA Code for Nurses" (Hamric, 1999, p. 106). The ANA Code provides statements of moral ideals rather than practical guidelines (e.g., commitment to caring for persons, client advocacy, maintaining competence, accepting responsibility for one's judgments and actions). Consequently, nurses have had limited guidance in how to practice ethically within the real world of resource allocation decisions.

Nurses also have neglected broader social justice issues associated with promoting the well-being and significant moral interests of marginalized or stigmatized groups (e.g., those with mental health problems; survivors of child abuse, sufferers of domestic and elder abuse; the poor; the homeless; the unemployed; the disabled; people from different cultural backgrounds; and homosexuals). It is important to avoid stigmatization and assigning "blaming the victim" pejorative labels to high-risk individuals.

Reflecting a paternalistic tradition, nurses have often used persuasion to "get" the client to follow a prescribed plan. Sugarman and Burk (1998) imply that when there are known effective therapies for a life-threatening disease (e.g., a treatable bacterial infection), exerting strong influence against therapeutic non-invasive modalities is appropriate, while influence is less appropriate for diseases in which there is no clearly effective conventional treatment (e.g., fibromyalgia). However, consistent with the principle of autonomy, respect for clients requires that all clients are completely informed of the risks and benefits of all treatment options and facilitated in their ability to make a choice. Last and Woolf (1996, p. 563) also point out that "when people have few or no other sources of pleasure or solace, clinicians have a responsibility to ensure that patients really will be better off after they have changed their behavior, not merely less prone to a particular risk factor" (Last & Woolf, 1996, p. 563).

Conventional normative ethics fails to account for important aspects of the moral experience of nurses, such as interconnection with others and responsibility in relationships. Additionally, conflicts between principles often seem impossible to resolve (Haddad, 1998). Haddad (1998, p. 382) points out that "societal ethics requires societal definitions of terminal illness, experimental treatment, and quality-of-life issues. Questions at this level always revolve around the common good rather than that of individuals."

A MODEL FOR PROFESSIONAL ETHICS

Given the concerns mentioned above, Bolletino (1998) has developed a professional ethics model that he labeled the law of the primacy of the patient. The law of primacy states that a client is to be viewed and treated as unconditionally inviolate. The law provides a definition of a client as 1) a total, multidimensional human being; 2) a unique individual; and 3) a person capable of structuring his or her own life. Elaborating, Bolletino (1998) explained that:

1. *The client is a total human being.* Each client needs to be seen and responded to as an individual with inseparable aspects: physical, psychological, emotional, intellectual, historical, relational, creative, social, and spiritual. "Practitioners' refusal or inability to extend their emotional boundaries can also be experienced by the client as a kind of abandonment. If practitioners maintain a 'professional' emotional detachment or remain uninvolved, or if they are cold, distant, joyless, or out of touch with themselves, the client is alone" (p. 15).

2. *The client is a unique individual.* "The individual is assessed, but not encountered (p. 12).... Viewing the [client] as a mechanism to be fixed, a statistic, a test result, an illness, a body part, a collection of symptoms, a diagnosis, or a member of any classification is anti-therapeutic and unethical (p. 13)... There is more and more evidence that when the biomedical model underlies professional practice, the resulting view of the [client] as something less than a whole person is anti-therapeutic. It is harmful, therefore unethical" (p. 15).

3. *The client has the ability to structure his or her own life.* "[Clients] are the leading authorities on themselves... practitioners are the authorities on diagnosis and care" (p. 13).

RELATIONAL NARRATIVE APPROACH TO PROFESSIONAL ETHICS

Instead of considering ethical principles as mutually exclusive alternatives, Gadow (1999, p. 57), proposes an ethical framework with "a triad of ethical layers: subjective immersion (ethical immediacy), objective detachment (ethical universalism), and intersubjective engagement (relational narrative) corresponding, respectively, to premodern, modern, and postmodern ethics" (see Box 6-2). In this framework, rather than the approaches being viewed as oppositional, they are instead considered to be intrinsically related and mutually enhancing, different perspectives that contribute to a better understanding of ethics as a whole. As with normative ethical frameworks, there is no assumption that any approach is necessarily superior.

Box 6-2

Categories of Philosophical Ethics

1. Ethical immediacy:
   - Reflects an unreflective and uncritical certainty about the good that reinforces certainty.
   - From a source that transcends the individual, such as religion, family, customs, or the ethos of a profession.
   - Based on an experience of certainty that needs and allows no explication.
   - A strength is solidarity if nurse and client share "an unquestioned view of the good and are united in their attempt to realize that good" (p. 60).
   - Prevents "fragmentation of the self that can result from self-questioning and critique. Immediacy serves to maintain the self and the group as a coherent, harmonious whole" (p. 60).

2. Ethical universalism:
   - Counters subjectivity with rational principles that are categorical and unconditional.
   - Based on equalizing reason and universality; "detachment provides the distance needed for objectivity" (p. 61).
   - Appreciates that principles can conflict in clinical situations. "Interpretation is required, and interpretations differ according to the perspectives of the people involved" (p. 62).
   - Does not allow modifications based on individual and contextual differences.

continued

Box 6-2 CONTINUED

3. Relational narrative

- Reflects personal responsiveness to the particular other. "The valuing of persons requires perception of each one's uniqueness, and perception involves engagement" (p. 63). "Being present with persons demonstrates a commitment for respecting and acknowledging individuals as experts of their own lives... Nurses do not try to change the person or the meaning of the situation" (Milton, 2000, p. 113).

- Based on intersubjectivity. Contrasts both with subjectivity of uncritical certainty and the objectivity of universal rules.

- There is "no uninterpreted basis [exists] from which to decide objectively among meanings" (p. 63).

Source: Adapted from Gadow, S. (1999). Relational narrative: The postmodern turn in nursing ethics. *Scholarly Inquiry for Nursing Practice: An International Journal, 13,* 57–69.

AN INTEGRATIVE MODEL FOR ETHICS

The majority of authors who write on the application of ethics to complementary and alternative medicine (CAM), integrative medicine, and nursing have tried to modify and apply normative bioethics to these new areas. However, Guinn (2001) argues that a new ethical understanding is needed that incorporates the "holistic, integrative, naturalistic, relational, and spiritual characteristics" of CAM (p. 69).

Guinn (2001) suggests that conventional bioethics is too narrow and limited, and therefore characterizes an incomplete understanding of health care ethics. He suggests that each of five core values: integrated humanity, ecological integrity, naturalism, relationalism, and spiritualism, reflect elements of both CAM and biomedicine, and that the principles of normative ethics are simply a subset within these values.

The concept of integrated humanity recognizes that people are not biological machines, but are a unified whole. Each person is considered to be inherently unique and special, and thus deserving of respect (embodies the conventional idea of autonomy). "Being respectful of [clients'] time and commitments, greeting them courteously, and providing them with comfortable surroundings all reflect an attitude of respect" (Guinn, 2001, p. 70). Each individual is viewed within relationship with others, the world, and "the transcendent" (p. 70).

The concept of ecological integrity reflects the fact that clients do not live in isolation. Social communities such as families and work, religious, economic, and political communities can create conditions that affect health. For example, a client with health insurance, ample financial resources, and a supportive family is much more likely to get adequate health care services than a client living alone in poverty. Nurses need to be sure that clients are aware of available social services, as well as to promote health services through social activism. However, as Guinn (2001) points out, the "dominance of the autonomous patient model" (p. 70) as the interaction between a client and his or her physician or nurse, and the principle of privacy, create limits on the ability to engage families or communities in client care.

The concept of naturalism is based on understanding of health within an "interactive existence within the natural world" (p. 70). There are three aspects of this value: normality, complexity, and dynamism. From this perspective, attention must be given to supporting natural and normal tendencies toward health. Health is complex, not based on simple cause-and-effect relationships, and therefore not amenable to reductionist empirical measurement. Given that any change in the environment alters health interrelationships, care cannot be reduced to commonalities, but rather must "reflect the unique and individual environment of each [client] and his or her reactions" (p. 71).

The concept of relationalism acknowledges that the client and the nurse are not isolated from each other, but rather enter into a relationship. In contrast to the current health care system, in which relationships between the client and professional caregivers is based on "dynamics of power and the disparities of power" (p. 71), relationships should be based on mutual respect. Guinn suggests that caregivers are justified in sharing their opinions as well as information in a relationship-based informed consent process. In addition, "the manner in which caregivers are treated by colleagues and the organization in which they work has a direct bearing on how [clients] are cared for as well" (p. 71).

The concept of spiritualism is based on the belief that health is significantly affected by a person's mental and spiritual aspects. Healing is more than relief of symptoms or imbalance in the body. This concept incorporates the spiritual dimension as an active force in the care of clients. Implications of this concept include consideration of the ethics of the placebo effect, which is real and has measurable outcomes. As Guinn (2001, p. 71) indicates, "An intention by the caregiver to create a placebo effect (by inducing the [client] to believe in a treatment that is not proven to be efficacious) violates the caregiver's duty of honesty to the [client]. Although the 'belief' might effect a cure, creating the belief would require lying."

According to Guinn (2001, p. 72), "the ideal of integrative ethics is to understand the dynamic health of the whole individual in the context of his or her life." Given this purpose, the core values of the integrative model have the potential to serve as an expanded ethical framework for integrative nursing. However, an ethical framework for practice is only one of the factors needed for the empowerment of nurses.

Power and Ethics

Empowerment and the idea that people can form a partnership with their health care provider are implicit in the concept of health promotion. Financial support for health promotion activities is required for a partnership to be successful. However, neither governments nor private insurance carriers have recognized or honored their obligation to provide sufficient financial support for health promotion and disease prevention. Some health promotion policies are clearly opposed for financial reasons. For example, stringent meat inspection for health protection may conflict with the economic interests of the food industry (Last & Woolf, 1996).

One of the powers granted to conventional biomedicine by society is the privilege of defining truth as it pertains to a number of health-related issues. This creates an obvious, if unconscious, temptation within conventional biomedicine "to use the power to secure its own economic dominance over potential competitors and to justify those practices in the name of scientific truth, to which only regular physicians (and, of course, never their competitors) have exclusive access" (Brody et al., 1999, p. 47). For example, responses to complementary and alternative medicine (CAM) have ranged from a perceived obligation to stifle harmful practices, to acceptance of nonharmful modalities, to encouragement of the use of beneficial interventions (Sugarman & Burk, 1998). Campaigns by organized medicine to protect "turf" by disparaging CAM interventions, have the effect of creating confusion and doubt in the minds of clients and nurses, effectively diminishing client access to potentially helpful noninvasive therapeutic interventions.

Physicians, even with good intentions, may not realize how their use of power affects people, as the exercise of power tends to be relatively invisible to a person in a more powerful position (Brody et al., 1999). Current theories in ethics are based on the assumption that any exercise of professional power can trespass on the client's vital rights and interests. Therefore, ethics demands that exercise of power be critically examined and justified—not only according to what physicians and nurses think is good for the client, but also in terms of the client's own free and informed choice. Greater influence, greater clinical expertise, more ethical concern, and having ethics education have been associated with greater willingness to act in an ethically troubling situation (Hamric, 1999).

Power is an important consideration for nurses and their clients. Since professional power includes the ability to exercise professional judgment and to influence others accordingly, nurses must balance their sense of purpose in caring for clients and "their contextual, role-dependent, and, especially in hierarchical structures, limited ability to fulfill that sense of purpose" (Haddad, 1998, p. 380). When nurses only consider the tasks to be accomplished and restrict care to "doctor's orders," the "hopes, wants, and desires" of those who receive nursing services go unnoticed (Milton, 2000, p. 114).

Power also needs to be considered in collaborative roles between nurses and other health care professionals. In the past decade, there has been renewed interest in pursuing professional collaboration at least in part due to 1) increased complexity of technology and acuity of patients in every type of practice setting from tertiary care to home care; 2) increased concern about the practical limits of financial resources with the inevitable impact on client care and patterns of reimbursement; 3) changes in consumer expectations of health care professionals (e.g., deepening mistrust due to fraud and abuse by health professionals); and 4) awareness of the influence, both positive and negative, that collaboration among health professionals has on client outcomes (Haddad, 1998).

Interprofessional collaboration is not just an issue of how individuals interact with one another. Institutional and societal structures, such as "structures of power, communication, status, relationship, autonomy, expression, and respect . . . create an environment that shapes behaviors such as ethical decision making" (Haddad, 1998, p. 379). However, in situations where nurses may lack status, an ethical framework can provide an alternative source of authority.

Legal Influences

Ethical considerations focus on personal values about right and wrong. In contrast, legal influences on practice are generalized regulations that must be adhered to for nursing practice within a professional license.

"Law is the body of rules and regulations that governs people's behavior as well as their relationships with others in the society and with the state" (Aiken, 1994, p. 3). Law uses coercion to achieve behavior in a nonvoluntary manner or to threaten punishment for noncompliance or inappropriate behavior (Rothschild, 2000). Civil law is concerned with punishment for wrongs against individuals. The wronged individual may bring legal action (a lawsuit) against the offender, seeking monetary compensation or the performance of a specific act. A tort is any private (civil) injury or wrongful act (except for breach of contract) committed against the person or property of another. There are different types of torts, such as:

- *Intentional torts* (for example, assault or battery). "An intentional tort is a wrong that results from a volition act committed with the intent to bring about certain consequences (or with the knowledge that the consequence was likely to occur) and was a substantial factor in bringing about the consequence" (Ely-Pierce, 1999, p. 80).

- *Quasi-intentional torts* (such as defamation or invasion of privacy). "Quasi-intentional torts are those torts in which the intent may not be as clear as with intentional torts. However, as with intentional torts, the wrongdoer still commits a volitional act, which brings about certain consequences" (Ely-Pierce, 1999, p. 80).

Health care providers are regulated under each state's police power, constitutional authority delegated to each state to protect the safety of its citizens. Previous court decisions have weighed police power more heavily than privacy, liberty, and free speech interests in the provision of and access to health care (Cohen, 1998). This power to protect citizens' health, safety, and welfare authorizes states to decide who may practice a profession such as nursing or medicine, and to establish licensing boards that admit or exclude persons from practice. Essential social values and culturally accepted models of health care are reflected in legal rules (Cohen, 1998). Regulation is supposed to prevent "indiscriminate practice of the healing arts by 'unskilled and unlicensed practitioners'" (Cohen, 1998, p. 24).

The intent of existing legal authority is to protect clients from dangerous or worthless treatments by relying on legal rules for matters such as licensing, scope of practice, and malpractice to sanction inappropriate provider behavior. Limited practice authority is granted by licensing statutes to nonmedical health care providers, and courts enforce medical practice acts strictly against providers who cross into "diagnosis" and "treatment." In addition, food and drug laws restrict the use of nutritional therapies to treat disease. Although such rules reflect a sound regulatory concern for preventing overreaching by providers, they also can result in "legislative, regulatory, and judicial ratification of biomedical dominance and biomedicine's attempt to monopolize professional healing" (Cohen, 1998, pp. 117-118). "Because licensure is a political process, the power to protect public health, safety, and welfare has been used to exclude or suppress from professional healing practice those persons and modalities outside the biomedical paradigm" (Cohen, 1998, p. 24).

LICENSURE LAWS

Licensure laws represent an example of a state's exercise of its police power. Licensure laws were originally intended to protect the consumer from unprepared or unscrupulous providers. However, medical licensing has been criticized as protecting the licensed, not the [client], by insulating physicians from the economic threat of other providers (Cohen, 1998). All states define the practice of medicine, in part, by using such words as diagnosis, treatment, prevention, cure, advise, and prescribe. These words are usually used in conjunction with disease, injury, deformity, and mental or physical condition. "The broad reach and interpretation of medical practice acts expresses biomedical dominance and the conceptual narrowing of professional healing practice to biomedical diagnosis and treatment" (Cohen, 1998, p. 31), providing a threat to all nonmedical healthcare providers, including professional nurses.

To address the "barriers to competition created by the all-encompassing scope in medical practice acts" (ANA, 1996), in 1996, the American Nurses' Association (ANA) developed a revised model practice act that places the primary responsibility for interpreting and enforcing the scope of nursing practice in the Board of Nursing, through regulations, advisory, and Board opinions. The Model Practice Act identifies nine skills that may be utilized in professional nursing performance.

However, a number of states have not followed the wording of the model practice act, retaining language that gives the State Board of Medicine the authority to influence nursing practice. For example, the Professional Nurse Law in the State of Pennsylvania defines the practice of professional nursing as "diagnosing and treating human responses to actual or potential health problems through such services as case finding, health teaching, health counseling, and provision of care supportive to or restorative of life and well-being, and executing medical regimens as prescribed by a licensed physician or dentist. *The foregoing shall not be deemed to include acts of medical diagnosis or prescription of medical therapeutic or corrective measures*, except as may be authorized by *rules and regulations jointly promulgated by the State Board of Medicine and the Board*, which rules and regulations shall be implemented by the Board" (Pennsylvania State Board of Nursing, 1999).

Licensure provides a number of benefits, including creating a minimum level of professional competence, elevating of the image of a profession, reassuring public and legislative concerns about quality control, preventing other professionals from gaining control over the licensed profession, and providing a recognized basis for hospital privileges, insurance reimbursement, and other professional opportunities (Cohen, 1998).

However, the breadth of medical practice acts puts at least thee groups at risk of prosecution for unlawfully practicing medicine (Cohen, 1998, p. 29):

1. Providers who lack licensure.

2. Licensed providers (including physicians and nurses) who employ or refer clients to providers practicing medicine unlawfully and therefore may be liable for "aiding and abetting" unlicensed medical practice.

3. Licensed providers, such as chiropractors and, in many states, licensed naturopaths, massage therapists, nurses, and others who are deemed to violate their legally authorized scope of practice by engaging in the diagnosis and treatment of disease. Nonmedical providers such as nurses "are limited to specific scope of practice authorized in their licensing laws and are expressly prohibited from practicing 'medicine'—from diagnosing, curing, and treating disease.... If a nonmedical provider makes an over broad claim and purports to treat or cure a disease in the medical sense, the provider not only is subject to potential tort law claims based on fraud and misrepresentation but also risks prosecution for the unlicensed practice of medicine" (Cohen, 1999, p. 52).

In many states, maintaining an office in which to receive, examine, and treat clients constitutes the practice of medicine. More than half the states include the use, administration, or prescription of drugs or medicine in the definition of the practice of medicine. Thus, broad definitions of the word drug pose problems for nurses who offer herbal and nutritional therapies as part of their professional practice (Cohen, 1998).

Nurses are legally prohibited from practicing medicine, but it is essential that nurses remember that statutes can be interpreted as prohibiting the nonphysician only from engaging in the diagnosis and treatment of biomedically defined pathology and not health promotion. "The prohibition applies to furnishing or purporting to furnish 'disease care' within the biomedical model, not 'wellness care' within the holistic healing model.... A delineation has been suggested between the furnishing of information, products, and/or services to encourage health (by nourishing, stimulating, and balancing vital energy) and purporting to cure disease as defined bio-medically" (Cohen, 1998, pp. 32-33). It is essential that nurses continue to lobby elected legislative representatives and appointed professional state board members to increase understanding of how professional nursing practice is distinct from medical practice. The ANA recommends that law be amended if physician assistants can supervise registered nurse practice, or if the Board of Medicine has control over nursing functions (as in the Pennsylvania statute).

NEGLIGENCE AND MALPRACTICE

Negligence and malpractice are related concepts given that malpractice is one form of professional negligence. Malpractice is the violation of the nurse's professional duty to act with reasonable care and in good faith. The standard of practice must be violated in order for the courts to find malpractice (Brody et al., 1999).

"Standard of care has been defined as 'that minimum level of care which the ordinary, reasonable prudent nurse, in the same or similar circumstances, would provide'.... The trend is toward a national standard" (Ely-Pierce, 1999, p. 81). "Standards of professional performance focus on the nurses' clinical performance, while standards of care focus on patient outcomes" (ANA, 1998, p. 3). The Nurse Practice Act defines nursing practice and establishes the standards for nurses in each state. The standards of care that are used for judgments of negligence may be derived from nurse practice acts; published court opinions; state statutes and administrative code books such as the patient's bill of rights and Centers for Medicare and Medicaid Services (previously the Health Care Financing Administration) regulations; guidelines, policies, and procedures for nursing care delivery published by national nursing organizations, state boards of nursing, credentialing bodies, and the Joint Commission on Accreditation of Healthcare Organizations; hospital policies; and authoritative nursing texts and journals.

Health care institutions, including hospitals, nursing homes, clinics, and managed care organizations, face at least two kinds of malpractice exposure when utilizing nurses who provide therapeutic noninvasive therapies. These are direct liability (for an act or omission of the institution, also known as corporate negligence) and vicarious liability (for an act or omission of the individual provider). "Under the doctrine of corporate negligence, courts have imposed direct liability on health care institutions for negligently failing to properly supervise health care professionals" (Cohen, 1998, p. 70).

Negligence is defined as "conduct lacking in due care; carelessness; a violation of the duty to use care; a wrong characterized by the absence of a positive intent to inflict injury but from which injury nevertheless results" (Ely-Pierce, 1999, p. 80). A negligence lawsuit is typically a civil case, in which a client, through tort law, attempts to right an injury that is claimed to have resulted from malpractice. The law defines nursing negligence as failure to exercise the degree of care that a reasonable nurse would exercise under the same or similar circumstances. According to Showers (2000), four things must be proved for a nurse to be found negligent:

- *Duty*. The nurse had a duty to provide care to the client and to follow an acceptable standard of care.

- *Breach*. The nurse failed to adhere to the standard of care.

- *Causation*. The nurse's failure to adhere to the standard of care caused the client's injuries.

- *Damages*. The client suffered injury as a result of the nurse's negligent actions.

Negligence claims are often alleged in the following situations (Aiken, 1994):

- Client falls
- Failure to monitor
- Failure to ensure client safety
- Improper performance of treatment
- Failure to respond to client
- Medication error
- Wrong dosage administered
- Failure to follow hospital procedure
- Improper technique
- Failure to supervise treatment

The important thing for the nurse to remember is to practice within his or her own level of competence. This may be especially important when performing noninvasive therapeutic therapies where a nursing standard of care has not been established. In as much as possible harm has the potential for a negligence claim, in a hospital setting Stone (1999, p. 49) takes a hard line in suggesting that "all potential risks of an intervention should be disclosed.... Nonconventional therapists should not alter the medication or treatment prescribed for patients by their medical practitioner." An established and agreed upon protocol, and the support and full knowledge of the line manager, would help to protect the nurse from a negligence claim.

In Box 6-3, Showers (2000) suggests other strategies that nurses can use for protection from a negligence action.

Box 6-3

Strategies to Protect from a Negligence Action

- Know your facility's policies on adverse incidents, and know your responsibilities and meet them.
- Follow your facility's procedures for completing an incident report.
- Treat each client as you would like to be treated.
- Delegate appropriately.
- Report any problems that may endanger your client.
- Know where drug references and other resources are located and make sure they are up-to-date.
- Maintain your competency through continuing education.
- If you don't understand an order or you're unfamiliar with a procedure, ask for help.
- When you document, keep the acronym FACT in mind; your notes should be **f**actual, **a**ccurate, **c**omplete, and **t**imely. Documentation in general can make or break your defense.
- Learn about other professionals who are available to help improve client care, such as diabetes counselors, respiratory therapists, and risk managers.

Source: Adapted from Showers, J. L. (2000). What you need to know about negligence lawsuits. *Nursing 2000, 30,* 45-48.

The client record should reflect what has occurred during the client's treatment. To avoid negligence claims, client assessment with concise, factual, accurate, and timely documentation and communication is essential (Trott, 1998). To effectively document, the nurse must:

- Write legibly.
- Use the standard date and time abbreviations to accompany the signature after each chart entry.

- Document without defaming the patient, previous nurses, or physicians. Deal with conflicts on a one-to-one basis. Defaming a person only reinforces a case and makes the nurse and the organization look bad from a legal and ethical standpoint.

- Document the client assessment as well as what the client has told the nurse.

- Document what has been done to protect the client and the client's response to the intervention.

The increasing use of computers in care settings, including the electronic recording of client record documentation, creates additional issues for nurses.

ENVIRONMENTAL LEGISLATION

Congress enacts statutes involving environmental protection. The goal of many environmental programs is to reduce human and environmental exposure to environmental contaminants to a level of acceptable risks to health and the environment (McGarity, 2004). There are three kinds of criteria that can be used to establish a legal standard: significant risks of harm from pollution, reasonable risk balancing, and a mixed strategy. The significant risks of harm from pollution criterion requires that risks posed by status quo exposures and alternative exposure levels must be assessed. Then, there has to be a determination of whether a given level of risk is "significant." This typically involves a host of incommensurable considerations, including the "robustness" of the data and the uncertainties in the risk predictions, the size of the exposed populations, the intensity of the exposures to particular individuals, the nature of the harm potentially induced by the exposure, the duration of the exposure, the value of the resources at risk, the degree to which the exposure is voluntary, the extent to which society tolerates similar risks in other contexts, and distributional considerations (McGarity, 2004, p. 535). The significant risk/protective goal does not involve a balancing of health and environmental risks against costs and other inconveniences entailed in reducing the risks.

The fundamental premise underlying the cost-benefit balancing goal is that society is willing to accept reasonable risks. The cost of reducing risks has been quantified and compared to the monetized benefit of the reduced risks. And, in a mixed strategy, the agency has to establish standards aimed at meeting both pollution reduction and acceptable risk goals, and further provide that the more stringent standard must be achieved. Our complex regulatory system allows regulations to meet varying goals; therefore, unidimensional approaches to setting environmental policy are unlikely to be successful.

ELECTRONIC HEALTH INFORMATION

Electronic devices and telemedicine are increasingly being used in health care. Telemedicine uses communications technology to deliver information and services between health care providers and clients who are geographically separated (Hodge et al., 1999).

There are many advantages for the systematic collection and use of electronic health data. Better data allow consumers to make more informed decisions about health plans, providers, diagnoses, products, and treatments. Clinical care is improved through faster and more accurate medical and nursing diagnoses, increased checks on diagnostic and therapeutic procedures, prevention of adverse drug interactions, instantaneous research, and the dissemination of expert information to areas traditionally undeserved. Increased access to accurate information can facilitate research and public health surveillance of morbidity and mortality across populations. Electronic security tools including personal access codes, encryption programs, and audit trails can more efficiently monitor health care fraud and abuse and protect data from unauthorized use and disclosures (Hodge et al., 1999).

Protecting the confidentiality of personally identifiable health data is critical. Specifically, e-mail poses privacy and security concerns. Hodge, Gostin, & Jacobson (1999) suggest that the nurse:

1. Obtain client informed consent before using e-mail for direct correspondence.

2. Explain and use security mechanisms.

3. Prohibit the forwarding of client e-mail without express authorization.

4. Inform clients about those having access to their messages and whether their messages will become part of their medical records.

5. Respond to messages responsibly.

6. Avoid references to third parties.

There is an increasing public interest in herbs and over-the-counter "natural" supplements. These areas are addressed by food and drug laws.

Food and Drug Regulation

Legal rules and decisions traditionally have emphasized the dangers of access to untested treatments, which in many cases includes therapeutic noninvasive therapies. The Access to Medical Treatment Act (AMTA) was introduced in Congress to increase clients' access to unapproved therapies, subject to certain safeguards, and to broaden providers' ability to offer nondangerous non-FDA-approved treatments. The legislation gives an individual "the right to be treated by a health care practitioner with any medical treatment (including a treatment that is not approved, certified, or licensed by the Secretary of Health and Human Services) that such individual desires or the legal representative of such individual desires, if the practitioner personally examines and agrees to treat the individual and the administration of the treatment is within the provider's authorized scope of practice." Furthermore, the treatment may be provided only if:

1. "There is no reasonable basis to conclude that the treatment itself, when used as directed, poses as unreasonable and significant danger to such individual.

2. In the case of a treatment requiring and lacking FDA approval, the individual receives written notice that the FDA has not approved, certified, or licensed the treatment, and that the individual uses such treatment at his or her own risk.

3. The provider notifies the patient in writing of the nature of the treatment, including, among other things, 'reasonably foreseeable side effects.'

4. No advertising claims are made as to efficacy.

5. The label of any drug, device, or food used in such treatment is not false or misleading.

6. The individual signs a written statement indicating informed consent as to items 1 through 4 and acceptance of the treatment" (Cohen, 1998, pp. 78-79).

The nurse who recommends nutritional and herbal health promotion therapies needs to be aware of food and drug laws. The Dietary Supplement Health Education Act (DSHEA) reaffirms that dietary supplements are "foods," thus exempting dietary supplements from the requirement of new drug or food additive approval. The statute defines "dietary supplements" to include products that contain, either individually or in combination, vitamins, minerals, herbs, or other botanicals, amino acids, or other products for use to supplement the diet by increasing total dietary intake (Cohen, 1998). However, the standard of care for nurses includes knowing the possible interactions of dietary supplements with traditional pharmaceuticals, as well as the contraindications of the use of various herbs with coexisting medical conditions.

IMPLICATIONS FOR PROFESSIONAL NURSES

Both federal and state legislative reform use disclosure and agreement rather than prohibition as the primary means of patient protection (Cohen, 1998). In practicing integrative health promotion, the nurse takes a detailed history, and thus tends to spend more personal time and have more emotional contact with clients. By structuring the provider-client relationship as a collaborative venture, the nurse can reduce the malpractice risk, while the client takes the responsibility for supporting the healing process (Cohen, 1998). "Integral health care entrusts the [client] with greater responsibility for prevention and self-care" (Cohen, 1998).

Generally, a nurse who incorporates noninvasive therapeutic modalities in health promotion practice is held to a standard of care appropriate to the profession (Cohen, 1998). Nurses who use these modalities are vulnerable to malpractice liability when they assume too much responsibility for the client's biomedical condition and fail to refer the client to an appropriate conventional physician. "The tort of misrepresentation is triggered when health care providers make claims exceeding the boundaries of professional training and skill.... [However], to show misrepresentation, a plaintiff must introduce evidence of intent to defraud, deceive, and/or misrepresent; deception alone is insufficient" (Cohen, 1998, p. 69).

Of concern when nurses utilize any therapeutic interventions within their practice is whether they are sufficiently competent to do so. Nurses should be wary of implementing new therapeutic approaches unless they have satisfactorily completed a training course recognized by a credible professional body which at the very least subscribes to a Code of Ethics and provides members with professional indemnity (Stone, 1999).

Just as individuals are responsible for an appropriate standard of care for their practice, health care institutions are also responsible for the standard of care administered by their employees. "The doctrine of vicarious liability (or respondeat superior) considers individual providers to be agents of the health care institution rather than independent contractors. In vicarious liability, negligent acts of the agent are attributable to, and considered to be acts of, the principal" (Cohen, 1998, p. 71).

Ideally, nurses practicing integrative health promotion should have levels of training, skill, and professionalism at least commensurate with that of peers practicing within the biomedical model. Professional organizations can reduce health care institutions' liability concerns by developing programs and criteria to ensure high standards in provider credentialing and care. Health care institutions can attempt to meet their duty to non-negligently retain and supervise individual nurse providers through:

- Periodic review and monitoring

- Ensuring that providers are delivering services within their legally authorized scope of practice

- Developing recognized protocols for collaborative practice between providers

- Peer review of services and practices and utilization review (Cohen, 1998)

From a legal perspective, when nurses decide whether to include noninvasive therapeutic therapies in their practice, four questions must be considered:

- How can the nurse be sure that the therapies being offered have the potential for benefit for a particular client, since many are still largely unsupported by a scientific research base?

- Can the therapy be potentially harmful for the particular client?

- Is the nurse competent to perform the modality?

- Has the client given fully informed consent?

Given appropriate answers to these questions, the potential for legal challenge should not prevent the nurse, in collaboration with the client, from incorporating non-invasive therapeutic therapies within an integrative health promotion practice.

Health law aims to create an environment in which health promotion, the protection of individual rights, and the general principles of equality and justice go hand in hand (Legemaate, 2002). However, healthful lifestyles are the result of opportunities available to people, and not a matter of free choice. Policy affects these opportunities (Rutton et al., 2003). "Policy is a plan or course of action selected from alternatives and intended to influence and determine decisions and actions" (Acosta, 2003, p. 2). Both public and private policies can have major impacts on health care outcomes. For example, health care system interventions that have demonstrated effectiveness include diabetes disease management and case management programs, tobacco cessation reminders and education for providers, reduction of out-of-pocket costs for vaccinations, and standing orders for vaccinations (Fielding et al., 2002).

A number of strategies can be used to promote health-related policies. Building a coalition of people and organizations working together to achieve shared goals is one of the most effective vehicles for grassroots impact. Other strategies include lobbying and advocacy. Lobbying is a particular kind of advocacy, which refers to activities in support of or opposition to legislation or regulations that are governed by one or more federal, state, or local laws. Examples of lobbying activities include:

- Writing to your elected official asking him or her to vote in favor of a specific bill.

- Asking members of your organization or the general public to contact elected officials to vote in favor of a specific bill.

- Testifying about your position in support of or opposition to a specific administrative regulation.

- Communicating your position supporting or opposing a proposed ballot initiative to a member of the general public.

- Engaging a lobbyist, public relations firm, or other individual or organization to undertake the activities listed above in support of a specific bill on your behalf (Acosta, 2003).

Acosta (2003) suggests that an extreme form of lobbying involves participating in a political campaign on behalf of or in opposition to a candidate for political office.

Advocacy is another strategy to affect policy change. Advocacy is much less restrictive than lobbying. Advocacy refers to all unregulated activities designed to influence public policy that do not fall under the lobbying definition. "The key difference between lobbying and advocacy is that advocacy entails communicating directly with policymakers and the public about an issue without requesting action on a specific legislative proposal" (Acosta, 2003, p. 5). Examples of advocacy include:

- Inviting elective officials to participate in a community forum to discuss the problem of traffic safety.

- Developing a publication that explains the problem of poor oral health in young children and developing general recommendations for policymakers, communities, and schools.

- Encouraging the community to call your organization for more information about the benefits of recycling and how to get more involved in preventing toxic dumping.

- Writing a press release explaining the high teen pregnancy rates in your county and how your program has succeeded in developing a new school-based health center that gives free sexuality education counseling to teens.

- Inviting your elected official to visit your program (Acosta, 2003).

This chapter has emphasized that the current standard for ethical decision making in biomedicine and nursing is normative ethics, based on abstract principles, impartiality, and universal application. In this perspective, the professional, viewed as the expert in health, has the obligation and the power to make ethical decisions. In contrast, integrative health promotion emphasizes individualized care and a nurse-client helping partnership with shared ethical decision making and power. There has also been an emphasis on the ethical and legal requirements for competence in professional nursing care, based on appropriate education and experience, with referral to medical practitioners when the goal is curative treatment of disease. Finally, given overwhelming global health concerns regarding the provision of justice, the valuing of autonomy as the predominant principle underlying ethical judgments in American culture must be questioned.

Chapter Key Points

- There are now challenges to the assumptions of impartiality and universality of traditional normative ethics.

- Any exercise of professional power can trespass on the client's vital rights and interests.

■ Ethical frameworks for judging decisions can be viewed as mutually exclusive (e.g., utilitarianism, liberalism, contextualism, or deontology) or as intrinsically related and mutually enhancing, different perspectives.

■ The principles of biomedical ethics are autonomy, nonmaleficence, beneficence, and justice.

■ Nurses must address broader social justice issues associated with promoting the well-being and significant moral interests of marginalized or stigmatized groups.

■ For a nurse to be found negligent, duty, breach, causation, and damages must be proved.

■ Malpractice exposure is reduced by structuring the provider and client relationship as a collaborative venture to health.

References

Acosta, C. M. (2003). Improving public health through policy advocacy. *Community-Based Public Health Policy Practice, 8*, 1-8.

Aiken, T. D. (1994). *Legal, ethical, and political issues in nursing*. Philadelphia: FA Davis

American Nurses' Association (1996). *Model practice act*. Washington, DC: American Nurses.

American Nurses' Association (1998). *Legal aspects of standards and guidelines for clinical nursing practice*. Washington, DC: American Nurses.

American Nurses' Association (2001). Code of ethics for nurses-Provisions. Retrieved on December 15, 2001, from http://www.ana.org/ethics/chcode.htm

Bolletino, R. C. (1998). The need for a new ethical model in medicine: A challenge for conventional, alternative, and complementary practitioners. *Advances in Mind-Body Medicine, 14*, 6-28.

Bournes, D. A. (2000). A commitment to honoring people's choices. *Nursing Science Quarterly, 13*, 18-23.

Braddock, C. H., Edwards, K. A., Hasenberg, N. M., Laidley, T. L., & Levinson, W. (1999). Informed decision making in outpatient practice. Time to get back to basics. JAMA, 282, 2313-2320.

Brody, H., Rygwelski, J. M., & Fetters, M. D. (1999). Ethics at the interface of conventional and complementary medicine. In W. B. Jonas, & J. S. Levin, *Essentials of complementary and alternative medicine* (pp. 46-56). Philadelphia: Lippincott.

Bunkers, S. S. (2001). On global health and justice: A nursing theory-guided perspective. *Nursing Science Quarterly, 14*, 297.

Clark, P. A. (2000). The ethics of alternative medicine therapies. *J Public Health Policy, 21*, 447-470.

Cohen, M. H. (1998). *Complementary and alternative medicine: Legal boundaries and regulatory perspectives*. Baltimore: Johns Hopkins University Press.

Cohen, M. H. (1999). Complementary and alternative medicine policy: The future of regulation. *Alternative and Complementary Therapies, 5*, 50-54.

Ely-Pierce, K. (1999). Legal issues for case managers: What you don't know can hurt you. *Family and Community Health, 22*, 78-9.

Fielding, J. E., Marks, J. S., Myers, B. W., Nolan, P. A., Rawson, R. D., & Toomay, K. E. (2002). How do we translate science into public health policy and law? *The Journal of Law, Medicine, & Ethics, 30* (Suppl. 3), 22-31.

Fry, S. T., & Duffy, M. E. (2001). The development and psychometric evaluation of the Ethical Issues Scale. *Journal of Nursing Scholarship, 33,* 273-277.

Gadow, S. (1999). Relational narrative: The postmodern turn in nursing ethics. *Scholarly Inquiry for Nursing Practice: An International Journal, 13,* 57-69.

Gilligan, C. (1982). *In a different voice: Psychological theory and women's development.* Cambridge, MA: Harvard University Press.

Gilligan, C. (1987). Moral orientation and moral development. In E. F. Kittay, & D. T. Meyers (Eds.), *Women and moral theory* (pp. 19-33). Totowa, NJ: Rowman and Littlefield.

Green, J. A. (1999). Collaborative physician-patient planning and professional liability: Opening the legal door to unconventional medicine. *Advances in Mind-Body Medicine, 15,* 83-94.

Guinn, D. E. (2001). Ethics and integrative medicine: Moving beyond the biomedical model. *Altern Ther Health Med, 7,* 68-72.

Guttman, N., & Ressler, W. H. (2001). On being responsible: Ethical issues in appeals to personal responsibility in health campaigns. *Journal of Health Communication, 6,* 117-136.

Haddad, A. (1998). The future of ethical decision making in health care. *Nursing Clinics North America, 33,* 373-384.

Hall, J. K. (1996). *Nursing ethics and law.* Philadelphia: W. B. Saunders.

Hamric, A. B. (1999). The nurse as a moral agent in modern health care. *Nurs Outlook, 47,* 106.

Hodge, J. G., Gostin, L. O., & Jacobson, P. D. (1999). Legal issues concerning electronic health information: Privacy, quality, and liability. JAMA, *282,* 1466-1471.

Johnstone, M. (1998). Advancing nursing ethics: Time to set a new global agenda? *Int Nurs Rev, 45,* 43.

Kuhse, H. (1997). *Caring: Nurses, women and ethics.* Oxford, UK: Blackwell.

Last, J. M., & Woolf, S. H. (1996). Ethical issues in health promotion and disease prevention. In S. H. Woolf, S. Jonas, & R. S. Lawrence (Eds.), *Health promotion and disease prevention in clinical practice* (pp. 554-568). Baltimore: Williams & Wilkins.

Legemaate, J. (2002). Integrating health law and healthy policy: A European perspective. *Health Policy, 60,* 101-110.

McGarity, T. O. (2004). The goals of environmental legislation. *Environmental Affairs, 31,* 529-554.

Milton, C. L. (2000). Beneficence: Honoring the commitment. *Nursing Science Quarterly, 13,* 111-115.

Nash, R. A. (1999). The biomedical ethics of alternative, complementary, and integrative medicine. *Alternative Therapies Health Medicine, 5,* 92-95.

Norton, L. (1995). Complementary therapies in practice: The ethical issues. *Journal of Clinical Nursing, 4,* 343-348.

Pellegrino, E. D. (1998). Emerging ethical issues in palliative care. JAMA, *279,* 1521-1522.

Pennsylvania State Board of Nursing. (1999). *Professional nurse law.* Harrisburg, PA: Department of State, Bureau of Professional and Occupational Affairs.

Rothschild, M. L. (2000). Ethical considerations in support of the marketing of public health issues. *American Journal of Health Behav, 24,* 26-35.

Rutten, A., Luschen, G., von Lengerke, T., Abel, T., Kannas, L., Diaz, J. A. R., Vinck, J., and van der Zee, J. Determinants of health policy impact: A theoretical framework for policy analysis. *Society for Preventive Medicine, 48,* 293-300.

Schwarz, J. K. (2000). Have we forgotten the patient? *American Journal of Nursing, 100,* 61, 64.

Showers, J. L. (2000). What you need to know about negligence lawsuits. *Nursing 2000, 30,* 45-48.

Stone, J. (1999). Using complementary therapies within nursing: Some ethical and legal considerations. *Complementary Therapies in Nursing & Midwifery, 5,* 46-50.

Sugarman, J., & Burk, L. (1998). Physician's ethical obligations regarding alternative medicine. *JAMA, 280,* 1623-1625.

Trott, M. C. (1998). Legal issues for nurse managers. *Nursing Management, 29,* 38-42.

BEYOND PHYSICAL ASSESSMENT 7

Abstract

The approach to assessment for many nurses is limited to physical skills, performed according to body system, to identify client's physical problems or potential problems. In contrast, in this chapter, it is assumed that the judicious use of holistic assessment techniques can identify client strengths and broaden the database from which clients and nurses develop health promotion plans. Therefore, a number of frameworks for assessment are presented, selected holistic categories of assessment are discussed, and, to supplement the typical Western biomedical physical assessment of body systems, two approaches (tongue and pulse assessment) commonly used in the Eastern traditions of Ayurveda and Chinese medicine are introduced. The chapter concludes with a brief discussion of procedures for disease screening

Learning Outcomes

By the end of this chapter the student will be able to:

- Identify a philosophy for health (as opposed to problem) assessment

- Describe the components of selected frameworks for assessment

- Discuss essential elements of functional ability, mental and nutritional status, and quality of life assessment

- Describe basic procedures for tongue and pulse assessment

Physical and Health Assessment

Physical assessment focuses on identification of clients' physical actual or potential problems in each body system. In contrast, health assessment is "a systematic collection of data about client health status, beliefs, and behaviors relevant to developing a health-protection-promotion plan" (Pender, 1996, p. 116). Health assessment is a collaborative process involving the nurse and the client that promotes mutual input into decision making and planning to improve the client's health and well-being. According to Pender (1996), the desired outcomes of health assessment include:

1. Identifying health assets

2. Identifying health-related lifestyle strengths

3. Determining key health-related beliefs

4. Identifying health beliefs and health behaviors that put the client at risk

5. Determining how the client wants to change to improve his or her quality of life

The initial health assessment provides a valuable baseline against which subsequent assessments can be compared. Health assessment should always take the whole person into account, including her or his general appearance, and should capitalize on the person's strengths.

Frameworks for Health Assessment

NURSING CONCEPTUAL MODELS

The many existing nursing models and theories provide diverse frameworks for assessment of health and organization of data (see Chapter 4, *The Meaning of Health: Models and Theories*, for a brief description of nine models and theories). Leddy (1998, p. 207) describes implications for data collection of these selected nursing models or theories. For example, within the context of Neuman's Health Care Systems model, the nurse would assess the client and the client's environment for intrapersonal, interpersonal, and extrapersonal stressors that might have an impact on the lines of resistance and defense. In contrast, within the context of Rogers' *Science of Unitary Human Beings*, the nurse would assess the mutual process and patterning of the human being-environment energy fields (see Table 7-1 for implications for data collection in selected nursing models organized by theoretical frameworks, and see Table 7-2 for selected assessment tools derived from nursing models and theories).

PENDER'S CATEGORIES FOR ASSESSMENT

Pender (1996, p. 116) proposes that important components of health assessment focusing on individual clients are:

- Functional health patterns
- Physical fitness evaluation

Table
7-1

Implications for Data Collection in Selected Nursing Models Organized by Theoretical Frameworks

NURSING MODELS	IMPLICATIONS FOR DATA COLLECTION
Systems Theory	
■ King	Perceptions of self, level of growth and development, level of stress, abilities to function in usual role, decision-making abilities, and abilities to communicate.
■ Neuman	Stressors, indications of disruption of the lines of defense, resistance factors.
Stress/Adaptation	
■ Roy	Adaptation level (related to three cases of stimuli), coping in relation to modes of adaptation, position on the health-illness continuum.
Caring	
■ Orem	Therapeutic self-care demand, presence of self-care deficits, ability of clients to meet self-care requisites.
■ Watson	Phenomenal field (self within space and motivational factors for health), values, needs for information, problem-solving abilities, developmental conflicts, losses, feelings about the human predicament.
Complexity	
■ Peplau	Physiologic and personality needs, illness symptoms, relationships with significant others, influences on establishment and maintenance of the nurse-client relationship.
■ Rogers	Characteristics of patterning, health potential, rhythms of life, simultaneous states of the individual and environment.
■ Parse	Thoughts and feelings about the situation, the synchronizing rhythms in human relationships, personal meanings, ways of being alike and different, and values.
■ Newman	Person-environment interactions, patterns of energy exchange, client's responses to symptoms, transforming potential, client's feelings and what he does because of those feelings, patterns of life.

Reprinted with permission from Leddy, S. K. (1998). *Leddy and Pepper's conceptual bases of professional nursing* (4th ed.). Philadelphia: JB Lippincott. © 1998 Lippincott Williams & Wilkins.

Table 7-2:   *Selected Assessment Tools Derived from Nursing Models and Theories: The King General Systems Model*

INSTRUMENT	CITATION	DESCRIPTION
Criterion-referenced measure of goal attainment (CRMGAT)	King, I. M. (1998). Measuring health goal attainment in patients. In C. F. Waltz & O. L. Strickland (Eds.), *Measurement of nursing outcomes. Vol 1. Measuring client outcomes.* (pp. 108–127). New York: Springer.	Used to assess, plan, and evaluate nursing in terms of the client's physical ability to perform activities of daily living (ADL), level of consciousness, hearing, vision, smell, taste, touch, speaking ability, listening ability, reading and writing abilities, nonverbal communication, and decision-making ability; response to the performance of ADL; and goals to be attained.
Assessment format	Swindale, J. E. (1989). The nurse's role in giving pre-operative information to reduce anxiety in patients admitted to hospital for elective minor surgery. *J Adv Nurs, 14,* 899–905.	Guides assessment of the minor surgery patient's anxieties, coping strategies, and nature of information needing.
Community health	Hanchett, E. S. (1998). *Nursing frameworks and community as client: Bridging the gap.* Norwolk, CT: Appleton & Lange.	Guides assessment of a community according to the dimensions of personal, interpersonal, and social systems.

continued

Table
7-2

Selected Assessment Tools Derived from Nursing Models and Theories *(continued)*: The Neuman Systems Model

INSTRUMENT	CITATION	DESCRIPTION
Neuman systems model assessment and intervention tool	Mirenda, R. M. (1986). The Neuman model in practice. *Senior Nurse, 5*, 26-27. Neuman, B. (1989). *The Neuman systems model* (2nd ed., pp. 3-63). Norwalk, CT: Appleton & Lange.	Guides client system assessment and permits documentation of goals, intervention plan, and outcomes from the perspective of both clients and caregivers.
Nursing assessment guide	Beckman, S. J., Boxley-Harges, S., Bruick-Sorge, C., & Eichenauer, J. (1998). Evaluation modalities for assessing student and program outcomes. In L. Lowry (Ed.), *The Neuman systems model and nursing education: Teaching strategies and outcomes* (pp. 149-160). Indianapolis, IN: Sigma Theta Tau International Center Press.	A modification of the Neuman systems model assessment and intervention tool.
Assessment and analysis	McHolm, F. A., & Geib, K. M. (1998). Application of the Neuman systems model to teaching health assessment and nursing process. *Nursing Diagnosis: Journal of Nursing Language and Classification, 9*, 23-33.	Guides health assessment and formulation of nursing diagnoses.

continued

Table 7-2

Selected Assessment Tools Derived from Nursing Models and Theories (continued): The Orem Self-Care Model

INSTRUMENT	CITATION	DESCRIPTION
Nursing history	Orem, D. E. (1995). Elements of a nursing history. In D. E. Orem (Ed.), *Nursing: Concepts of practice* (5th ed., pp. 422–430). St. Louis, MO: Mosby.	Guides the assessment of changes in a patient's therapeutic self-care demand and the patient's self-care agency as well as the patient's conditions and pattern of living.
Structured data collection	Laschinger, H. S. (1990). Helping students apply a nursing conceptual framework in the clinical setting. *Nurse Educator, 15,* 20–24.	Guides assessment of patients in relation to the self-care framework.
Nursing assessment tool	Fernandez, R., & Wheeler, J. I. (1990). Organizing a nursing system through theory-based practice. In G. G. Meyer, M. J. Madden, & E. Lawrenz (Eds.), *Patient care delivery models* (pp. 63–83). Rockville, MD: Aspen.	Guides the nursing history and assessment in the areas of the basic conditioning factors and universal self-care requisites.

continued

Table 7-2

Selected Assessment Tools Derived from Nursing Models and Theories (continued): Rogers' Science of Unitary Human Beings

INSTRUMENT	CITATION	DESCRIPTION
Nursing assessment of patterns indicative of health	Madrid, M., & Winstead-Fry, P. (1986). Rogers' conceptual model. In P. Winstead-Fry (Ed.), *Case studies in nursing theory* (pp. 73-102). New York: National League for Nursing.	Guides assessment of pattern, including relative present, communication, sense of rhythm, connection to environment, personal myth, and system integrity.
Power as knowing participation in change	Barrett, E. A. M. (1990). An instrument to measure power as knowing-participation-in-change. In O. Strickland, & C. Waltz (Eds.), *The measurement of nursing outcomes. Vol. 4. Measuring client self-care and coping skills* (pp. 159-180). New York: Springer.	Measures the person's capacity to participate knowingly in change by means of semantic differential ratings of the concepts awareness, choices, freedom to act intentionally, and involvement in creating changes.
Nursing process format	Falco, S. M., & Lobo, M. L. (1995). Martha E. Rogers. In J. B. George (Ed.), *Nursing theories. The base for professional nursing practice* (4th ed., pp. 229-248). Norwalk, CT: Appleton & Lange.	Guides use of a Rogerian nursing process, including nursing assessment, nursing diagnosis, nursing planning for implementation, and nursing evaluation according to the principles of integrality, resonancy, and helicy.

continued

Table 7-2 Selected Assessment Tools Derived from Nursing Models and Theories (continued): The Roy Adaptation Model

INSTRUMENT	CITATION	DESCRIPTION
Nursing manual: Assessment tool according to the Roy adaptation model	Cho, J. (1998). *Nursing manual: Assessment tool according to the Roy adaptation model*. Glendale, CA: Polaris.	Guides assessment of behaviors and stimuli for the physiological, self-concept, role function, and interdependent adaptive modes.
Typology of indicators of positive adaptation	Roy, C., & Andrews, H. A. (1999). *The Roy adaptation model* (2nd ed., pp. 79-81). Stanford, CT: Appleton & Lange.	A list of tthe indicators of positive adaptation for individuals and groups in the physiological/physical, self-concept/group identity, role function, and interdependent adaptive modes.
Nursing diagnostic	Roy, C., & Andrews, H. A. (1999). *The Roy adaptation model* (2nd ed., pp. 139, 161, 184, 214, 247, 279, 305, 340, 372, 417, 462, 503). Stanford, CT: Appleton & Lange.	A list of generic nursing diagnoses within the context of indicators of positive adaptation, common adaptation problems, and NANDA nursing diagnoses for all aspects of the physiological/physical adaptive mode, and the self-concept/group identity, role function, and interdependent adaptive modes.

continued

Table 7-2

Selected Assessment Tools Derived from Nursing Models and Theories (continued): The Watson Theory of Human Caring

INSTRUMENT	CITATION	DESCRIPTION
Caring behaviors assessment	Harrison, B. P. (1998). Development of the caring behaviors assessment based on Watson's theory of caring. *Master's Abstracts International, 27,* 95.	Measures nurse caring behaviors in terms of the carative factors.
Caring assessment tool	Duffy, J. R. (1992). The impact of nursing caring on patient outcomes. In D. Gaut (Ed.), *The presence of caring in nursing* (pp. 113–136). New York: National League for Nursing.	Measures nurses' caring activities.
Caring behaviors inventory	Wolf, Z. R., Giordino, E. R., Osbourne, P. A., & Ambrose, M. S. (1994). Dimensions of nurse caring. *Image: Journal of Scholarship, 26,* 107–111.	Measures nurses' caring behaviors within the context of the carative factors.

continued

Table 7-2

Selected Assessment Tools Derived from Nursing Models and Theories (continued): The Leddy Human Energy Model

INSTRUMENT	CITATION	DESCRIPTION
Person-environment participation scale (PEPS)	Leddy, S. K. (1995). Measuring mutual process: Development and psychometric testing of the person-environment participation scale. *Visions: Journal of Rogerian Nursing Science, 3,* 20–31.	Measures the person's experience of continuous human-environment mutual process by means of semantic differential ratings of 15 bipolar adjectives representing the content areas of comfort, influence, continuity, ease, and energy.
Leddy healthiness scale	Leddy, S. K. (1996). Development and psychometric testing of the the Leddy healthiness scale. *Research in Nursing and Health, 19,* 431–440.	Measures the person's perceived purpose and power to achieve goals by means of Likert scale ratings of 26 items representing meaningfulness, ends, choice, challenge, confidence, control, capacity, capability to function, and connections.

Source: Adapted from Fawcett, J. (2000). *Analysis and evaluation of contemporary nursing knowledge: Nursing models and theories.* Philadelphia: F. A. Davis; Leddy, S. K. (1998). *Leddy and Pepper's conceptual bases of professional nursing.* Philadelphia: Lippincott Williams & Wilkins.

- Nutritional assessment
- Health risk appraisal
- Life stress review
- Spiritual health assessment
- Social support systems review
- Health beliefs review
- Lifestyle assessment

GORDON'S FUNCTIONAL HEALTH PATTERNS

Gordon's (1995) typology of 11 functional health patterns provides another framework for assessing individuals, families, and communities. "By examining the specific functional patterns and the interaction among the patterns, the nurse can accurately determine and diagnose actual or potential problems, intervene more effectively, and achieve outcomes that promote health and well-being.... A major goal in assessing each pattern is to determine the client's knowledge of health promotion, ability to manage health-promoting activities, and the value that the individual ascribes to health promotion" (Edelman & Mandle, 1998, pp. 121, 125).

The patterns included in Gordon's typology include:

1. *The Health Perception-Health Management Pattern* describes the client's perceived pattern of health and well-being and how health is managed:

   - How has general health been
   - Most important things done to keep healthy
   - Relevance of health status to current activities and future planning
   - Health and safety practices (health risk management)
   - General health care behavior
   - Belief in ability to influence one's own health through lifestyle changes
   - Previous patterns of adherence or compliance and use of the health care system
   - Knowledge of availability of health services
   - Patterns indicating at what point health care is sought
   - Accessibility to health care through financial resources, health insurance, and transportation factors

2. *The Nutritional-Metabolic Pattern* describes pattern of food and fluid consumption relative to metabolic need and pattern indicators of local nutrient supply:

   - Patterns of food and fluid consumption
   - Typical food and fluid intake
   - Appetite

- Weight loss or gain
- Daily eating times
- Types and quantity of food and fluids consumed
- Particular food preferences
- Use of nutrient or vitamin supplements, caffeine, or alcohol
- Food allergies
- How foods are prepared
- Are there adequate financial resources for an adequate diet
- Breast feeding and infant feeding patterns
- Condition of skin, hair, nails, mucous membranes, and teeth

3. *The Elimination Pattern* describes patterns of bowel, bladder, and skin excretory function:

- Perceived regularity
- Use of routines or laxatives for bowel elimination
- Devices employed to control excretion
- Changes in time-pattern, mode of excretion, quality, or quantity

4. *The Activity-Exercise Pattern* describes patterns of exercise, activity, leisure, and recreation:

- Activities of daily living requiring energy expenditure (e.g., hygiene, cooking, shopping, eating, working, and home maintenance)
- Sufficient energy for desired or required activities
- Type, quantity, and quality of exercise including sports
- Activities of high importance or significance for leisure (recreation)

5. *The Sleep-Rest Pattern* describes patterns of sleep, rest, and relaxation:

- Perception of the quality and quantity of sleep and rest
- Generally rested and ready for daily activities after sleep
- Perception of energy level
- Aids to sleep such as medications or nighttime routines

6. *The Cognitive-Perceptual Pattern* describes sensory-perceptual and cognitive patterns:

- Adequacy of vision, hearing, taste, touch, or smell
- Compensation or prostheses utilized for disturbances
- Pain perception and how pain is managed
- Any change in memory lately
- Easiest way to learn things
- Cognitive functional abilities such as language, memory, and decision making

7. *The Self-Perception-Self-Concept Pattern* describes self-concept patterns and perceptions of self:

- Attitudes about himself or herself
- Perception of cognitive, affective, or physical abilities
- Body image
- Identity
- General sense of worth
- General emotional pattern
- Pattern of body posture and movement, eye contact, voice and speech pattern

8. *The Role-Relationship Pattern* describes a pattern of role engagements and relationships:

- Individual's perception of major roles and responsibilities
- Satisfaction or disturbances in family, work, or social relationships
- How does family usually handle problems

9. *The Sexuality-Reproductive Pattern* describes patterns of satisfaction or dissatisfaction in sexuality:

- Reproductive pattern
- Female's reproductive stage and any perceived problems
- Perceived satisfaction or disturbances in sexuality

10. *The Coping-Stress-Tolerance Pattern* describes general coping patterns and effectiveness of the patterns in terms of stress tolerance:

- Reserve or capacity to resist challenge to self-integrity
- Modes of handling stress
- Family or other support systems
- Any big changes or crisis in the last year or two
- Perceived ability to control and manage situations
- How problems are handled

11. *The Value-Belief Pattern* describes patterns of values, goals, or beliefs that guide choices or decisions:

- What is perceived as important in life
- Quality of life
- Perceived conflicts in health-related values, beliefs, or expectations
- Importance of religion
- Important plans for the future

Selected Categories for Assessment

THE HEALTH HISTORY

Regardless of which approach is used for assessment and organization of data, the first step in the process is to interview the client and determine the health history.

At the core of the data collection process is the nurse-client interview, a highly specialized, purposeful, goal-directed interaction. Thus, the first step is to become expert at interviewing skills and techniques. The nurse also must know what information is needed from the client (Rychlee, 2000). "The purpose of the health history is to collect subjective data, what the person says about himself or herself. The history is combined with the objective data from the physical examination and laboratory studies, and [subjective data from other assessments] to form the data base. The data base is used to make a judgment or a diagnosis about the health status of the individual.... For the well person, the history is used to assess his or her lifestyle, including such factors as exercise, diet, risk reduction, and health promotion behaviors" (Jarvis, 2000, p. 80). Box 7-1 lists areas usually included in a health history.

The following categories of assessment have been selected as examples of the many types of assessment that are available to the nurse who seeks a holistic, multidimensional representation of client health patterns.

Box 7-1

Areas for Health History Questions

The "health" history usually proceeds according to questions in the following areas:

1. Biographical data

2. Reason for seeking care. Which concern prompted the person to seek help now?

3. Present health or history of present illness. For well person, this is a short statement about the general state of health; for the ill person this is a chronological record of the reason for seeking care. Eight critical characteristics of symptoms include:

   - *Location.* Be specific.

   - *Character or quality.* Burning, sharp, dull, aching.

   - *Quantity or severity.* How does the symptom affect daily activities.

   - *Timing.* Onset, duration, and frequency.

continued

Box 7-1 continued

- *Setting.* What brings on the symptom?
- *Aggravating or relieving factors.* What seems to help?
- *Associated factors.*
- *Patient's perception.* Meaning of the symptom.

4. Review of systems. Examples of health promotion questions:

- *Skin.* Amount of sun exposure.
- *Eyes.* Last vision check; glasses or contacts?
- *Ears.* Hearing loss; how loss affects daily life.
- *Mouth and throat.* Pattern of daily dental care; use of prostheses; last dental checkup.
- *Breast.* Performs self-examination; last mammogram.
- *Respiratory.* Last chest x-ray.
- *Cardiovascular.* Last Electrocardiogram.
- *Peripheral vascular.* Any long-term sitting or standing? Avoid crossing legs at knees.
- *Gastrointestinal.* Antacids or laxatives?
- *Genitals.* Testicular self-examination? Last gynecological exam and Pap smear.
- *Musculoskeletal.* How much walking each day? Any limits on range of motion?
- *Mental.* Interpersonal relationships; coping patterns.

ASSESSMENT OF HEALTH

Dimension Scales

One common approach to health assessment is to evaluate "multiple dimensions" of health (Young, 1997). For example, Keegan and Dossey (1987) developed dimension scales for self-assessment of physical, mental, social, emotional, and spiritual dimensions of the individual. No theoretical basis for these scales is apparent. Examples of items include "have a good level of energy" (physical); "trust others easily" (social); and "have a relationship with a higher power" (spiritual). Items are scored as occurring most of the time, often, sometimes, or seldom. The separate dimension scores can be used to compile a total self-assessment score. The individual items can also be used by the client and the nurse to identify particular strengths and weaknesses in each dimension. Reliability and validity of these scales have not been established.

The Leddy Healthiness Scale

There are scales to measure well-being (psychological) and health status (medical), but investigators have been slow to develop instruments to measure health within a holistic or unitary perspective. One exception is the Leddy Healthiness Scale (LHS) (Leddy, 1996), which measures healthiness, defined as "a process characterized by perceived purpose, connections, and the power to achieve goals" (Leddy, 1997). As a resource that influences the ongoing patterning reflected in health, healthiness reflects a human being's perceived involvement in shaping change experienced in living. The LHS was derived from the Human Energy Model (Leddy, 1998; 2004).

The LHS is a 26-item, 6-point Likert type scale. Items measure meaningfulness, connections, ends, capability, control, choice, challenge, capacity, and confidence. The items are summed for a healthiness score. The LHS has demonstrated internal consistency reliability and construct validity. In studies with the LHS (Leddy, 1996, 1997; Leddy & Fawcett, 1997), healthiness has been found to be moderately and negatively related to fatigue and symptom experience in women with breast cancer, and moderately and positively related to mental health, health status, and satisfaction with life in a sample of healthy people. The LHS is available in Appendix A at the end of this book.

The Wellness Inventory

Another example of an approach to holistic assessment is the Wellness Inventory, developed by Travis and Ryan (1988), which provides "an integrated overview of all human life functions," including wellness and:

1. Self-responsibility and love
2. Breathing
3. Sensing
4. Eating
5. Moving
6. Feeling
7. Thinking
8. Playing or working
9. Communicating
10. Sex
11. Finding meaning
12. Transcending

The authors believe that the "harmonious balancing of these life functions results in good health and well-being" (p. xxix), but no theoretical framework was identified as the basis for the Wellness Inventory.

The Wellness Inventory consists of 120 Likert-type questions abridged from the 380 question Wellness Index. Items are ranked on a 3-part scale consisting of yes, usually, sometimes, and no, rarely; and are then summed by dimension for use in self-evaluation or wellness assessment with clients. Examples of items from the Wellness Inventory/Index include: "How I live my life is an important factor in determining my state of health," and "I look to the future as an opportunity for further growth." No information is available about reliability, validity, or psychometric testing of the Inventory. See the additional information at the end of the chapter for information about how to obtain the Wellness Inventory.

FUNCTIONAL ASSESSMENT

"Functional status refers to the entire domain of functioning.... It is defined as a multidimensional concept characterizing one's ability to provide for the necessities of life; that is, those activities people do in the normal course of their lives to meet basic needs, fulfill usual roles, and maintain their health and well-being.... Necessities include, but are not limited to, physical, psychological, social, and spiritual needs that are socially influenced and individually determined" (Leidy, 1994, p. 197). Functional status is often mistakenly interpreted only in the physical domain (Haas, 1999), but Leidy (1994) identifies four dimensions of functional status: capacity, performance, reserve, and capacity utilization.

Functional capacity "is defined as one's maximum potential to perform those activities people do in the normal course of their lives to meet basic needs, fulfill usual roles, and maintain their health and well-being" (Leidy, 1994, p. 198). Functional capacity, which consists of strengths and resources that provide individuals with the potential for activity, may refer to any domain, including physical, cognitive, psychological, social, spiritual, and sociodemographic areas.

Functional performance "is defined as the physical, psychological, social, occupational, and spiritual activities that people actually do in the normal course of their lives to meet basic needs, fulfill usual roles, and maintain their health and well-being.... The value an individual places on an activity or task and his or her need or desire to perform it are important components of performance" (Leidy, 1994, pp. 198, 200).

In a study of functional status from the client's perspective, Leidy and Haase (1999, p. 68) found that "people who are ill face an ongoing challenge of preserving their personal integrity, defined as a satisfying sense of wholeness, as they encounter a variety of physical changes that can interfere with day-to-day activity.... Qualities most salient to integrity are a sense of effectiveness, or 'being able,' and of connectedness, or 'being with.' The major categories of activity included household maintenance, movement, family activities, social activities, work, altruistic avocation, and recreation."

Effectiveness was characterized in the Leidy and Haase (1999) study as a sense of being able, expressed through the physical body and through the perception of competence, contribution, and purpose in daily activities, including self-care, family roles and tasks, and work. A second characteristic of effectiveness was energy. Energy contributed to an ability to perform various activities with spontaneity and ease, while connectedness, or being with, was defined as "a sense of significant, shared, and meaningful relationship with other people, a spiritual being, nature, or aspects of one's inner self" (Leidy & Haase, 1999, pp. 70-72).

Functional reserve "is the difference between capacity and performance" while functional capacity utilization (FCU) "refers to the extent to which functional potential is called upon in the selected level of performance.... As FCU increases, exertion increases, performance approaches capacity, and reserve is diminished" (Leidy, 1994, p. 199).

Leidy (1994) suggests that assessment of functional status should include the following aspects:

- *Self-esteem or self-concept.* Value belief system, personal strengths.

- *Activity and exercise.* Leisure activities, exercise pattern.

- *Sleep/rest.* Patterns; any sleep aids used.

- *Nutrition and elimination.* Recall of food and beverages for 24 hours; use of laxatives.

- *Interpersonal relationships and resources.* Social roles; support systems.

- *Coping and stress management.* Current stressors, methods used to relieve stress.

- *Personal habits.* Tobacco, alcohol, street drugs? Any desire to quit?

- *Environment and hazards.* Safety; involvement in community services.

- *Occupational health.* Likes and dislikes about job; any environmental hazards?

- *Perception of health.* Health goals; what is expected from health professionals?

The author is unaware of any one instrument that assesses all of these areas of functional status.

MENTAL ASSESSMENT

Mental assessment includes consideration of emotional and cognitive functioning, including:

- *Consciousness.* Awareness of surroundings, ability to think coherently.

- *Language.* Communication of thoughts and feelings.

- *Mood and affect.* Prevailing feelings that color one's emotional life.

- *Orientation.* Awareness of the objective world in relation to the self.

- *Attention.* Power of concentration without distraction.

- *Memory.* Recent and remote.

- *Abstract reasoning.* Pondering a deeper meaning beyond the concrete and literal.

- *Thought process.* Logical train of thought.

- *Thought content.* Specific ideas, beliefs, and the use of words.

- *Perceptions.* Awareness through the senses.

The Mental Health Index

The Mental Health Index (MHI) measures cognitive functioning, the balance between positive and negative affect, and the extent of psychological distress. The MHI is an established, 17-item, 6-point Likert type scale that was developed as part of the Medical Outcomes Study (Stewart & Ware, 1992). The items are scored on a range from "all of the time" to "none of the time" (in the past 4 weeks). Examples of items on the MHI include "felt loved and wanted," "been anxious or worried," and "been in firm control of your behavior, emotions, feelings, thoughts?"

The Perceived Well-Being Scale

Reker and Wong (1984) developed the perceived well-being scale (PWB) to measure physical and psychological well-being. Psychological well-being was defined as "the presence of positive emotions such as happiness, contentment, joy, and peace of mind and the absence of negative emotions such as fear, anxiety, and depression, but no theoretical framework has been identified for this definition. The PWB contains 14 items, scored on a 7-point, strongly agree to strongly disagree Likert scale. Six of the items comprise the psychological well-being subscale. Examples of items include, "no one really cares whether I am dead or alive," "I feel that life is worth living, and "I am often bored." This instrument has documented internal consistency reliability, stability, and validity.

NUTRITIONAL ASSESSMENT

Nutritional assessment reviews the degree of balance between nutrient intake and nutrient requirements. Nutrition screening is a quick and easy way to identify individuals at nutrition risk. If at risk, they should undergo a comprehensive nutritional assessment. Guided by the biomedical model, some of the possible considerations are:

- Eating patterns; food preferences
- Consistency with major dietary guidelines
- Usual weight
- Changes in appetite, taste, smell, chewing, and swallowing
- Recent surgery, trauma, burns, and infection
- Chronic illnesses
- Vomiting, diarrhea, and constipation
- Food allergies or intolerance
- Medications and/or nutritional supplements
- Self-care behaviors
- Alcohol or illegal drug use
- Exercise and activity patterns
- Family history

Assessment of nutritional intake may be based on one of several paper and pencil instruments such as a food frequency questionnaire (FFQ), or dietary recall diary or questionnaire, which may be supplemented with standardized measurements such as the body mass index (BMI), body weight, and/or blood laboratory tests. A typical FFQ asks the client to report the frequency with which many foods and beverages are eaten, over some time period ranging from 1 day to 1 year. Many FFQs ask about typical portion sizes. Consequently, the FFQ requires long-term recall and estimation of both frequency and quantity information. For research in which reliability is an issue, clients need to be trained to correctly estimate portion sizes. Most FFQs can be self-administered in one client contact, requiring an average of 30 minutes for completion. A variant of one of two published FFQs (Block et al., 1986; Willett et al., 1987) is often used, although a number of investigators develop their own questionnaires, making it difficult to assess reliability and concurrent validity. Additionally, it has been asserted that FFQs measure attitude and subjective inferences about the nature of the habitual diet more than memory for what was actually consumed (Drewnowski, 2001).

Food records and diaries also have problems. Clients have to be taught how to self-monitor and score their food and beverage intake. Staff burden is considerable, as several contacts with the client may be needed, and records are often incomplete and need to be supplemented with additional information. Most often, a 24-hour recall is requested, but a record of up to 4 days is commonly used. When compared with energy expenditure using doubly labeled water, evidence indicates that systemic error in the reporting of true dietary intake exists with use of either a FFQ or dietary recall (Trabulsi & Schoeller, 2001).

Recently, Soderhamn and Soderhamn (2002) published a nutritional form for the elderly (NUFFE) to identify actual and potential undernutrition among older clients. The original version of the instrument is in the Swedish language. The instrument is a summated three-point ordinal scale (from zero to two) with 15 items. There are two questions about weight loss and changes in dietary intake; nine questions related to appetite, food and fluid intake and eating difficulties; and four questions about obtaining food products, company at meals, activity, and number of drugs. Initial internal consistency reliability and validity are reported.

SPIRITUAL ASSESSMENT

Although there are many definitions of spirituality, each of them seems to focus on finding meaning and purpose in life and/or developing awareness of and allegiance to something sacred (Patton, 2001). According to Patton (2001), meaning in a person's life will provide a sense of peace and serenity, enhance self-understanding and insight, increase energy, promote hope and encouragement, and preserve a sense of integrity. Areas that provide meaning and purpose in the client's life can be identified by asking questions such as what gives your life meaning? What gives you a sense of serenity and peace? What provides joy and fulfillment? Or, what is your source of strength and hope?

The JAREL spiritual well-being scale (Hungelmann et al., 1989; 1996), based on the initials of the first names of the four scale developers, is an often used Likert-type instrument with 21 items scored according to a six-point scale from strongly agree to strongly disagree. Examples of items include "prayer is an important part of my life," "I accept life situations," and "I find meaning and purpose in my life." Reliability and validity data have not been reported. The authors suggest that the scores in each of three identified instrument factors (faith/belief, life/self responsibility, and life-satisfaction/self-actualization) can be used to identify needs or concerns.

QUALITY OF LIFE ASSESSMENT

Quality of life (QOL) as been described as "primarily a subjective sense of well-being encompassing physical, psychological, social, and spiritual dimensions" (Haas, 1999, p. 219). According to Haas (1999), indicators of QOL include: satisfaction with life, a subjective indicator; well-being, a subjective assessment concerned with all dimensions of life; and functional status, focused on objective indicators and concerned with all dimensions of life. In contrast, in their precede-proceed model of health promotion planning, Green and Krewer (1991) propose quality of life and health as outcomes of health promotion. The PRECEDE-PROCEED model is discussed in Chapter 8.

Raphael and colleagues suggest that quality of life encompasses "the degree to which a person enjoys the important possibilities of his/her life. The enjoyment of important possibilities is relevant to three major life domains: being, belonging, and becoming" (Raphael et al., 1997, p. 120).

Being reflects "who one is" and has three subdomains: physical being encompasses physical health, personal hygiene, nutrition, exercise, grooming, clothing, and general appearance. Psychological being includes the person's psychological health and adjustment, cognition, feelings, and evaluations concerning the self, such as self-esteem and self-concept. Spiritual being refers to one's personal values, standards of conduct, and spiritual beliefs.

Belonging concerns the person's fit with his or her environments and also has three subdomains: physical belonging describes the person's connections with the physical environments of home, workplace, neighborhood, school, and community. Social belonging includes links with social environments and involves acceptance by intimate others, family, friends, co-workers, and neighborhood and community. Community belonging represents access to public resources, such as adequate income, health and social services, employment, educational and recreational programs, and community events and activities.

Becoming refers to the activities carried out in the course of daily living, including those to achieve personal goals, hopes, and aspirations. Practical becoming describes day-to-day activities, such as domestic activities, paid work, school, or volunteer activities, and seeing to health or social needs. Growth-becoming activities promote the maintenance or improvement of knowledge and skills, and adapting to change. Leisure becoming includes activities carried out primarily for enjoyment that promote relaxation and stress reduction.

The relative importance or meaning attached to each particular dimension and the extent of the person's enjoyment influence the extent of a person's QOL. "The domains of QOL may serve as a determinant of health; improvement in the domains may be seen as a desired goal of health-promotion activities; assessment within the domains can serve as an indicator of needs" (Raphael et al., 1997, p. 121).

In contrast, Browne, McGee, and O'Boyle (1997, p. 738) suggest that "needs (as opposed to wants) are the most important determinant of quality of life. Domains normally included are physical health status and functional ability, psychological status and well-being, social interactions and economic status.... Above a basic standard of living, individually determined criteria, based more on wants than needs, become important in determining quality of life.... Certain needs are assumed to be more important than others" (p. 739). Each individual has his or her own definition of what constitutes a good or poor quality of life. More specifically, individuals define life domains in different ways, use different criteria to evaluate the domains, and place differing emphases on their importance to overall life quality.

Assessment Techniques from Eastern Traditions

The intent in the following section is to supplement the typical Western biomedical physical assessment of body systems with an introduction to two approaches (tongue and pulse assessment) commonly used in the Eastern traditions of Ayurveda and Chinese medicine. It is assumed that the judicious use of holistic techniques can broaden the database from which the client and nurse develop a health promotion plan.

Ohashi (1991, p. 15) describes four approaches to assessing the "health and character" of another person. These approaches clearly indicate how Eastern approaches differ from the typical Western assessment techniques.

- *Bo Shin.* Seeing or observing "with your entire being." Be open to the client's vibration and don't become preoccupied with details (p. 16).

- *Setsu Shin.* Touching or feeling "the core" or "inner being" of the client (p. 17), "using the hands as if they were knives" (p. 18).

- *Mon Shin.* Asking questions for information, listening for what is not being said. Gain the client's trust. Know your limits by not probing too deeply.

- *Bun Shin.* Listening to the quality of the client's voice and smelling odors given off by imbalance (e.g., ammonia from a high protein diet smells foul, fat smells rancid, and hormonal imbalance smells slightly burnt).

Two of the major Eastern health care belief systems are Ayurveda and Chinese medicine.

AYURVEDIC ASSESSMENT

One branch of Ayurveda is known as *Maharishi Ayur-Veda* (MAV). According to this tradition, the very first step in the development of disease is *pragya-aparadh*, a change in awareness deep inside. This results in being cut off from one's own innermost nature. As a result, "mistakes" are induced in three areas: diet, regimen, and mental activity. MAV diagnostic techniques reveal the individual's state of balance and weak points. Disease can be detected so early that symptoms have not yet become evident (Sharma & Clark, 1998).

Classic Ayurvedic texts describe three main modalities of diagnosis: sight, speech, and touch. Sight includes careful examination for details of imbalance, which can be revealed in the eyes, tongue, and other physical structures. Speech refers to a process of questioning the client about complaints, history, and causative factors. Touch involves many aspects including palpation and pulse assessment.

Pulse Assessment

In Ayurveda, the body is considered to be a pattern of information and intelligence. Information about the body as a whole is carried in the cardiovascular system in the form of fluid vibratory waves. Any imbalance creates a particular wave function, which can be identified by an experienced diagnostician. "The main value of pulse [assessment] is in revealing imbalances in the doshas and subdoshas, and the early stages of disease that result from such imbalances" (Sharma & Clark, 1998, pp. 55). (See Chapter 2 for a review of doshas).

Sharma and Clark (1998) describe the relationship of pulse assessment to Ayurvedic doshas. The radial artery of the right wrist of males and the left wrist of females is used to take the pulse using the clinician's index, middle, and ring fingers. The relative strength and characteristic style of pulsation under each finger relates to a specific dosha. The pattern of the Vata pulse is compared to the motion of a snake: light, quick, rough, thin, and rapidly undulating; Pitta's pulse pattern is compared to a frog: sharp, cutting, and jerky; and Kapha's pulse pattern is compared to the motion of a swan: heavy, full, slow, soft, and graceful. Pulsation in the wrong finger indicates dislocation of the doshas. The pulse at the surface of the skin (the vikriti) reflects imbalances present in the physiology, while the pulse felt at one-half of the artery's thickness (the prakriti), reflects the underlying nature. "Also, different parts of the fingertip relate to different subdoshas; and different techniques reveal information about the dhatus" (1998, p. 55).

To learn pulse assessment, the nurse should monitor his or her own pulse. By doing so many times a day over a prolonged time, the nurse can become more alert to the subtle information carried by the pulse. In the course of a day, of a year, and of different types of activities, the three doshas vary in their predominance and their states of balance. "As you monitor your own pulse, you become more alert to what, and how, your body is doing" (Sharma & Clark, 1998, pp. 55-56).

ASSESSMENT IN CHINESE MEDICINE

Western biomedicine medicine regards symptoms of disease to be reactions to noxious stimuli, as "errors to be "corrected" with drugs and surgery. These methods do nothing to eliminate the root cause of the symptoms. On the contrary, they only further weaken the client's system, eventually giving rise to even worse symptoms and more severe disease (Reid, 1995).

In contrast, traditional medical belief systems "view symptoms of disease as normal responses to abnormal stimuli, as alarm signals indicating a defect in the environment or a mistake in lifestyle that must be corrected at the root source" (Reid, 1995, p. 90). Traditional healing methods such as herbal medicine, diet, fasting, therapeutic exercise, acupuncture, and massage eliminate the basic causes of disease by removing toxins from the body, restoring vital functions, and re-establishing optimum balance and harmony among the "various organ energies of the human energy system" (p. 90). If successful, all abnormal symptoms naturally disappear and the client is cured. The problem will not recur if the client then takes preventive measures to eliminate the environmental or lifestyle factors that initially caused the problem (Reid, 1995).

Western diagnosis often involves evaluation of a battery of laboratory tests and machine measurements. Chinese diagnosis emphasizes methods that rely solely on the clinician's own sense perceptions, judgment, intuition, and experience. The clinician identifies what is seen, heard, smelled, and felt, asking questions about activities and events that cannot be observed directly, and listening to the client's feelings and complaints (Beinfield & Korngold, 1991). "Using himself as the instrument, the [clinician] takes the measure of the [client]: focusing mind and perception upon the gestalt of posture, stature, emotional and behavioral expression; upon specific attributes of the tongue, pulse, and complexion; and finally upon the areas and quality of pain or discomfort, restriction or freedom of movement, overall vigor and weakness. . . . The intent is to know not only the nature of the problem, but the nature of the [client]" (Beinfield & Korngold, 1991, p. 70).

In Chinese medicine, any part of the body (pulse, tongue, eye, ear) gives information about the whole. "Any aspect of a human being can become a window or lens for revealing the state of the person" (Beinfield & Korngold, 1991, p. 70). The objective is to formulate a picture of healthy and distorted patterns of function, with each set of diagnostic parameters providing one dimension of the total picture. Causes are really descriptions of underlying relationships rather than descriptions of material agents or pathogens.

Beinfield and Korngold (1991) describe several holistic methods used for assessment in Chinese medicine. These methods, in many cases quite different than Western traditions, include:

1. *Observing.* Complexion, eyes, tongue, nails, hair, gait, stature, affect, quality of excretions, and secretions.

2. *Listening and smelling.* Sound of voice and breath, odor of breath, skin, excretions, and secretions.

3. *Questioning.* Current complaints, health history, family health history, patterns of sleep, appetite, weight, elimination, menses, and stress.

4. *Touching.* Texture, humidity, temperature, elasticity of skin; strength and tone of muscles; flexibility, range of motion of joints; sensitivity of diagnostic points; and radial pulse assessment and evaluation.

Observation is based on visual analysis. The color and tone of the client's complexion, eyes, ears, tongue, hair, skin, and nails provide direct reflections of the condition of the related internal organs. Observing the way she or he walks, talks, breathes, and moves his or her arms and legs can assess the client's energy and spirit. "Chinese physicians carefully observe what they call *chee seh,* literally the 'color of energy,' which is reflected in facial complexion, the color of the earlobes, and the condition of the facial apertures, signs which clearly indicate the state of the [client's] vitality and resistance" (Reid, 1995, p. 88).

Listening is based on auditory and olfactory analysis in Chinese diagnosis. Odors of the client's breath and bodily secretions, and sounds of the client's breath, voice, cough, heartbeat, and stomach and bowels help determine the nature and location of the disease and the type of energy imbalance involved (Reid, 1995).

Touching is based on tactile analysis of the client's skin and supporting structures, palpation of the internal organs, and acupressure massage of the major energy meridians in order to determine which organs are affected by the disease. "Particular vital points along the meridians, known as 'alarm points', become very tender and painful to touch when their associated organs are ailing, and nerve ganglia along the spine become tight and knotted when the organs they control are weak or dysfunctional" (Reid, 1995, p. 88).

Generally, Chinese medicine recognizes emotions, climate, and lifestyle as the primary sources of pathogenic stress. "Sudden changes in weather or prolonged exposure can leave the body vulnerable to attack by wind, heat, dampness, dryness, and cold. Intense, persistent or suppressed emotional reactions such as anger, joy, anxiety, sorrow, or fear can cause a disruption of the circulation of qi and blood. Misuse of the body through overwork, overuse of the senses, or prolonged sitting, lying, or standing wastes the qi and injures the blood. Overindulgence in or neglect of dietary and sexual needs depletes vital essence" (Beinfield & Korngold, 1991).

Pulse Assessment

Ayurveda relates pulse assessment to the dosha constitution. In contrast, in Chinese medicine, pulse assessment is based on the principle that qi and blood circulate together as a single entity. The movement of blood allows the clinician to infer the activity of qi, moisture, and blood. The movement of blood in the arteries produces the pulse, but the force of qi initiates the movement (Beinfield & Korngold, 1991).

In pulse assessment three positions on each wrist are felt along the radial artery, at positions corresponding to "metabolic zones known as the triple-burner or three-heater. The position closest to the thumb corresponds to the chest and upper body (the heart and lung). The middle position corresponds to the upper abdomen (the stomach, spleen, gallbladder, and liver). The position farthest from the wrist corresponds to the lower abdomen (the kidney, bladder, small intestine, and large intestine)" (Beinfield & Korngold, 1991, p. 74).

The strength, rate, rhythm, and size of the pulse express the integrity of the qi and blood and the functional activity of the five organ networks. "A healthy pulse is regular, with four to five beats per cycle of respiration and a smooth, flowing feeling as it rises and falls. It is both elastic and resilient, evoking a sense of relaxed and vigorous rhythm and harmony" (Beinfield & Korngold, 1991, p. 74).

As many as 32 pulse qualities are described in the classical texts, each indicating a particular type of disturbance. For example, "if the pulse is 'floating'—that is, it can be felt with light pressure but fades away as the pressure increases—it indicates an adverse climate (wind, cold, heat, dampness, or dryness) has penetrated the surface from the outside. If the pulse is floating and rapid, or floating and strong, this reflects the influence of these adverse climates in conflict with the vigorous defensive qi of the body. The 'sinking' pulse is its counterpart. It is perceived only with deeper pressure and feels like a stone settling in water. Since it is relatively hidden or buried, it indicates that the problem exists at the deeper internal level" (Beinfield & Korngold, 1991, p. 77).

A frail and weak pulse generally indicates problems of a yin nature, while a strong and full pulse indicates problems of a yang nature. If one system is hyperactive and another is underactive, a full and forceful pulse may be felt in one position with a soft and weak pulse in another. A tense and erratic pulse can be generated by either excess or deficiency and is produced by stagnation. "Heat can be generated by a lack of yin as well as an excess of yang or fire. Most people are not diagnosed as having problems of a purely yin or yang nature, and often more than one organ network is involved in their disorder" (Beinfield & Korngold, 1991, p. 77).

Tongue Assessment

The tongue can be evaluated by observing its color, texture, moisture, size, and shape. "A healthy tongue fits comfortably in the mouth and is smooth, moist, bright, pink, and firm, with a thin white fur that covers the upper surface. Changes in the body of the tongue generally reflect long-term dysfunction of the viscera, whereas changes in the fur reflect short-term disturbances of digestion, fluid balance, and heat regulation" (Beinfield & Korngold, 1991, p. 71). Twenty-four different conditions based on the color, tone, texture of the tongue, and tongue fur have been distinguished in Chinese medical practice (Reid, 1995).

Each part of the tongue corresponds to the condition or state of an organ network. "To see the condition of the heart network one looks at the extreme tip of the tongue, whereas to gauge the state of the lung, one looks near the tip. So a very red-tipped tongue indicates not only the general presence of heat, but heat affecting these two networks. A tongue that is purplish indicates poor circulation, particularly associated with the stagnation of qi or blood in the liver. And greasy yellow fur in the center of the tongue reports damp heat in the spleen and stomach" (Beinfield & Korngold, 1991, p. 73).

The intrinsic strength and functional capacity of the individual is reflected in the quality of the fur and color of the tongue, as is the progress of illness. However, many external factors can also affect the appearance of the tongue, such as smoking, coffee, alcohol, and the use of pharmaceutical drugs. Under these conditions, the tongue may reflect the effect of these agents rather than give a true picture of the underlying state (Beinfield & Korngold, 1991).

Although the usual emphasis for assessment in nursing has been on physical methods to identify health problems and symptoms of disease, the emphasis in this chapter has been on multiple approaches to the assessment of health, including strengths and resources. Most health assessment measures are atheoretical and dimensional (e.g., functional ability, mental status, nutritional status, spiritual beliefs, quality of life), based on the disease perspective that health is additive. Much more theoretical work needs to be done as the basis for holistic measures (e.g., pulse and tongue assessment) that are consistent with a unitary perspective of health.

Screening for Disease

Screening and counseling for risk factors in order to prevent disease, an application of primary prevention, will be discussed in Chapter 8, *Promoting Individual Behavior Change.* Screening for disease conditions, an application of secondary prevention, aims to detect diseases in an early stage, in order to prevent the morbidity and costs associated with disease progression. Screening procedures include special tests or standardized examinations, usually with asymptomatic clients, to identify high-risk persons, who can then be referred for follow-up diagnosis and possible treatment. Based on a systematic review of evidence of clinical effectiveness, the U.S. Preventive Services Task Force (1996) developed detailed clinical recommendations on the appropriate use of screening interventions for many common clinically significant conditions, with existing, potentially effective preventive interventions. For a screening test to be considered effective, two major elements were required:

"The test must be able to detect the target condition earlier than without screening and with sufficient accuracy to avoid producing large numbers of false-positive and false-negative results; and screening for and treating persons with early disease should improve the likelihood of favorable health outcomes compared to treating [clients] when they present with signs or symptoms of the disease" (U.S. Preventive Task Force, 1996, p. xiii).

Task Force recommendations are summarized in Tables 7-3 to 7-6.

Table
7-3

Screening Interventions for the General Population by Age

AGE	SCREENING INTERVENTION
Birth to 10 years	Height and weight
	Blood pressure
	Vision screen (age 3 to 4 years)
	Hemoglobinopathy screen (birth)
	Phenylalanine level (birth)
	T4 and/or TSH (birth)
Ages 11 to 24 years	Height and weight
	Blood pressure
	Papanicolaou test (females)
	Chlamydia screen (females <20 years)
	Rubella serology or vaccination hx (females >12 years)
	Assess for problem drinking
	Blood pressure
	Height and weight
	Total blood cholesterol (men ages 35 to 64); (women ages 45 to 64)
Ages 25 to 64 years	Papanicolaou test (women)
	Fecal occult blood and/or sigmoidoscopy (>50 years)
	Mammogram (women ages 50 to 69)
	Assess for problem drinking
	Rubella serology or vaccination hx (women of child bearing age)
Age 65 and older	Blood pressure
	Height and weight
	Fecal occult blood and/or sigmoidoscopy
	Papanicolaou test (women)
	Mammogram (women >69 years)
	Assess for problem drinking
	Assess for hearing impairment
	Vision screening

continued

| Table 7-3 | ***Screening Interventions for the General Population by Age (continued)*** |

AGE	SCREENING INTERVENTION
Pregnant women	Blood pressure
	Hemoglobin/hematocrit
	Hepatitis B surface antigen
	RPR/VDRL
	Chlamydia screen (<25 years)
	Rubella serology or vaccination hx
	D typing, antibody screen
	Offer CVS (<13 weeks) or amniocentesis (15 to 18 weeks) (age >35 years)
	Offer hemoglobinopathy screening
	Assess for problem or risk drinking
	Offer HIV screening

Source: U.S. Preventive Services (1996). *Guide to clinical preventive services.* Baltimore: Williams and Wilkins.

Truglio-Londrigan and O'Connor (1998) discuss ethical issues associated with the use of screening procedures. Of considerable concern is the possibility for misinterpretation of the results by the client. Clients should be aware of the possibility of false-positive or false-negative results and clearly informed that the results of screening tests are not diagnostic. In addition, consideration should be given to the obligation to clients who have received a false-positive result, resulting in expense for further testing, stigmatization by a disease considered to be socially or personally unacceptable, and/or anxiety while waiting for the results of further testing. What is the ethical obligation to persons who may receive a false-negative result and lose the opportunity for early intervention? What about borderline cases?

The periodic health examination provides an obvious opportunity for implementing screening procedures. However, it should be stressed that only clinically effective screening tests should be used and only when interventions are available that could improve outcomes for clients who test positive for the disease. It is vital that screening activities be followed by appropriate referral and follow-up counseling.

Table 7-4

Interventions for which There Is Insufficient Evidence to Recommend for or Against Screening Asymptomatic Persons

DISEASE OR PROBLEM	SCREENING TEST
Coronary artery disease	Resting electrocardiography (ECG) Ambulatory ECG Exercise ECG *Routine screening is not recommended as part of the periodic health visit or pre-participation sports examination for children, adolescents, or young adults. There is lack of evidence that earlier detection of CAD leads to better outcomes. The only interventions proven to reduce coronary events in asymptomatic persons are modifications of risk factors such as smoking, high cholesterol, and elevated blood pressure.*
Abdominal aortic aneurysm	Abdominal palpation or ultrasound
Skin cancer	Visual skin examination *There is insufficient evidence to recommend for or against sunscreen use for the primary prevention of skin cancer or counseling patients to perform periodic skin self-examination. Avoidance of sun exposure, specially between 10 am to 3 pm, and the use of protective clothing.*
Oral cancer	Visual examination *Discontinue all forms of tobacco and consumption of alcohol.*
Diabetes mellitus or gestational diabetes	*Routine ultrasound in the second trimester in low-risk pregnant women.*
Glaucoma	
Preterm labor	*Home uterine activity monitoring (HUAM) in high-risk pregnancies*

continued

Table
7-4

Interventions for which There Is Insufficient Evidence to Recommend for or Against Screening Asymptomatic Persons (continued)

Osteoporosis in postmenopausal women	Bone densitometry *Women should be counseled about hormone prophylaxis, smoking cessation, regular exercise, and adequate calcium intake.*
Idiopathic scoliosis in asymptomatic adolescents	
Dementia	Standardized instruments *Evaluate mental status in persons who have problems performing daily activities.*
Depression	Standardized questionnaires *Be alert for depressive symptoms in persons at high risk of depression.*
Suicide risk	*Be alert to signs of suicidal ideation in persons with established risk factors. Be alert to depression and use of alcohol and other drugs.*
Family violence	Screening instruments *Ask questions about physical abuse.*
Drug abuse	Standardized questionnaires or biologic assays *Question adolescents and adults while taking a history.*

Source: U. S. Preventive Services. (1996). *Guide to clinical preventive services.* Baltimore: Williams and Wilkins.

Table 7-5	***Interventions for which Screening of Asymptomatic Persons Is Recommended***

DISEASE	SCREENING TEST
High blood cholesterol (men ages 35 to 65 and women ages 45 to 65)	An interval of 5 years has been suggested. All adults, adolescents, and children over age 2 years, including those with normal cholesterol levels, should receive periodic counseling regarding dietary intake of fat and saturated fat.
Hypertension (all children and adults)	If hypertension is confirmed, should receive counseling regarding physical activity, weight reduction, and dietary sodium intake.
Breast cancer (women ages 50 to 69)	Mammography alone or mammography and annual clinical breast examination (CBE) every 1 to 2 years. There is insufficient evidence to recommend for or against the use of screening CBE alone or the teaching of breast self-examination.
Colorectal cancer	Annual fecal occult blood testing or sigmoidoscopy.
Cervical cancer (ages 50 and older)	Papanicolaou (Pap) testing for all women who are or have been sexually active and who have a cervix every 3 years up to age 65.
Height and weight measurements for obesity	Body mass index (body weight in kilograms divided by the square of height in meters) can be used as the basis for further assessment. All clients should be counseled to promote physical activity and a healthy diet.
Iron deficiency anemia measurements for obesity	Hemoglobin or hematocrit for pregnant women and high-risk infants. Encourage breast feeding. Insufficient evidence for routine use of iron supplements for healthy infants or pregnant women.
Elevated lead levels	Measuring blood lead at least once at age 12 months for all children at increased risk of lead exposure.

continued

Table
7-5

Interventions for which Screening of Asymptomatic Persons Is Recommended (continued)

DISEASE	SCREENING TEST
Hepatitis B	Surface antigen (HbsAg) for all pregnant women at their first prenatal visit. May be repeated in the third trimester for women at increased risk of HBV infection during pregnancy.
Tuberculosis	Tuberculin skin testing.
Syphilis	Serologic screening for all pregnant women and persons at increased risk of infection. Counseling is suggested to prevent sexually transmitted diseases.
Gonorrhea (*Neisseria gonorrhoeae*)	For asymptomatic women at high risk of infection. All high-risk women should be screened during pregnancy. Not recommended for the general adult population.
Human immunodeficiency virus (HIV)	Periodic screening for all persons at increased risk of infection. Infants born to high-risk women if the mother's antibody status is not known.
Chlamydial infection (Chlamydia trachomatis)	For all sexually active female adolescents, high-risk pregnant women, and other asymptomatic women at high risk of infection. Not recommended for the general population.
Asymptomatic bacteruria	Urine culture for all pregnant women. Insufficient evidence for diabetic or ambulatory elderly women.
Rubella	History of vaccination or by serology for all women of childbearing age at their first clinical encounter. Susceptible nonpregnant women should be offered rubella vaccination; susceptible pregnant women should be vaccinated immediately after delivery. An alternative for nonpregnant women of childbearing age is vaccination without screening.

continued

Table 7-5

Interventions for which Screening of Asymptomatic Persons Is Recommended (continued)

Disease	*Screening Test*
Visual impairment or diminished visual acuity (elderly)	Vision screening with Snellen visual acuity chart. Detection of amblyopia and strabismus is recommended once for all children prior to entering school, preferably between ages 3 and 4. Older adults should be periodically questioned about their hearing and counseled about the availability of hearing aid devices. Insufficient evidence for asymptomatic adolescents and working-age adults or older adults using audiometric testing.
Preeclampsia	Blood pressure measurement for all pregnant women at the first prenatal visit and periodically throughout the remainder of pregnancy.
D (formerly Rh)	Blood typing and antibody screening for all pregnant women at their first prenatal visit. Repeat antibody screening at 24 to 28 weeks gestation is recommended for unsensitized D-negative women.
Down syndrome	Chromosomal studies of amniocentesis or chorionic villus sampling (CVS) for pregnant women at high risk if there are adequate counseling and follow-up services. Serum multiple marker testing can be used for all low-risk pregnant women and as an alternative to amniocentesis or CVS for high-risk women.
Neural tube defects	Maternal serum a-fetoprotein (MSAFP) measurement with adequate counseling and follow-up services. Daily multivitamins with folic acid to reduce the risk of neural tube defects are recommended for all women who are planning or capable of pregnancy.
Sickle hemoglobinopathies	Neonatal screeening to identify infants who may benefit from antibiotic prophylaxis to prevent sepsis. Requires comprehensive counseling and treatment services.

continued

Table
7-5

Interventions for which Screening of Asymptomatic Persons Is Recommended (continued)

DISEASE	SCREENING TEST
Phenylketonuria (PKU)	Measurement of phenylalanine level on a dried-blood spot specimen for all newborns prior to discharge from the nursery. Infants who are tested before 24 hours of age should receive a repeat screening test by 2 weeks of age.
Congenital hypothyroidism	Thyroid function tests on dried-blood spot specimens for all newborns in the first week of life.
Problem drinking (all adults and adolescents)	Standardized screening questionnaires and/or careful history of alcohol use counsel about the dangers of operating a motor vehicle.

Source: U.S. Preventive Services (1996). *Guide to clinical preventive services.* Baltimore: Williams and Wilkins.

Table
7-6

Interventions for which Routine Screening of Asymptomatic Persons Is not Recommended

DISEASE	SCREENING TEST
Peripheral arterial disease	Should screen for hypertension and hypercholesterolemia and counsel regarding the use of tobacco, physical activity, and nutritional risk factors for atherosclerotic disease.
Prostate cancer	Digital rectal examinations, serum tumor markers (e.g., prostate-specific antigen) or transrectal ultrasound.
Lung cancer	Chest radiography or sputum cytology. All patients should be counseled against tobacco use.
Ovarian cancer	Ultrasound, measurement of serum tumor markers, or pelvic examination.

continued

Table 7-6	*Interventions for which Routine Screening of Asymptomatic Persons Is not Recommended (continued)*

DISEASE	SCREENING TEST
Pancreatic cancer	Abdominal palpation, ultrasonography, or serologic markers.
Bladder cancer	Urine dipstick, microscopic uninalysis or urine cytology; stop smoking.
Thyroid cancer or thyroid disease	Neck palpation or ultrasonography.
Genital herpes simplex	Viral culture or other tests.
Routine electronic fetal monitoring	For low-risk women in labor. Insufficient evidence for high-risk pregnant women.

Source: U.S. Preventive Services. (1996). *Guide to clinical preventive services*. Baltimore: Williams and Wilkins.

Chapter Key Points

- The nurse collects data from a variety of assessment sources to identify health assets and strengths to improve the client's health and well-being.

- There are many different nursing approaches to the organization of assessment processes including nursing conceptual models or theories and functional health patterns.

- Assessment of client parameters such as functional ability, mental and nutritional status, and quality of life can add vital information for the health database.

- The judicious use of techniques such as tongue and pulse assessment can broaden the database from which the client and nurse develop a health promotion plan.

- Clinically effective screening procedures can provide early detection of disease, reducing morbidity and cost. However, consideration must be given to ethical concerns, appropriate referral, and follow-up counseling.

References

Beinfield, H., & Korngold, E. (1991). *Between heaven and earth: A guide to Chinese medicine*. New York: Ballantine.

Block, G., Hartman, A. M., Dresser, C. M., Carroll, M. D., Gannon, J., & Gardner, L. (1986). A data-based approach to diet questionnaire design and testing. *American Journal of Epidemiology, 24*, 453-469.

Browne, J. P., McGee, H. M., & O'Boyle, C. A. (1997). Conceptual approaches to the assessment of quality of life. *Psychology and Health, 12*, 737-751.

Drewnowski, A. (2001). Diet image: A new perspective on the food frequency questionnaire. *Nutrition Review, 59*, 370-372.

Edelman, C. L., & Mandle, C. L. (1998). *Health promotion throughout the lifespan* (4th ed.). St. Louis: Mosby.

Frankish, C. J., Milligan, C. D., & Reid, C. (1998). A review of relationships between active living and determinants of health. *Soc Sci Med, 47*, 287-301.

Gordon, M. (1995). *Manual of nursing diagnosis: 1995-1996*. St. Louis: Mosby.

Green, L. W. & Kreuter, M. W. (1991). *Health promotion planning. An educational and environmental approach* (2nd ed.). Mountain View, CA: Mayfield Publishing.

Haas, B. K. (1999). Clarification and integration of similar quality of life concepts. *Journal of Nursing Scholarship, 31*, 215-220.

Hungelmann, J. A., Kenkel-Rossi, E., Klassen, L., & Stollenwerk, R. M. (1989). Development of the JAREL spiritual well-being scale. In R. M Carrol-Johnson (Ed.), *Classification of nursing diagnoses: Proceedings of the eighth conference, North American Diagnosis Association* (pp. 393-398). Philadelphia: Lippincott.

Hungelmann, J., Kenkel-Rossi, E., Klassen, L., & Stollenwerk, R. (1996). Focus on spiritual well-being: Harmonious interconnectedness of mind-body-spirit. Use of the JAREL spiritual well-being scale. *Geriatric Nursing, 17*, 262-266.

Jarvis, C. (2000). *Physical examination and health assessment* (3rd ed.). Philadelphia: W. B. Saunders.

Keegan, L. & Dossey, B. (1987). *Self-care: A program to improve your life*. Temple, Texas: Bodymind Systems.

Leddy, S. K. (1996). Development and psychometric testing of the Leddy healthiness scale. *Research in Nursing and Health, 19*, 431-440.

Leddy, S. K. (1997). Healthiness, fatigue, and symptom experience in women with and without breast cancer. *Holistic Nursing Practice, 12*, 48-53.

Leddy, S. K. (1998). *Leddy and Pepper's conceptual bases of professional nursing* (4th ed.). Philadelphia: Lippincott.

Leddy, S. K. (2004). Human energy: A conceptual model of unitary nursing science. *Visions: The Journal of Rogerian Nursing Science, 12*, 14-27.

Leddy, S. K. & Fawcett, J. (1997). Testing the theory of healthiness: Conceptual and methodological issues. In M. Madrid (Ed.), *Patterns of Rogerian Knowing* (pp. 75-86). New York: NLN.

Leidy, N. K. (1994). Functional status and the forward progress of merry-go-rounds: Toward a coherent analytical framework. *Nursing Research, 43*, 196-202.

Leidy, N. K., & Haase, J. E. (1999). Functional status from the patient's perspective: The challenge of preserving personal integrity. *Research in Nursing and Health, 22*, 67-77.

Ohashi, W. (1991). *Ohashi's book of oriental diagnosis*. New York: Penguin.

Patton, G. L. (2001, September-October). Spirituality assessment in health care. *Health Progress*, 15-18.

Pender, N. J. (1996). *Health promotion in nursing practice* (3rd ed.). Norwalk, CT: Appleton & Lange.

Raphael, D., Brown, I., Renwick, R., & Rootman, I. (1997). Quality of life: What are the implications for health promotion? *American Journal of Health Behavior, 21*, 118-128.

Reid, D. (1995). *The complete book of Chinese health and healing: Guarding the three treasures*. Boston: Shambhala.

Reker, G. T., & Wong, P. T. P. (1984). Psychological and physical well-being in the elderly: The perceived well-being scale. *Canadian Journal on Aging, 3*, 23-32.

Rychlee, A. L. (May 8, 2000). Assessment: The critical first step in the nursing process. *Advance for Nurses Greater Philadelphia, 2*, 31.

Sharma, H., & Clark, C. (1998). *Contemporary Ayurveda: Medicine and research in Maharishi Ayurveda*. Philadelphia: Churchill Livingstone.

Soderhamn, U., & Soderhamn, O. (2002). Reliability and validity of the nutritional form for the elderly (NUFFE). *J Adv Nurs, 37*, 28-34.

Stewart, A. L., & Ware, J. E., Jr. (1992). *Measuring functioning and well-being. The medical outcomes study approach*. Durham, NC: Duke University Press.

Trabulsi, J., & Schoeller, D. A. (2001). Evaluation of dietary assessment instruments against doubly labeled water, a biomarker of habitual energy intake. *American Journal of Physiol Endocrinol Metabolism, 281*, E891-899.

Travis, J. W., & Ryan, R. S. (1988). *Wellness workbook* (2nd ed.). Berkley, CA: Ten Speed Press.

Truglio-Londrigan, M., & O'Connor, J. M. (1998). Screening. In C. L. Edelman, & C. L. Mandle, *Health promotion throughout the lifespan* (4th ed., pp. 195-221). St. Louis: Mosby.

U.S. Preventive Services Task Force. (1996). *Guide to clinical preventive services* (2nd ed.). Baltimore: Williams & Wilkins.

Willett, W. C., Reynolds, R. D., Cottreil-Hoehner, S., Sampson, L., & Browne, M. L. (1987). Validation of a semi-quantitative food frequency questionnaire: Comparison with a 1-year diet record. *Journal of the American Diet Association, 87*, 43-47.

Young, A. (1997). Self-assessments. In B. M. Dossey, *Core curriculum for holistic* (pp. 136-142). Gaithersburg, MD: Aspen.

THE DISEASE WORLDVIEW

Section II, *The Disease Worldview*, includes two chapters that emphasize health protection (risk reduction) and individual behavior change approaches to health promotion. Chapter 8, *Promoting Individual Behavior Change*, describes a number of theories of health behavior change, with strategies for promoting behavior change of individuals. And, Chapter 9, *Global Health: The Ecocentric Approach*, proposes strategies for nursing involvement in environmental, societal, and global health issues.

PROMOTING INDIVIDUAL BEHAVIOR CHANGE

Abstract

Influences on health occur at individual, interpersonal, community, environmental, and health care system levels. This chapter emphasizes psychological theories of individual health behavior change and strategies for promoting behavior change of individuals, recognizing that adoption of healthful lifestyle behaviors and decreasing or stopping harmful behaviors is not easy for most people.

Learning Outcomes

- Describe selected social cognitive models and theories of influences on individual behavior change
- Identify ways for the nurse to promote health through an individual's lifestyle changes

Influences on Behavior Change on Individuals

Adopting healthful lifestyle behaviors and decreasing or stopping harmful behaviors is not easy for most people and do not occur automatically. Currently, "most trends for obesity and weight management, tobacco use, physical activity, and diet are going in the wrong direction" (Orleans, 2000, p. 76). For example, the prevalence of obesity in the United States has risen from 25% in the 1960s to about 33% of the population today (Jeffery et al., 2000). Declines in physical activity levels begin at age 6 and continue over the life span, and about 70% of adults over age 45 get no regular exercise (Marcus et al., 2000). Additionally, only 25% of adult Americans meet the goal of 30% or less of calories from fat, and sodium intake is increasing (Kumanyika et al., 2000).

Health care providers who want to facilitate health promotion need an understanding of how and why people change behavior. A number of complex models have used social cognitive theories to explain individual level health behavior change. Social cognitive theories assume that personal, social, and environmental influences interact to affect behavior and changes in behavior. Some of the social cognitive models and theories most often cited in the literature are listed in Box 8-1.

Box 8-1

Selected Social Cognitive Models and Theories

- *Transtheoretical Model* (Prochaska, & DiClemente, 1984). Proposes that stages and processes of change, decisional balance, and self-efficacy influence the stopping of an addictive behavior or the adopting of a healthy behavior.

- *Modified Health Belief Model* (Rosenstock et al., 1988). Proposes that perception of susceptibility and seriousness affect a person's perceived threat of disease, which combined with the balance between perceived benefits and barriers of action affect the likelihood of a preventative health action being taken.

- *Revised Health Promotion Model* (Pender, 1996). Depicts individual characteristics and experiences and behavior-specific cognitions and affect that influence health promoting behavior.

- *Self-efficacy Theory* (Bandura, 1986). Concerned with people's judgments of their capabilities to execute given levels of performance and to exercise control over events.

- *Theory of Reasoned Action* (Fishbein & Ajzen, 1975). Emphasizes the effects of attitude and subjective norms on behavioral intention and actual behavior.

- *Theory of Planned Behavior* (Ajzen, 1985). Adds perceived behavioral control to the effects of attitude and subjective norms on behavioral intention and actual behavior.

continued

BOX 8-1 CONTINUED

- *Theory of Locus of Control* (Rotter, 1954). Proposes that people either believe that their action controls an outcome (internals), or that they are controlled by forces other than themselves (externals), such as chance or powerful others.

- *Theory of Health Locus of Control* (Wallston, 1976). Proposes a disposition to act in health-related situations based on perceptions of control over health status and valuing of health as an end in itself or as a means to a different end.

- *Common Sense Model* (Leventhal, 1980). Proposes that common sense beliefs, or representations, about identity, cause, timeline, consequences, and cure or control of illness guide how people cope with health problems by directing attention to information and serving as bases for selecting coping strategies.

The scientific literature has viewed the various models and theories as competitive. As a result, studies have compared the ability of constructs within a theory or model to explain or predict behavior change. The emphasis has been on determination of the "best" predictor theory or model. However, it has become clear that there is a great deal of overlap of constructs among the various theories and models. In addition, it appears that a complex network of constructs may predict only a portion of each behavior and vary from one behavior to the other. In most studies, much of human behavior remains unaccounted for (AbuSabha & Achterberg, 1997).

Another approach is to study the constructs that appear across models and theories. The intent is to move toward an understanding of how the influences on a specific behavior and across a variety of behaviors might be combined for the greatest explanatory power. The following section will explore a number of constructs that have demonstrated potential to explain or predict behavior change.

STAGES OF CHANGE

Stages and processes of change are two of the four constructs in the transtheoretical model (TTM). Six basic assumptions of this stage model are (Laitakari, 1998, p. 32):

1. Change in health behavior happens through distinct stages or steps.

2. Change takes place optimally in a certain order of stages.

3. The completion of the previous stages promotes the reaching of the subsequent stages.

4. There are factors that promote adoption (e.g., "processes" or "supporting-factors") specific to each stage.

5. The stage-specific factors can be mobilized through intervention methods (e.g., "techniques") to speed up the process of adoption.

6. Relapse is possible from each stage, but relapse can be used to provide valuable information to help the individual to make a new attempt to change.

A consistent series of five stages of behavior change have been documented across 12 different health-related behaviors (Prochaska et al., 1992; Prochaska et al., 1994a). The same pattern of change among TTM variables across stages was documented in a cross sectional study of high school and undergraduate university students and employed adults (Rodgers et al., 2001):

- *Precontemplation.* The stage at which there is no intention to change behavior in the foreseeable future. Resistance to recognizing or modifying a problem is the hallmark of precontemplation.

- *Contemplation.* The stage at which people are aware that a problem exists and are seriously thinking about overcoming it but have not yet made a commitment to take action. There is weighing of the pros and cons of the problem and the solution to the problem. Serious consideration of problem resolution is the central element of contemplation.

- *Preparation.* A stage that combines intention and behavioral criteria. Individuals in this stage are intending to take action in the next month and have unsuccessfully taken action in the past year. The hallmark of preparation is decision-making.

- *Action.* The stage in which individuals modify their behavior, experiences, or environment in order to overcome their problems. Modification of the target behavior to an acceptable criterion and significant overt efforts to change are the hallmarks of action.

- *Maintenance.* The stage in which people work to prevent relapse and consolidate the gains attained during action. Stabilizing behavior change and avoiding relapse are the hallmarks of maintenance.

Instead of an orderly progression through the stages, relapse and recycling through the stages occur quite frequently. During relapse, individuals regress to an earlier stage. Typically 40% of a population with an unhealthy behavior would be categorized in the precontemplation stage, 40% would fall in the contemplation stage, and 20% would self-assess in the preparation stage (Fava et al., 1995).

Laitakari (1998) suggests many benefits associated with a stage model. One benefit is the realism of this approach. It is clear that one learning experience or environmental modification is usually not sufficient for the adoption of a new behavior. A planned series of learning experiences or environmental changes in an atmosphere of mutual trust may be needed to support fully the change or adoption process. The nurse must not try to manipulate an individual's behavior in a predetermined direction.

Another benefit is the enhancement of a person-centered approach. Instead of standard interventions, each individual is assessed and given feedback about his or her apparent readiness for change, within the context of supportive environmental and social factors. In addition, the stage model provides order and direction to health education and health promotion efforts. Instead of taking the longitudinal process of behavior change for granted, stage-specific experiences can be planned, while respecting the individual's responsibility for independent decision making. Finally, the concept of a stage is fairly easily understood and seen as meaningful by both lay persons and professionals.

PROCESSES OF CHANGE

Ten different processes that explain how change occurs have received empirical and theoretical support across various theories (Prochaska et al., 1992). These processes of change are matched with representative interventions in Table 8-1.

As a start toward matching particular interventions to key individual client characteristics, particular processes can be applied or avoided at each stage of change, as listed below (Prochaska et al., 1992, p. 1109):

- *Precontemplation stage*. Change processes are used significantly less than by people in any of the other stages. Precontemplators process less information about problems, devote less time and energy to re-evaluation, experience fewer emotional reactions to the negative aspects of problems, are less open with significant others about problems, and do little to shift their attention or environment in the direction to overcoming problems.

- *Contemplation stage*. People are most open to consciousness-raising techniques such as observations, confrontations, and interpretations, and dramatic relief experiences which raise emotions and lower negative affect if the person changes. People are also more likely to reevaluate their values and problems and their effect on the persons with whom they are closest.

- *Preparation stage*. People use counterconditioning and stimulus control to begin reducing situations in which triggers for negative behavior occur.

- *Action stage*. People rely increasingly on support and understanding from helping relationships. They increasingly believe that they have autonomy and willpower.

- *Maintenance stage*. Involves an assessment of the conditions that promote relapse, and development of alternative (and non self-defeating) responses. Most important is a conviction that maintaining change is highly valued by the person and at least one significant other.

Stages and processes of change have been studied in smoking cessation, stopping cocaine use, weight control, high-fat diets, adolescent delinquent behaviors, safer sex, condom use, sunscreen use, radon gas exposure, exercise acquisition, mammography screening, and physician's preventive practices with smokers (Prochaska et al., 1994). One recent longitudinal study of stage transition for exercise found the strongest support in the action/maintenance stage retention, with limited impact on progression from the precontemplation and preparation stages (Plotnikoff et al., 2001). However, in a study of smokers using three outcomes (habit strength, positive evaluation strength, and negative evaluation strength), movement from the stages of precontemplation, contemplation or preparation was accurately predicted 1 year later, with 36 of the 40 predictions confirmed (Velicer et al., 1999). Rodgers and colleagues found that the behavioral processes were more sensitive than the cognitive processes

Table 8-1	***Titles, Definitions, and Representative Interventions of the Processes of Change***

PROCESS	DEFINITIONS AND INTERVENTIONS
Consciousness raising	Increasing information about self and problem: observations, confrontations, interpretations, bibliotherapy
Self-re-evaluation	Assessing how one feels and thinks about oneself with respect to a problem: value clarification, imagery, corrective emotional experience
Self-liberation	Choosing and commitment to act or belief in ability to change: decision-making therapy, New Year's resolutions, logotherapy techniques, commitment-enhancing techniques
Counterconditioning	Substituting alternatives for problem behaviors: relaxation, desensitization, assertion, positive self-statements
Stimulus control	Avoiding or countering stimuli that elicit problem behaviors: restructuring one's environment (e.g., removing alcohol or fattening foods), avoiding high risk cues, fading techniques
Reinforcement management	Rewarding oneself or being rewarded by others for making changes: contingency contracts, over and covert reinforcement, self-reward
Helping relationships	Being open and trusting about problems with someone who cares: therapeutic alliance, social support, self-help groups
Dramatic relief	Experiencing and expressing feelings about one's problems and solutions: psychodrama, grieving losses, role playing
Environmental re-evaluation	Assessing how one's problem affects physical environment: empathy training, documentaries
Social liberation	Increasing alternatives for nonproblem behaviors available in society: advocating for rights of repressed; empowering policy interventions

Reprinted from Prochaska, J. O., DiClemente, C. C., & Norcross, J. C. (1992). In search of how people change. *Am Psychol, 47,* 1108. © 1992 by the American Psychological Association. Reprinted with permission.

for distinguishing between stages of exercise behavior (Rodgers et al., 2001). The most important implications of the stages and processes of change research is that each client's readiness for change must be evaluated before any interventions are attempted. Then, specific interventions need to be tailored to the individual client's stage of readiness for change.

DECISIONAL BALANCE

Part of the decision to move toward action is thought to be based on the relative weight given to the pros and cons of changing behavior. According to Prochaska, Velicer, Rossi, Goldstein, Marcus, and Rakowski (1994a), the pros, incentives, or perceived benefits are advantages or positive aspects of changing behavior (i.e., facilitators of change). The cons, or perceived barriers, to action are the disadvantages or negative aspects of changing behavior (i.e., barriers to change).

Benefits and barriers of behavior change have been incorporated into at least five multidimensional models of health behavior (Leddy, 1997). Perceived barriers have been found to be the most powerful of the dimensions of the health belief model (Becker et al., 1977) in explaining various health behaviors (Janz & Becker, 1984). The advantages outweighing disadvantages have been identified as one of eight critical variables in the theory of reasoned action (Fishbein & Ajzen, 1975; Fishbein et al., 1991). Benefits and barriers also have been empirically supported as predictors of health behaviors in the majority of studies using the health promotion model (Pender, 1996), with barriers receiving the strongest support and benefits receiving moderate support. In the use of the transtheoretical model (Prochaska & DiClemente, 1984), incentives (i.e., pros) have accounted for more of the variance in the movement through behavior change stages, whereas barriers (i.e., cons) have remained relatively stable across the stages of change (Prochaska et al., 1994b). Measures of decisional balance also have demonstrated predictive utility for smoking cessation (Prochaska et al., 1985) and exercise readiness (Marcus & Owen, 1992) in studies based on multiattribute utility theory (Carter, 1990).

A meta-analysis of 24 retrospective studies demonstrated significantly large effect sizes for both benefits and barriers for health-related behaviors (Harrison et al., 1992). However, given that "relapse is the norm for most behavior change attempts" (Prochaska et al., 1994), focusing interventions to increase the incentives as well as decrease the barriers for health behavior change for the individual appears to be essential.

SELF-EFFICACY

Bandura (1977) developed the concept of self-efficacy to describe beliefs about how capable a person feels about performing specific tasks in specific behavioral situations. Self-efficacy theory proposes that confidence in one's ability to perform a given behavior is strongly related to one's actual ability to perform that behavior. Although a person's efficacy expectations will vary greatly depending on the particular task and context, perceived self-efficacy is believed to influence all aspects of behavior (Strecher et al., 1986) including:

- Acquisition of new behaviors (e.g., a sexually active young adult learning how to use a particular contraceptive device)

- Inhibition of existing behaviors (e.g., decreasing or stopping cigarette smoking)

- Disinhibition of behaviors (e.g., resuming sexual activity after a myocardial infarction)
- Choices of behavioral settings
- Amount of effort to be expended on a task
- Length of time of persistence in the face of obstacles
- Emotional reactions (e.g., anxiety and distress)
- Thought patterns (e.g., ruminating about personal deficiencies rather than thinking about accomplishing a task)

According to Bandura (1977), efficacy expectations vary in magnitude (ordering of tasks by difficulty), strength (certainty of ability to perform a task), and generality (degree to which expectations about one task apply to other tasks). In addition, Bandura et al. (1987) linked judgment of capability to perform with perceived ability to exercise control over events. In a modification of Bandura's concept, the transtheoretical model operationalizes self-efficacy as both confidence in changing a problem behavior, and situational temptation to engage in the problem behavior (Prochaska et al., 1994a).

Marcus, Selby, Niaura, and Rossi (1992) found that exercise self-efficacy was significantly related to stage in the change process, with precontemplators scoring the lowest and those in maintenance scoring the highest in self-efficacy. Plotnikoff and colleagues (2001), in a longitudinal study, also found moderate to strong support of exercise self-efficacy as a predictor of forward stage transition. In smoking cessation studies, confidence is an important predictor of stage movement to action and maintenance, while temptation is an important predictor of relapse (Prochaska et al., 1994). Self-efficacy has been shown to be related to many other health behaviors, including contraceptive behavior, cardiac rehabilitation, weight loss, and nutrition (AbuSabha & Achterberg, 1997). Increased self-efficacy in people with cancer has also been associated with increased adherence to treatment, increased self-care behaviors, and decreased symptoms (Lev, 1997).

LOCUS OF CONTROL

Locus of control has been confused with self-efficacy. Locus of control is based on the belief that people view the ability to attain a particular outcome as either within their control (internals), where their action determines the outcome, or outside their control (externals), where reward is controlled by forces other than one's self (Rotter, 1954). Levenson (1974) extended external's beliefs into two beliefs: chance expectations such as fate or luck and control by powerful others such as family members or physicians. While self-efficacy is task specific, locus of control is believed to be domain specific (e.g., health domain, social domain), which is much more general. However, locus of control has limited stability across time or different domains.

Studies have shown that people with an "internal" locus of control take responsibility for their own actions and engage more readily in health-promoting behaviors (AbuSabha & Achterberg, 1997). However, when used alone, the effect of locus of control on behavior is small. Wallston (1992, p. 194) suggests "a rapprochement" of Rotter's and Bandura's social learning theories, substituting a generalized expectancy of perceived control for locus of control, and incorporating perceived competence. The revised formulation states that "people must value health as an outcome, believe that their health actions influence their health status, and concurrently believe that they are capable of carrying out the necessary behaviors in order to have a high likelihood of engaging in a health-directed action" (Wallston, 1992, p. 195). The perceived health competence construct appears to hold promise as a predictor of adherence behavior (Christensen et al., 1996).

HEALTH BELIEFS

A belief is the conviction of truth (or falsehood) of an association between two concepts. Belief may be based on observation, for example, the experience of feeling energized after exercise would support a belief that exercise increases vitality. Scientific evidence may also support belief, for example, much research supports a link between exercise and reduction of myocardial disease. Some of the specific health beliefs that have been found to influence behavior include:

- *Perceived susceptibility.* A person's belief of being vulnerable to a particular health problem.

- *Perceived severity.* A person's belief that the health problem has potential serious consequences.

- *Perceived consequences* (may also be called outcome expectations). A person's beliefs regarding the consequences (positive or negative) of performing a specific health behavior.

- *Perceived benefits.* A person's belief that taking action toward improving health behavior will prevent illness or improve health. This is an example of a positive consequence.

- *Value of health.* A measurement of the importance that a person places on outcome expectations.

- *Perceived barriers.* A person's belief that certain personal or environmental factors make it difficult or impossible to take action toward improving health behavior.

- *Perceived threat.* A combination of personal susceptibility and seriousness of a particular health problem.

- *Perceived self-efficacy.* A person's beliefs about how capable they feel about performing a specific task in a specific behavioral situation.

Health beliefs have been incorporated into a number of health behavior models. Beliefs are the fundamental building blocks in the theory of reasoned action, as "the totality of a person's beliefs serves as the informational base that ultimately determines his attitudes, intentions, and behaviors" (Fishbein & Ajzen, 1975, p. 14). However, in a review of 10 years of studies related to the health belief model (Rosenstock, 1966), Janz and Becker (1984) concluded that only two of the belief components, perceived barriers and perceived susceptibility, explained or predicted preventive behaviors. Studies of the health promotion model (Pender, 1996) have supported perceived benefits and perceived self-efficacy in addition to perceived barriers.

THE PRECEDE-PROCEED MODEL

A dominant planning model in health education is the Predisposing, Reinforcing, and Enabling Constructs in Educational/Ecological Diagnosis and Evaluation (PRECEDE), coupled with Policy, Regulatory, and Organizational Constructs in Education and Environmental Development (PROCEED). Through a series of diagnostic steps, the PRECEDE-PROCEED planning model facilitates consideration of both individual and environmental factors that influence health and health behaviors. The model begins at the end, focusing on the outcome of interest, and works backward to determine how best to achieve that outcome. Factors that predispose, enable, or reinforce the behavioral and environmental determinants then become the targets of change (Kegler & Miner, 2004).

In the PRECEDE-PROCEED model, a health promotion program is seen as an intervention whose purpose it is to decrease illness or enhance quality of life through change or development of health-related behavior and conditions of living. The PRECEDE framework takes into account the multiple factors that shape health status and helps to arrive at a highly focused subset of those factors as targets for intervention. PRECEDE also generates specific objectives and criteria for evaluation. The PROCEED framework provides additional steps for developing policy and initiating the implementation and evaluation process (Green & Kreuter, 1991, p. 22). However, neither PRECEDE nor PROCEED provides substantive guidance on how to actually intervene.

The PRECEDE framework directs initial attention to outcomes rather than inputs. It encourages asking why before how. In phase 1 the hopes and problems of concern to the target population are assessed, and in phase 2, the specific health goals or problems that may contribute to the social goals or problems noted in phase 1 are identified. Phase 3 consists of identifying the specific health-related behavioral and environmental factors that could be linked to the health problems chosen as most deserving of attention. The PRECEDE model then groups them (phase 4) into predisposing, reinforcing, and enabling factors. Phase 5 involves assessment of the organizational and administrative capabilities and resources for the development and implementation of a health promotion program, while phases 6-8 are involved with evaluation. PROCEED highlights the important role of environmental factors as determinants of health and health behaviors (see Figure 8-1 for the PRECEDE-PROCEED model).

OTHER INFLUENCES ON HEALTH BEHAVIOR

Pender (1996), in the revised health promotion model (HPM), has proposed a complex combination of individual characteristics and experiences, behavior-specific cognitions, and behavioral outcomes. Influences that have not been discussed earlier include:

- *Prior related behavior.* Having performed the same or a similar behavior in the past.

- *Personal factors.* Prediction of behavior is shaped by the nature of the target behavior.

- *Activity-related affect.* Subjective feelings before, during, and after a behavior.

- *Interpersonal influences.* Cognitions concerning behaviors, beliefs, or attitudes of others.

- *Situational influences.* Perceptions and cognitions about the context for behavior.

- *Commitment to a plan of action.* Intent to carry out a specific action including intended strategies.

- *Competing demands and preferences.* Alternative behaviors that become competing courses of action to an intended health-promoting behavior.

Support has previously been found for many of the behavior-specific cognitions, including perceived benefits, perceived self-efficacy, and perceived barriers (Pender, 1996). The vari-

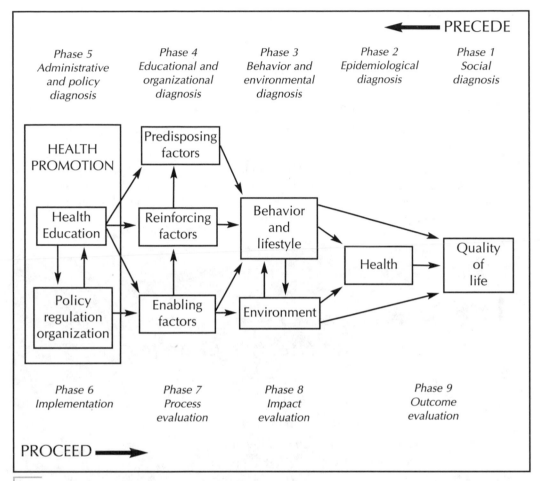

PRECEDE

Phase 5
Administrative
and policy
diagnosis

Phase 4
Educational and
organizational
diagnosis

Phase 3
Behavior and
environmental
diagnosis

Phase 2
Epidemiological
diagnosis

Phase 1
Social
diagnosis

HEALTH
PROMOTION

Predisposing
factors

Health
Education

Reinforcing
factors

Behavior
and
lifestyle

Health

Quality
of
life

Policy
regulation
organization

Enabling
factors

Environment

Phase 6
Implementation

Phase 7
Process
evaluation

Phase 8
Impact
evaluation

Phase 9
Outcome
evaluation

PROCEED

Figure 8-1. PRECEDE-PROCEED model of health promotion planning. Reprinted with permission from Green, L. W., & Kreuter, M. W. (1991). *Health promotion planning. An educational and environmental approach* (2nd ed.). Mountain View, CA: Mayfield Publishing. Reproduced with permission of the McGraw-Hill Companies.

ables of activity-related affect, commitment to a plan of action, and immediate competing demands and preferences are new variables. The entire revised model is undergoing testing.

Strategies for Promoting Behavior Change

The idea of changing health behavior is uncomfortable for many people. Deeply ingrained habits, even harmful ones, can be difficult to change, and most people have difficulty making even minor changes. According to Westberg and Jason (1996, pp. 147-148), people tend to resist change because of beliefs that a change of behavior may:

■ Require giving up pleasure (e.g., eating high-fat ice cream)

- Be unpleasant (e.g., doing certain exercises)

- Be overtly painful (e.g., discontinuing addictive substances)

- Be stressful (e.g., facing social situations without alcohol)

- Jeopardize social relationships (e.g., engaging in unprotected adolescent sex)

- Not seem important anymore (e.g., in the case of older individuals)

- Require alteration in self-image (e.g., in the case of a hard-working executive learning how to play)

As a result, giving up long-standing habits and attitudes is not easy for most people.

Given that health behavior change is difficult for most people, Box 8-2 suggests ways for the individual to promote "what it takes" to make meaningful, lasting changes in lifestyle. However, these are pragmatic suggestions rather than based on theory.

Box 8-2

Suggested Ways for the Individual to Promote Lifestyle Changes

- Endorse the need for change
- Have "ownership" of the need for change
- Feel that there is more to gain than lose
- Develop an enhanced sense of self-worth
- Identify realistic goals and workable plans
- Seek gradual change rather than a "quick fix"
- Have patience
- Address starting new behaviors instead of just focusing on what behaviors should be stopped
- Practice new behaviors
- Seek the support of family, friends, colleagues, or health professionals
- Gain positive reinforcement for the desired behavior
- Have a strategy for monitoring progress and making needed changes
- Seek constructive, personalized feedback to strengthen motivation for change
- Have a mechanism of follow-up to reduce backsliding

Source: Adapted from Westberg, J., & Jason, H. (1996). Fostering healthy behavior: The process. In S. H. Woolf, S. Jonas, & R. S. Lawrence (Eds.), *Health promotion and disease prevention in clinical practice* (pp. 145-162). Baltimore: Williams & Wilkins.

Health-related behaviors are either protective in nature (e.g., exercise, good nutrition, and stress management) or negatively impact health (e.g., smoking, drinking, and sedentary lifestyle). Learning how to help people adopt and sustain healthy attitudes and habits is a challenge for health professionals. "There are no miracle drugs available for helping people change long-standing patterns of living. Simply telling people to stop smoking, eat less fat, have safe sex, exercise more, discontinue their abusive practices, or reduce their life stresses seldom works" (Westberg & Jason, 1996, p. 146). Clients often do not follow the advice of nurses or physicians, particularly when authoritarian "orders" are given. Clients must be actively involved as collaborative partners who assess their own current health and develop and monitor their own long-term health plans. The health professional can best promote and sustain change by educating, facilitating, and advising.

According to Prochaska and colleagues (1994a), some of the most frequently replicated strategies and techniques to help clients modify their behavior include consciousness raising, self-re-evaluation, environmental re-evaluation, self-liberation, social liberation, helping relationships, stimulus control, counterconditioning, and reinforcement management. These strategies and techniques have been linked with movement along stages of change (transtheoretical model) in one of few theory-based interventions for behavior change.

CONSCIOUSNESS RAISING

During the contemplation stage of behavior change, consciousness raising occurs as the individual seeks information. The health care provider can share potential information resources so that the individual can be actively involved. The client's perceived incentives and barriers to change can be clarified, and the provider can help explain and interpret often conflicting or unclear information. In addition, the knowledge and interest of family members can be assessed. It may be helpful for the individual to talk with others who have successfully made the contemplated changes.

SELF- AND ENVIRONMENTAL RE-EVALUATION

As movement occurs toward the preparation and action stages of change, the individual engages in self- and environmental re-evaluation. The individual considers how the current problem behavior (or lack of positive behavior) affects the physical and social environment and personal standards and values. Questions that might be asked include: Will I like myself better as a (thinner, nonsmoking, less-stressed) person? Is my environment supportive of the proposed changes? Do I believe that I am able to make and continue the changes needed? The assumption is that changes will not occur unless they are congruent with a person's self-concept.

SELF- AND SOCIAL LIBERATION

A strategy that can assist with self- and social liberation is cognitive restructuring. "Cognitive restructuring focuses on client's thinking, imagery, and attitudes toward the self and self-competencies as they affect the change process" (Pender, 1996, p. 171). The provider can help clients clarify the messages they give themselves about their health and health-related behaviors. Certain beliefs can be irrational compared with actual reality. Positive affirmations and imagery, repeated several times a day, can help clients to believe that they have the power to think positively and make desired lifestyle changes.

HELPING RELATIONSHIPS

Helping relationships with family members, friends, colleagues, or health care professional can be critical in helping to move the individual through the preparation, action, and maintenance stages of change. A self-help group is a strategy that has been found to be very helpful for modeling, support, and reinforcement of desired behavior.

STIMULUS CONTROL

Stimulus control, emphasizing activities that precede the desired behavior, can be helpful during the action and maintenance stages of change. The activities, which must be personally relevant for the individual client, might include a postcard reminder for mammography screening, a personal call from the provider to encourage continued exercise, or a scheduled group meeting to practice relaxation. To encourage the development of a desirable behavior habit it may be helpful to promote the behavior in the same setting or context and time on a daily basis. For example, the client can be encouraged to exercise in a consistent place, early each morning before other activities intervene.

COUNTERCONDITIONING

Counterconditioning to break an undesirable association between a stimulus and a response can be desirable during the later part of the action stage and during the maintenance stage. Undesirable associations can occur and create a negative emotional response to the behavior. For example, many people indicate that exercising can become boring. The provider can encourage a varied routine, walking outside whenever the weather permits, and at least occasional exercise with a partner to counteract boredom.

REINFORCEMENT MANAGEMENT

Reinforcement management is an effective strategy, especially during the preparation and action stages of change. "It is based on the premise that all behaviors are determined by their consequences. If positive consequences occur, the probability is high that the behavior will occur again. If negative consequences occur, the probability is low for the behavior's being repeated" (Pender, 1996, p. 172). Immediate reinforcement of the desired behavior is important, especially in the early phases of change. Personalized attention and positive verbal feedback are helpful. Eventually, a desirable consequence of the behavior can become an intrinsic reward. For example, a weekly scale reading indicating decreasing weight can be a reward in itself for continuing on a weight reduction diet.

The object of these strategies is to decrease barriers and increase incentives to change of behavior. Barriers to change include lack of knowledge, skills, perception of control, facilities, materials, clear goals, social support, time, and motivation. In comparison, according to Leddy (1997), incentives to change behavior include expectation of benefit, sense of personal responsibility, enjoyment of the activity, previous experience, guilt for not changing behavior, and support from family, peers, or professionals. The choice of appropriate strategies to foster incentives and reduce barriers and thereby promote behavior change should be based on an individualized and collaborative assessment by the provider and the client.

Given that maintenance and relapse involve repeated cycles of abstinence and relapse (Orleans, 2000), a shift in focus from relapse prevention to relapse management is needed.

MOTIVATIONAL INTERVIEWING

Another intervention technique that has been proposed is motivational interviewing—a style of relating that focuses on increasing client readiness for change in behavior. Motivational interviewing has been defined as "a directive, client-centered counselling style for eliciting behavior change by helping clients to explore and resolve ambivalence" (Rollnick & Miller, 1995, p. 326). Assuming that the motivation to change cannot be imposed, but comes from the client, this approach relies upon identifying and mobilizing the client's intrinsic values and goals in order to stimulate change in behavior. Believing that direct persuasion is not an effective method for helping a client to resolve ambivalence about behavior, the nurse's goals when using this approach are to facilitate the expression of ambivalence, clarify and resolve the impasse, and guide the client toward an acceptable resolution that triggers change in behavior. Specific behaviors that are characteristics of a motivational interviewing style include:

- Relating in a partnership relationship in contrast to taking expert/recipient roles
- Being quiet and eliciting rather than using a persuasive, aggressive, or confrontational style
- Developing discrepancies by engaging in a discussion between present behavior and valued goals
- Using reflective listening to understand the client's frame of reference
- Expressing empathy, acceptance, and affirmation
- Eliciting and selectively reinforcing the client's own self-motivational statements regarding expressions of problem recognition and desire, intention, and ability to change
- Monitoring the client's degree of readiness to change
- Supporting self-efficacy
- Affirming the client's freedom of choice and self-direction
- Providing meaningful personal feedback

LEVELS OF INTERVENTION

Successful individual intervention strategies include the use of self-regulatory skill training (e.g., goal setting, self-monitoring, feedback and social support, and relapse prevention or preparation training), with ongoing support and guidance. Worksite interventions involving combinations of competition, individual and group goal setting, and management support can help change health behaviors. Interventions involving point-of-choice information have had a positive effect in at least three health behavior areas (i.e., smoking, nutrition, and physical activity). Policy/legislative level of impact strategies aimed at deterring cigarette smoking have met with success. Such policies include smoke-free building and transportation regulations, and statewide increases in cigarette taxation. Interventions that include a social-environmental approach are believed to be more sustainable and cost-effective over the long term (Ory, Jordan, & Bazzarre, 2002, pp. 506-507).

PATIENT-CENTERED COUNSELING MODEL

The patient-centered counseling model (Rosal et al., 2001) has been shown to facilitate change and long-term maintenance in dietary behavior by assessing client needs and then tailoring an intervention to the client's stage in the process of change. Objectives for the nurse of the model are to increase the client's awareness of risks of current behavior, provide information, increase the client's confidence in her or his ability to make changes in behavior, and enhance skills needed for long-term maintenance of the behavior change. The steps in the model include a complete behavioral assessment, personalized advisement based on the client's health concerns and stated reasons for wanting to change behavior, assistance in change based on stage of readiness for change, goal setting, re-assessment of self-efficacy, a behavioral contract, and arrangement for follow-up to prevent relapse and promote maintenance of the behavior change.

Counseling to Reduce Disease Risk Factors

Based on a systematic review of evidence of clinical effectiveness (see Chapter 7, *Beyond Physical Assessment*), the U.S. Preventive Services Task Force (1996) has recommended counseling interventions to reduce a number of disease risk factors.

PREVENTING TOBACCO USE

The task force recommends that all children, adolescents, and adults be counseled to stop using any tobacco products. Strategies to increase the effectiveness of counseling against tobacco use include (U.S. Preventive Services Task Force, 1996):

- Direct, face-to-face advice and suggestions
- Reinforcement
- Office reminders
- Self-help materials
- Community programs for additional help in quitting
- Drug therapy (nicotine patch or gum)

PROMOTING PHYSICAL ACTIVITY

"Evidence exists that physical activity and fitness reduce morbidity and mortality for at least six chronic conditions: coronary heart disease, hypertension, obesity, diabetes, osteoporosis, and mental health disorders" (U.S. Preventive Services Task Force, 1996, p. 611). Unfortunately, studies that have demonstrated benefits from counseling provide little information about long-term compliance and have limited generalizability. However, despite the limited direct evidence that clinician counseling can increase the long-term physical activity of asymptomatic clients, the relative risk for sedentary individuals supports devoting time and effort to counseling for all children and adults. The emphasis should be on regular, moderate intensity physical activity (see Chapter 13, *Re-establishing Energy Flow: Physical Activity and Exercise*).

PROMOTING A HEALTHY DIET

The effectiveness of nutritional counseling in changing dietary habits has been demonstrated in a number of clinical trials. Therefore, the task force recommends counseling children over the age of 2 and adults to limit dietary intake of fat, especially saturated fat, and cholesterol, maintain caloric balance in their diet, and emphasize foods containing fiber. The task force found that there was insufficient evidence to recommend for or against counseling the general population to reduce dietary sodium intake or increase dietary intake of iron, beta-carotene, or other antioxidants. Women should be encouraged to consume recommended amounts of calcium and should be encouraged to breastfeed their infants (see Chapter 16, *Regenerating Energy: Nutrition*).

PREVENTING MOTOR VEHICLE INJURIES

Although little is known about how effective clinician counseling is in altering these behaviors, all clients and the parents of young children should be counseled to use occupant restraints (lap and shoulder safety belts and child safety seats), to wear helmets when riding motorcycles and bicycles, and to refrain from driving while under the influence of alcohol or other drugs.

PREVENTING HOUSEHOLD AND RECREATIONAL INJURIES

Unintentional injuries including falls, poisonings, drowning, fires and burns, mechanical suffocation and aspiration, and firearm injuries were the fifth leading cause of death in 1993 (U.S. Preventive Services Task Force, 1996). Evidence from controlled trials indicates that counseling the parents of young children can increase safety-related behaviors. On the other hand, no trials of counseling in elderly adults have demonstrated significant reductions in serious fall injuries. It appears that the most effective measures to control injuries are passive interventions such as window guards in high-rise apartments, nonflammable sleepwear, automatic sprinkler systems, and child-resistant packaging to prevent poisoning. Counseling is most effective in combination with other compliance inducing measures such as safety regulations.

PREVENTING LOW BACK PAIN

Low back pain is one of the most expensive health problems in industrialized countries (U.S. Preventive Task Force, 1996). However, there is insufficient evidence to recommend for or against counseling clients to exercise to prevent low back pain. Alternatively, education such as information on back biomechanics, preferred lifting strategies, optimal posture, exercises to prevent back pain, and stress and pain management has been effective in reducing employment-related injuries and relieving chronic low back pain. These comprehensive educational strategies might also be effective in the clinical setting.

PREVENTING DENTAL AND PERIODONTAL DISEASE

Risk reduction for dental and periodontal disease has been recommended through counseling clients about:

- Regular visits to a dental care provider

- Daily flossing

- Daily teeth-brushing with a fluoride-containing toothpaste

- Appropriate use of fluoride for caries prevention

- Chemotherapeutic mouth rinses for plaque prevention

Additionally, parents should be counseled not to put infants and children to bed with a bottle. Data suggest that many persons, especially those in minority groups or those having low socioeconomic status, lack adequate knowledge about how to prevent oral diseases. However, the effectiveness of clinician counseling to change any of these behaviors has not been adequately evaluated.

PREVENTING HIV INFECTION AND OTHER SEXUALLY TRANSMITTED DISEASES

All adolescent and adult clients should be advised about risk factors for human immunodeficiency virus (HIV) infection and other sexually transmitted diseases (STDs), and counseled appropriately about effective measures to reduce the risk of infection. Counseling should be tailored to individual risk factors, needs, and abilities of each client. Risk reduction has been shown to be effective, although the effectiveness of clinician counseling in a primary care setting is uncertain. There is consistent evidence that both men and women have changed high-risk sexual behavior in response to information about HIV and other STDs, provided through public education and clinician encounters.

PREVENTING UNINTENDED PREGNANCY

Periodic counseling about effective contraceptive methods is recommended for all women and men at risk for unintended pregnancy. Hormonal contraceptives, barrier methods used with spermicides, and IUDs can be recommended as the most effective reversible means of preventing pregnancy in sexually active persons. Sexual abstinence, the maintenance of a mutually faithful monogamous sexual relationship, and consistent use of condoms are important measures to reduce the risk of STDs (U.S. Preventive Task Force, 1996). Counseling should be based on information from a careful sexual history and should be individualized based on preferences, abilities, and risks of each client. Empathy, confidentiality, and a nonjudgmental, supportive attitude are especially important when discussing issues of sexuality with adolescents.

Promoting the Maintenance of Health Behavior Change

While there has been some progress in the development of short-term interventions to change risk behaviors (e.g., tobacco use, improper diet, and insufficient exercise), there has been much less progress in promoting maintenance of the behavior change; and relapse remains the norm, with most successfully treated individuals reverting to their old high-risk behaviors within 6 to 12 months of treatment (Orleans, 2000). Most of the interventions have targeted individual behavior change aimed at persons who possess the risk factor. However, it has been proposed (McKinlay, 1995) that given "a social system that encourages, rewards, and profits from at-risk behaviors" (Orleans, 2000, p. 79), interventions also need to be aimed at defined populations involving organizational channels such as schools, worksites, and communities, as well as interventions aimed at public policy and environments "designed to subvert or redirect strong societal and industry counterforces at the broadest population levels" (Orleans, 2000, p. 77), such as:

- Economic incentives such as excise taxes on high-fat or tobacco products

- Protection from environmental hazards such as reduced access to dangerous products

- Reduced exposure to advertising such as through counter-advertising campaigns

The implication is that success in maintaining long-term behavior change requires broad-spectrum approaches at all levels. However, very little is known about the mechanisms responsible for the most effective maintenance strategies, such as extended contact with a support person, telephone, support, or supplying appropriate foods in diet and weight loss programs. Most existing maintenance interventions are not effective, and "even the most promising interventions are limited in impact and poorly understood" (Orleans, 2000, p. 82). Theory-based intervention research is badly needed.

The emphasis in this chapter has been on understanding a variety of constructs such as stages and processes of change, decisional balance, self-efficacy, and health beliefs that are being applied across various models and theories to foster individual behavior change. However, although the focus of many interventions has been on the initiation of behavior change, the high rate of relapse indicates that more attention needs to be paid to the maintenance of behavior change. Additionally, despite the emphasis of most behavior change interventions at the level of the individual, it appears that broad spectrum approaches, with interventions focused at the social environment, policy, and individual levels, are most effective.

Chapter Key Points

- A number of constructs that appear across models and theories, including stages and processes of change, decisional balance, self efficacy, locus of control, and health beliefs have demonstrated potential to explain or predict individual behavior change.

■ Frequently replicated strategies and techniques to help clients modify their behavior include motivational interviewing, consciousness raising, self-re-evaluation, environmental re-evaluation, self-liberation, social liberation, helping relationships, stimulus control, counter-conditioning, reinforcement management, and counseling.

■ Success in maintaining long-term behavior change requires broad-spectrum interpersonal, community, environmental, and health care system approaches as well as individual interventions.

References

AbuSabha, R., & Achterberg, C. (1997). Review of self-efficacy and locus of control for nutrition- and health-related behavior. *Journal of the American Diet Association, 97*, 1122-1132.

Ajzen, I. (1985). From intentions to actions: A theory of planned behavior. In J. Kuhl, & J. Beckmann (Eds.), *Action-control: From cognition to behavior* (pp. 11-39). Hidelberg, Germany: Springer.

Bandura, A. (1977). Self-efficacy: Toward a unifying theory of behavioral change. *Psychological Review, 84*, 191-215.

Bandura, A. (1986). *Social foundations of thought and action: A social cognitive theory*. Englewood Cliffs, NJ: Prentice Hall.

Bandura, A., O'Leary, A., Taylor, C. B., Gauthier, J., & Gossard, D. (1987). Perceived self-efficacy and pain control: Opioid and non-opioid mechanisms. *Journal Personality and Social Psychology, 53*, 563-571.

Becker, M. H., Haefner, D. P., Kasl, S. V., Kirscht, J. P., Maiman, L. A., & Rosenstock, I. M. (1977). Selected psychosocial models and correlates of individual health-related behaviors. *Med Care, 15*(Suppl.), 27-46.

Carter, W. B. (1990). Health behavior as a rational process: Theory of reasoned action and multiattribute utility theory. In K. Glanz, F. M. Lewis, & B. K. Rimer (Eds.), *Health behavior and health education* (pp. 63-91). San Francisco: Jossey-Bass.

Christensen, A. J., Wiebe, J. S., Benotsch, E. G., & Lawton, W. J. (1996). Perceived health competence, health locus of control, and patient adherence in renal dialysis. *Cognitive Therapy and Research, 20*, 411-421.

Fava, J. L., Velicer, W. F., & Prochaska, J. O. (1995). Applying the transtheoretical model to a representative sample of smokers. *Addiction Behavior, 20*, 189-203.

Fishbein, M., & Ajzen, I. (1975). *Belief, attitude, intention and behavior: An introduction to theory and research*. Reading, MA: Addison-Wesley.

Fishbein, M., Bandura, A., Triandis, H. C., Kanfer, F., & Becker, M. (1991). *Factors influencing behavior and behavior change: Final report of theorist's workshop on AIDS-related behaviors*. Washington, DC: National Institute of Mental Health, National Institutes of Health.

Green, L. W., & Kreuter, M. W. (1991). *Health promotion planning. An educational and environmental approach* (2nd ed.). Mountain View, CA: Mayfield Publishing.

Harrison, J. A., Mullen, P. D., & Green, L. W. (1992). A meta-analysis of studies of the health belief model with adults. *Health Education Research, 7*, 107-116.

Janz, N.K., & Becker, M. H. (1984). The health belief model: A decade later. *Health Education Quarterly, 11*(1), 1-47.

Jeffery, R. W., Drewnowski, A., Epstein, L. H., Stunkard, A. J., Wilson, G. T., Wing, R., et al. (2000). Long-term maintenance of weight loss: Current status. *Health Psychology, 19*(Suppl), 5-16.

Kegler, M. C., & Miner, K. (2004). Environmental health promotion interventions: Considerations for preparation and practice. *Health education & behavior, 31*, 510-525.

Kumanyika, S. K., Van Horn, L., Bowen, D., Perri, M. G., Rolls, B. J., Czajkowski, S. M., et al. (2000). Maintenance on dietary behavior change. *Health Psychology, 19*(Suppl), 42-56.

Laitakari, J. (1998). On the practical applicability of stage models to health promotion and health education. *American Journal of Health Behavior, 22*, 28-38.

Leddy, S. K. (1997). Incentives and barriers to exercise in women with a history of breast cancer. *Oncol Nurs Forum, 24*, 885-890.

Lev, E. L. (1997). Bandura's theory of self-efficacy: Applications to oncology. *Scholarly Inquiry for Nursing Practice, 11*(1), 21-37.

Levenson, H. (1974). Activism and powerful others: Distinctions within the concept of internal-external control. *J Pers Assess, 38*, 377-383.

Leventhal, H., Meyer, D., & Nerenz, D. (1980). The common sense representation of illness danger. In S. Rachman (Ed.), *Contributions to medical psychology* (pp. 7-30). New York: Pergamon Press.

Marcus, B. H., Dubbert, P. M., Forsyth, L. H., McKenzie, T. L., Stone, E. J., Dunn, A. L., et al. (2000). Physical activity behavior change: Issues in adoption and maintenance. *Health Psychology, 19*(Suppl), 32-41.

Marcus, B. H., & Owen, N. (1992). Motivational readiness, self-efficacy and decision-making for exercise. *Journal of Applied Social Psychology, 22*(1), 3-16.

Marcus, B. H., Selby, V. C., Niaura, R. S., & Rossi, J. S. (1992). Self-efficacy and the stages of exercise behavior change. *Research Quarterly for Exercise and Sport, 63*, 60-66.

McKinlay, J. B. (1995). The new public health approach to improving physical activity and autonomy in older populations. In E. Heikkinen (Ed.), *Preparation for aging* (pp. 87-103). New York: Plenum Press.

Orleans, C. T. (2000). Promoting the maintenance of health behavior change: Recommendations for the next generation of research and practice. *Health Psychology, 19*(Suppl), 76-83.

Ory, M. G., Jordan, P. J., & Bazzarre, T. (2002). The behavior change consortium: Setting the stage for a new century of health behavior-change research. *Health Education Research, Theory and Practice, 17*, 500-511.

Pender, N. J. (1996). *Health promotion in nursing practice* (3rd ed.) Stamford, CT: Appleton & Lange.

Plotnikoff, R. C., Hotz, S. B., Birkett, N. J., & Courneya, K. S. (2001). Exercise and the transtheoretical model: A longitudinal test of a population sample. *Prev Med, 33*, 441-452.

Prochaska, J. O., & DiClemente, C. C. (1984). *The transtheoretical approach: Crossing traditional boundaries of change*. Homewood, IL: Dow Jones-Irwin.

Prochaska, J. O., DiClemente, C. C., & Norcross, J. C. (1992). In search of how people change. *Am Psychol, 47*, 1102-1114.

Prochaska, J. O., DiClemente, C. C., Velicer, W. F., Ginpil, S., & Norcross, J. C. (1985). Predicting change in smoking status for self-changers. *Addictive Behavior, 10*, 395-406.

Prochaska, J. O., Velicer, W. F., Rossi, J. S., Goldstein, M. G., Marcus, B., Rakowski, W. et al. (1994a). Stages of change and decisional balance for 12 problem behaviors. *Health Psychology, 13*, 39-46.

Prochaska, J. O., Redding, C. A., Harlow, L. L., Rossi, J. S., & Velicer, W. F. (1994b). The transtheoretical model of change and HIV prevention: A review. *Health Education Quarterly, 21*, 471-486.

Rodgers, W. M., Courneya, K. S., & Bayduza, A. L. (2001). Examination of the Transtheoretical model and exercise in 3 populations. *Am J Health Behav, 25*, 33-41.

Rollnick, S., & Miller, W. R. (1995). What is motivational interviewing? *Behavioral and Cognitive Psychotherapy, 23*, 325-334.

Rosal, M. C., Ebbeling, C. B., Lofgren, I., Ockene, J., Ockene, I. S., & Hebert, J. R. (2001). Facilitating dietary change: The patient-centered counseling model. *J Am Diet Assoc, 101*, 332-338, 341.

Rosenstock, I. M. (1966, July). Why people use health services. *Milbank Q, 44*, 94-127.

Rosenstock, I. M., Strecher, V. J., & Becker, M. H. (1988). Social learning theory and the health belief model. *Health Education Quarterly, 15*, 175-183.

Rotter, J. B. (1954). *Social learning and clinical psychology* (Vol. 80). Englewood Cliffs, NJ: Prentice-Hall.

Strecher, V. J., DeVellis, B. M., Becker, M. H., & Rosenstock, I. M. (1986). The role of self-efficacy in achieving health behavior change. *Health Education Quarterly, 13*, 73-91.

U.S. Preventive Services Task Force. (1996). *Guide to clinical preventive services* (2nd ed.). Baltimore: Williams & Wilkins.

Velicer, W. F., Norman, G. J., Fava, J. L., & Prochaska, J. O. (1999). Testing 40 predictions from the transtheoretical model. *Addictive Behavior, 24*, 455-69.

Wallston, K. A. (1992). Hocus-pocus, the focus isn't strictly on locus: Rotter's social learning theory modified for health. *Cognitive Therapy and Research, 16*, 183-199.

Wallston, K. A., Maides, S. A., & Wallston, B. S. (1976). Health related information seeking as a function of health related locus of control and health value. *Journal of Research in Personality, 10*, 215-222.

Westberg, J., & Jason, H. (1996). Fostering healthy behavior: The process. In S. H. Woolf, S. Jonas, & R. S. Lawrence (Eds.), *Health promotion and disease prevention in clinical practice* (pp. 145-162). Baltimore: Williams & Wilkins.

GLOBAL HEALTH

The Ecocentric Approach

Abstract

In this chapter the interrelations between human beings and their environments within a global perspective are explored. The assumptions that humans are the most important of all the species, and that the world's resources are inexhaustible and available for the taking have raised serious concerns about environmental health, and ethical questions about the nature of our obligations to future generations and to other organisms on the planet. In addition, health professionals have traditionally been concerned almost exclusively with individual risk factors for diseases, ignoring social, economic, and political structures that are the underlying causes for health problems. Strategies are proposed for nursing involvement in environmental, societal, and global health issues.

Learning Outcomes

By the end of the chapter the student should be able to:

- Discuss the ecocentric approach to environmental health

- Discuss the ethical implications of the view that the world's resources are inexhaustible and available for the taking

- Describe social, economic, and political structures that are the underlying causes of health problems

- List examples of toxic exposure, exploitation of natural resources, pollution, deforestation, and climactic change, and their effects on the environment

- List examples of societal health concerns such as childhood health problems, infectious diseases, accidents, poor access to food, illiteracy, lack of clean water, migration, multinational business interests, poverty, and overpopulation and family planning
- Explain how empowerment to promote global health can be facilitated

Ecocentric Worldview of Health

The ecocentric worldview of health "assumes that everything is connected to everything else, that the whole is greater than the sum of its parts, that meaning is dependent on context, that biological and social systems are open, and that humans and nonhumans are one within the same organic system" (Kleffel, 1996, pp. 2-4). In the ecocentric approach, "environment is a factor that predisposes, enables, and reinforces individual and collective behavior" (Green et al., 1996, p. 272). Therefore, health promotion can achieve effective results by empowering people to influence the behavioral and environmental conditions that affect health.

This chapter will present medical, public health, and epidemiologic approaches to health. Much of this content seems to focus on the negative and on risks to health. However, the tenets of primary preventive health care can be applied at the global, societal, and environmental levels (Lane & Rubinstein, 1996, p. 418).

Global (International) Health

Global affairs encompass relations beyond governments and includes individuals and groups within societies that interact across national boundaries, in contrast to intergovernmental relations between states and their governments traditionally defined as international affairs. The process by which human societies move from international to global relations is called globalization (Lee, 1998). Some authors have more biased views such as "international health refers to the flow of advice, health professionals, and health technology from the wealthier nations to the poorer" (Lane & Rubinstein, 1996, p. 397). A global perspective provides "a holistic view of the complex interactions between the cultures, economic systems, political organizations, and ecology of the planet itself" (Helman, 1994, p. 338).

The current global context has been described as "one of clashing worldviews, economic instability, environmental crises, and declining health" (Hegyvary, 2001, p. 304). Health status and general well-being are static, if not deteriorating, for a large proportion of the world's population, and there are widening disparities in the burden of disease and access to health resources (Leuning, 2001).

"The Western worldview has been shaped over centuries through the power of the scientific method, analytical philosophy, industrialization, urbanization, democratization, liberalism, and capitalism. The modern perspective emphasizes capitalism, the pursuit of rational economic self-interest, and the nation-state framework of international relations" (Benatar, 1998, p. 295). However, "an overemphasis on economic thinking (and underemphasis on social and economic rights), has also been associated with erosion of spirituality, loss of a sense of community, and division of the world (and many countries) into a small, rich core and a large, poor periphery" (Benatar, 1998, p. 296). Exploitation of people and nature in the pursuit of what is considered to be progress, "contributes to the widening national and global disparities (in health, wealth, and human rights) that now jeopardize human health and survival" (Benatar, 1998, p. 295).

Serious global health problems exist. For example, although in 1996 the global average life expectancy at birth reached 65 years, chronic diseases were responsible for more than 24 million deaths a year, or almost half of the global total. The problems of chronic diseases will exacerbate as the population of those aged 65 and above increases globally by more than 80% by 2020. Additionally, "poor countries inherit the problems of the rich, including not merely illness but also the harmful effects of tobacco, alcohol and drug use, and of accidents, suicide and violence" (WHR, 1997, pp. 248-249, 258).

Governments are no longer the sole agents in the global-health arena. Beyond national programs, the global-health systems now contain:

■ *The private or commercial sector.* Including multinational corporations.

■ *The independent sector and nongovernmental organizations.* Such as universities, private foundations, and relief and advocacy organizations.

■ *The multilateral sector.* Including multinational organizations such as the World Health Organization (WHO), and the United Nations (UN) development agencies; regional health organizations; and the World Bank and regional development banks.

■ *The bilateral sector.* Which involves various government and overseas development agencies that are funded by single governments or regional partners.

This pluralism brings a strong need, and opportunity, for active national engagement in global health issues (Howson et al., 1998). However, countries do not have equal financial resources. One distinction that has been made is between developed, or relatively wealthy countries, and poorer countries that are considered underdeveloped.

DEVELOPED AND UNDERDEVELOPED COUNTRIES

Seventy-seven percent of the world's population lived in developing countries at the end of the 20th century (Benatar, 1998), where health care has become increasingly inaccessible to growing numbers of vulnerable individuals, families, and communities. The concept of underdeveloped "holds the West to be the 'developed' goal to which other countries must aspire, and in doing so devalues more than half of the world.... There are no nonpejorative terms" (Lane & Rubinstein, 1996, pp. 398-399). This view assumes that wealthier (developed) countries have the money, talent, and knowledge and, therefore, should do the planning and direction to solve the health problems of the poorer countries. It is also assumed that Western health care institutions and approaches will work in solving health problems in less developed countries, and that health care will improve the health of the recipients.

However, in developed countries, economic globalization has been accompanied by an "emphasis on individual responsibility, the downsizing of governments, and the role of the 'market' as the favored policy instrument. Thus, policies to reduce state expenditure have placed tremendous pressure on publicly funded health and welfare services.... Typically, the public-health sector receives less than 5% of the total health care budget and, from a policy perspective, is overshadowed by the demands of acute medical-care services and the power of the pharmaceutical industry" (Beaglehole & Bonita, 1998, pp. 591-592). It will be a challenge for developed countries to foster a commitment to shared benefits of national wealth, as well as the establishment of strong and continuing practitioner-community partnerships despite dominant ideologies of individual responsibility and reliance on market forces (Beaglehole & Bonita, 1998).

Dichotomizing countries on the basis of economic concepts such as developed or underdeveloped raises a number of moral questions related to health and health care. Given that "worldwide free-market forces are increasingly structuring health as a commodity rather than as an entitlement" (Austin, 2001, p. 9), does the achievement of health development need an economic rationale, or is it of value in itself? How can health-related resources be distributed based on need (justice) rather than ability to pay? Does the work of a global health organization depend on the question "what's in it for me?" or is there still room for benevolence? (Lee, 1998). Are "enduring traditions of humanitarian concern" and "compelling reasons of enlightened self-interest" still valid incentives (Howson et al., 1998)? Can a "holistic harmony" global perspective be fostered, emphasizing nature, society, neighborhood, and mutual aid rather than the autonomous individual (Austin, 2001, p. 14)? What is the right thing to do (Austin, 2001)?

When "health is viewed as a standard, a basic, and essential part of human experience that encompasses human dignity, human rights, as well as an individual's personal beliefs and values related to health" (Leuning, 2001, p. 298), the emphasis shifts to the degree to which human rights and human dignity are honored, and the strengthening of a community or nation's political will to uphold these standards. At all levels of global-health systems, nurses can seek opportunities to be involved in dialogues addressing these issues. Nurses can focus on basic human rights and dignity as well as health needs through political advocacy, education, and access to care for those, for example, displaced by war or terrorism, women and children, and people with HIV-AIDS.

GLOBAL HEALTH DEVELOPMENT

"The main variations in health status among countries result from environmental, socioeconomic, and cultural factors, and medical care is of secondary importance. Poverty is the most important cause of preventable death, disease, and disability" (Beaglehole & Bonita, 1998, p. 590). Given that many of the health problems of the developing world result from inequality and poverty, the greatest improvement in health would be accomplished by fostering education and literacy, the provision of adequate food, clean water, sanitation, housing, employment, and freedom from war (Beaglehole & Bonita, 1998; Lane & Rubinstein, 1996).

Lane and Rubinstein (1996) express concern with shortsighted planning that results from programs that attribute success only on the basis of easily measured outcomes. Examples of this include the number of children vaccinated, the number of oral rehydration solution packets distributed, or planning tied to short-term cycles, such as the fiscal year, rather than to time periods that reflect realistic program spans. Given that health improvements that result from clean water, adequate housing, or fair wages are much more difficult to measure, they tend to be discounted in priority. "Concerns of the First World provide the major imperatives for action" (Lane & Rubinstein, 1996, p. 421), but exportation of technology and development based on rational, scientific principles reflects a basic ethnocentrism (Lane & Rubinstein, 1996).

Health care alone may not be the best method of improving the health of people internationally, particularly when their health problems stem directly from poverty (Lane & Rubinstein, 1996). Some health projects have actually worsened the health of the people they were trying to help, while many projects have failed to improve health. Despite medical intervention programs, both the diseases of deprivation such as malaria and tuberculosis, and the diseases of development such as hypertension, diabetes, and alcoholism, have increased (Kaseje, 1995).

The principles of primary health care can be applied at the global level. "The basic components of primary health care are community involvement, appropriate health technology, and reorientation of health services... toward country-wide health programs. It includes an emphasis on preventive medicine and employs community health workers to serve the needs of their communities" (Lane & Rubinstein, 1996, p. 418). Although organization for global health is international, actual activities and programs take place at the community level. Therefore, empowerment is very relevant to enhancement of global health. This content will be discussed in depth in Chapter 11, *Empowering Community Health*.

EMPOWERMENT FOR GLOBAL HEALTH

An empowered community is one in which "individuals and organizations apply their skills and resources in collective efforts to meet their respective needs" (Israel et al., 1994, p. 153). Community organization describes the process of organizing people around problems or issues that are larger than group members' own immediate concerns. Robertson & Minkler (1994) suggest helpful strategies to increase community problem-solving abilities, or "community competence":

- Assisting individuals and communities in articulating both their health problems and the solutions to address those problems.

- Providing access to information. Education is critical in envisioning choices and solutions to problems.

- Supporting indigenous community leadership.

- Assisting the community in overcoming bureaucratic obstacles to action.

"A community empowerment model emphasizes participation, caring, sharing, responsibility to others, and conceives of power as an expanding commodity" (Israel et al., 1994, p. 154). People need to listen to each other, identify their commonalities, and construct new strategies for change (Wallerstein & Bernstein, 1988). Therefore, elements of community empowerment include "a social action process, people being 'subjects' of their own lives, connectedness to others, critical thinking, personal and social capacity building, and transformed power relations" (Wallerstein & Bernstein, 1988, p. 145).

According to Neighbors and colleagues (1995), recommendations to empower individuals and groups include:

- Beginning with an analysis of perceived needs of the target group rather than the needs and expectations of the program planners

- Focusing explicitly on neighborhood issues and community resources

- Incorporating factors from the family and neighborhood level

- Giving culturally sensitive health messages phrased within the context of self-help and self-reliance

- Providing specific skill-oriented training

- Using the expertise of the members of a target group who understand their culture and health problems, and most important, knowing what solutions are likely to work in their communities

Many of the needs at the community level are related to societal health problems, which will be discussed in the next section.

Societal (Public) Health Concerns

Public health is the traditional title for the medically related discipline dealing with the health of society. The basic causes of many major worldwide societal health problems can be found in similar sociopolitical and ecological influences. A critical question is whether "public-health professionals [should] be concerned with the fundamentals of health such as employment, housing, transport, food and nutrition, and global trade imperatives, or should attention be restricted to individual risk factors for diseases" (Beaglehole & Bonita, 1998, p. 591)?

Beaglehole and Bonita (1998) emphasize that, until now, much of health promotion has been based on the health education model, which focuses on a high-risk approach to primary prevention rather than a population approach. Modern public health is focused on health-services research, evidence-based health care, and the search for new risk factors at the individual level to improve the effectiveness and efficiency of medical services. The challenge for public-health practitioners is to justify and promote global concerns while addressing health inequalities and proceeding with evidence-based, disease-specific public health programs. Some of the major worldwide societal health problems are discussed in the following section, with a particular emphasis on problems in "developing" countries.

CHILDHOOD HEALTH PROBLEMS

Major leading worldwide killers are communicable, perinatal, and nutritional disorders largely affecting children. "Ninety-eight percent of all deaths in children younger than 15 years are in the developing world.... Injuries, which account for 10% of global mortality, are often ignored as a major cause of death" (Murray & Lopez, 1997, p. 1269). "Of more than 52 million deaths in 1996 worldwide, over 17 million were ascribable to infectious and parasitic diseases; more than 15 million to circulatory diseases; over 6 million to cancers; and about 3 million to diseases of the respiratory system. About 40 million deaths occurred in the developing world" (WHR, 1997, p. 252).

Many children are unvaccinated due to factors such as maternal time constraints and competing priorities; socioeconomic factors; lack of knowledge and education; low motivation; fears and negative community opinion; and insufficient accessibility, availability, acceptability, and affordability of health services. Immunization requires numerous visits to the health facility, even though there is no illness (Coreil, 1997, p. 187).

In addition, issues related to breast-feeding have a significant impact on infant health. Coreil (1997, p. 187) describes multiple detrimental feeding practices such as "discarding colostrum, giving prelacteal feeds before breast milk comes in, introducing supplemental food too early or too late, preparing breast milk substitutes improperly, and using weaning foods with inadequate nutritional value." A variety of sociocultural variables such as social networks, urbanization, women's work patterns, household income, maternal health and nutrition, and the advertising of commercial infant formulas influences infant feeding practices.

INFECTIOUS DISEASES

High infant deaths in the least developed countries are due largely to malnutrition and infections, which kill about 17 million people a year and afflict hundreds of millions of others. "In terms of setting global health priorities, therefore, the poor stand to benefit much more than the rich from a continued emphasis on infectious diseases" (WHR, 1997, pp. 248, 250). The leading infectious causes of infant and childhood death are diarrhea, respiratory illnesses, malaria, measles, and neonatal tetanus. Infections in some developing countries are promoted by poverty and a warm climate (Bradley, 1994). "Malaria and tuberculosis are the main diseases of global concern, and treatment is complicated by resistance, lack of resources, and poverty" (Wait, 1998, p. 435).

Emerging new and reemerging old diseases include resistant strains of tuberculosis, *Streptococcus pneumoniae*, and *Staphylococcus aureus*, as well as new and potentially fatal viruses including HIV, hantavirus, Legionnaires' disease, and Ebola virus. The resurgence of infectious diseases is facilitated by the increased mobility of the world's population, inappropriate and indiscriminate use of antimicrobials, and rapid urbanization (Howson et al., 1998). The spread of HIV-AIDS has reached global pandemic proportions, affected by the fact that many women have little influence on the risk behavior of their male partners (Coreil, 1997). In addition, major chronic parasitic diseases such as malaria, schistosomiasis, onchocerciasis, trypanasomiasis, leischmaniasis, filiriasis, dracunculiasis, and the intestinal parasites cause debility, loss of productivity, and shortened life spans for both children and adults (Lane & Rubinstein, 1996). Many of the parasitic diseases could be prevented with access to clean drinking and bathing water.

ACCIDENTS

Many cities in the developing world have traffic congestion that rivals that in the industrialized world. For example, in much of rural India, a two-lane, dirt, pockmarked road with cows roaming at will is used by speeding motorists who lean on their horn instead of brakes. Accidents, particularly motor vehicle accidents, are common. In addition, the use of open fires or small kerosene stoves for cooking and heating contributes to frequent burn accidents, particularly for women and children (Lane & Rubinstein, 1996). The smoke from an open fire in an underventilated area also contributes to respiratory illnesses, particularly in infants.

ACCESS TO FOOD

Nutritional status is the most important determinant of health (Lane & Rubinstein, 1996). But, "dietary inadequacy often results from unequal distribution of food within a country and between countries, which occurs even when adequate food stores exist" (Lane &

Rubinstein, 1996, p. 406). The technology that has produced high-yield hybrid foods (e.g., grains such as corn and wheat) also contributes to a cycle in which the expense of necessary fertilizer and pesticides, which the developing countries are often forced to purchase from the West, forces many small farmers off their land. Then, the land is bought by agribusinesses and used to produce cash crops. "In many parts of the world, land tenure remains nearly feudal, with a small percentage of landlords owning the fields on which tenant farmers grow crops" (Lane & Rubinstein, 1996, p. 407).

Lane and Rubinstein (1996, p. 407) explain how the diets of farmers and their families have been hurt by the shift from subsistence agriculture to growing cash crops. Under the influence of European colonialism, nonfood items such as cotton or coffee were grown for export, often on the best land. Farmers then had to grow their families' food on smaller and poorer plots of land, purchase the remainder of the food needed for their families, and purchase seeds, fertilizer, and pesticides to grow the next year's cash crop. "The families' diet, which may have been relatively abundant and varied during subsistence farming, suffers, and the most vulnerable members of each family, the children and childbearing women, suffer the most."

ILLITERACY

Illiteracy is often high, and in some countries a majority of women are illiterate. "In no society are women treated equally to men, and women, children, and older people are at greatest risk of poverty" (Beaglehole & Bonita, 1998, p. 590). Illiteracy has an indirect impact on health. For example, being unable to read directions on a medicine container may result in over- or underdosing. Increasing female literacy is associated with a decrease in the birthrate and decreased infant mortality rates (Lane & Rubinstein, 1996).

LACK OF CLEAN WATER

In many countries, "piped water and sanitation are luxuries of the urban middle and upper classes" (Lane & Rubinstein, 1996, p. 408). Diseases associated with inadequate water supplies include:

- *Water-borne diseases*, which occur when drinking water is contaminated with fecal organisms, such as cholera, typhoid, amoebiasis, hepatitis A, polio, and diarrhea.

- *Water-washed diseases*, such as skin and eye infections which increase when wash water is inadequate.

- *Water-based diseases*, such as schistosomiasis, in which the infectious agent is present in the water and penetrates the skin during washing,. "The most ubiquitous water-borne disease, diarrhea, is the leading cause of death in children under 5 in developing countries" (Lane & Rubinstein, 1996, p. 408).

MIGRATION

Migration, especially rural-to-urban migration and the flight from war and natural disasters, has been increasing every year (Lane & Rubinstein, 1996). As a result, 20% to 50% of the population live without basic sanitation in crowded, makeshift housing. "In Third World cities, rural-to-urban migrants have swelled the squatter settlements. Most of these residents were farmers who lost their land due to poverty and must now purchase all of their food. With high unemployment and lack of literacy and job skills to survive in a city, they and their children may starve due to lack of money" (Lane & Rubinstein, 1996, p. 407). The health effects of migration include:

- Physiological stresses such as crowding, inadequate food, inadequate water, and inadequate sewage disposal can both lower resistance to disease and expose migrants to tuberculosis, parasitism, diarrhea, and respiratory illnesses (Lane & Rubinstein, 1996).

- Psychological stresses such as grief, anxiety, stress, insecurity, marital breakdowns, depression, alcoholism, smoking, domestic violence, and drug addiction contribute to both physical and mental illness (Helman, 1994).

- Sociocultural stresses such as language barriers and resettlement may lead to such economic, family, and social problems as alcoholism (Lane & Rubinstein, 1996).

- Direct problems of poverty include unemployment, low income, limited education and literacy, inadequate diet, lack of breast feeding, and prostitution.

- Environmental problems result from poor housing, overcrowding, inadequate sanitation and water supplies, lack of waste disposal, air pollution, traffic accidents, the siting of hazardous industries nearby, and lack of land for growth of food.

MULTINATIONAL BUSINESS INTERESTS

Globalization is being driven by the search for inexpensive labor and new markets for trade by transnational countries (Beaglehole & Bonita, 1998). "Businesses often place profits above other considerations, including the health of unsuspecting consumers" (Lane & Rubinstein, 1996, p. 412). Examples of exploitation, especially in developing countries, include:

- The international trade in "illegal products and contaminated foodstuffs, inconsistent safety standards, and the indiscriminate spread of medical technologies... [and the] sale of prescription drugs that have not been approved by national drug-monitoring bodies" (Wait, 1998, p. 436).

- Infant formula intensely promoted for economic reasons, even though breast milk is healthier than formula, and it is free and sterile. However, the formula is so expensive that mothers have been forced to dilute the strength of the mixture, and one-fourth to one-third of family income might be needed just to purchase formula. Lack of refrigeration and contamination of the water used to mix formula, and the fact that formula confers no immunoprotection are other concerns.

- Outdated drugs, including antibiotics have been dumped in the Third World. In addition to their lack of effectiveness in treating infections, this practice has led to the proliferation of "super" bacteria, immune to most available antibiotics.

- Cutting down the rainforest increased malaria because it gave the mosquito more open pools of stagnant water in which to breed (Lane & Rubinstein, 1996).

■ The extraction of vast quantities of material and human resources from poor developing countries to rich industrialized nations. "The 1 billion people residing in industrialized countries use 10 times the resources and produce 10 times the waste per capita of the 4 billion people residing in developing countries" (Benatar, 1998, pp. 296-297). A major contributor to environmental degradation is the continued overconsumption of the world's resources by wealthy countries (Beaglehole & Bonita, 1998).

POVERTY

Poverty has been growing in many parts of the world. Sociopolitical conditions, including inadequate food, clean water, stress associated with migration, war, multinational business interests, and large-scale development projects both cause some health problems and make a number of existing problems worse (Lane & Rubinstein, 1996). "About a fifth of the world's population, 1.3 billion people, live on a daily income of less than US$1. Although most of the world's poor live in South and East Asia, sub-Saharan Africa has the fastest growing proportion of people who live in poverty" (Beaglehole & Bonita, 1998, p. 590). More than 10 million abandoned or orphaned African children live on their own (Howson et al., 1998).

Many of the poorer nations devote a disproportionate share of their economy to maintaining a military force, leading to disruption of human services, social supports, food distribution, and health care (Lane & Rubinstein, 1996). In addition, unemployment and underemployment contributes to poverty as the "best and brightest emigrate to seek their fortunes in other countries.... Brain drain disproportionately affects the ranks of physicians and nurses, the loss of whom directly affects a country's health care" (Lane & Rubinstein, 1996, p. 405).

OVERPOPULATION AND FAMILY PLANNING

At present, global population growth is about 90 million persons per year, with about 90% of future growth projected to occur in developing countries (Beaglehole & Bonita, 1998). It is worth noting that in nearly all other animal species, when population increases have been as explosive as current human growth, a point has been reached where environmental factors such as disease, food supply, and predators caused a rapid decline in numbers (Smith, 1994). For humans, however, environmental factors have not been able to constrain population, and growth is continuing to accelerate.

In the 1960s through the 1980s, many of the population programs "concentrated on population control at the expense of human dignity and rights" (Lane & Rubinstein, 1996, p. 414). Maternal mortality can be lowered by as much as 25% through spacing of births, prevention of unsafe abortions, and prevention of maternal nutritional deficiencies due to frequent breast feeding (Coreil, 1997). Excluding China, the prevalence of modern contraceptive use in the developing world is 32% (1997). However, some religions disapprove of all artificial forms of birth control, and the cost or availability of artificial forms of birth control may be limited.

In most cases, the meaning of family planning is closely related to the value given to children. In many cultures, having a child is the visible sign of adult status; and for many men, the birth of a son is the ultimate proof of their virility (Helman, 1994). Women often do not have the power to make decisions about fertility. Additionally, cultural beliefs about the body impact on family planning. Examples of such beliefs include a woman can't get pregnant except when uterus is "open" during menstruation, decreased menstrual blood may leave more "poison," and an intrauterine contraceptive device might move and "get lost" (Helman, 1994). Having many children ensures future economic and social security for the family. An important role for nurses is to "enhance the capacity of poor home-based caregivers, most of whom are women, to take part effectively in decision making and action for health?" (Kaseje, 1995, p. 210).

The global prevalence of all the leading chronic diseases is increasing, with the majority occurring in developing countries and projected to increase substantially over the next 2 decades, driven by urbanization, trade, foreign investment, and promotional marketing. Cardiovascular disease is already the leading cause of mortality in developing countries. Between 1990 and 2000 mortality from ischemic heart disease in developing countries was expected to increase by 120% for women and 137% for men. Predictions for the next 2 decades include a near tripling of ischemic heart disease and stroke mortality in Latin America, the Middle East, and sub-Saharan Africa. The global number of individuals with diabetes in 2000 was estimated to be 171 million (2.8% of the world's population), a figure projected to increase in 2030 to 366 million (6.5%), 298 million of whom will live in developing countries. Cancer incidence increased 19% between 1990 and 2000 mainly in developing countries. Death and disability due to chronic obstructive pulmonary disease are increasing across most regions. Risks for chronic disease are also escalating. Smoking prevalence and obesity levels among adolescents in developing countries have risen over the past decade and portend rapid increases in chronic diseases (Yach et al., 2004, p. 2616).

The emphasis on communicable diseases has excluded consideration of chronic diseases in low-middle and middle income with the up-to-date evidence about the burden and impacts of chronic diseases. Tackle chronic diseases upstream. Governments can play a role by altering economic incentives for businesses and individuals. Expanding markets for fruits and vegetables will allow developing countries to gain from increased export earnings and consumption. Raising the tobacco excise tax to levels that will decrease consumption effectively will increase government revenue and reduce the burden of disease (Yach et al., 2004, p. 2621).

SOCIETAL HEALTH STRATEGIES FOR THE FUTURE

According to Roemer and Roemer (1990, p. 1191), "the solution to poor quality government services is not to privatize them but rather to heighten the priority and enhance the support of governmental activities for advancement of health." Global leadership and a true global health plan are needed, for which financial resources are vital. However, "the total annual UNICEF budget of $1 billion is equivalent to the expenditures for less than 9 hours of health care in the U.S.... [and] the per capita U.S. annual contribution to UNICEF is $0.62 while the average Norwegian contributes $13.12" (Foege, 1998, p. 1932).

Private companies, such as pharmaceutical companies, have also provided a significant investment of resources. For example, Merck has supplied ivermectin (Mectizan) to treat river blindness (onchocerciasis); Glaxo Wellcome has supplied Malarone, combining atovaquone and progguanil to treat malaria; American Cyanamid (Abate) and Precision Fabrics Group have provided temephos, a larvicide and nylon filter material to strain drinking water and eradicate guinea worms; and SmithKline Beecham Pharmaceuticals has supplied alben-dazole to combat lymphatic filariasis (elephantiasis) (Foege, 1998).

Another societal strategy is to reduce population growth. "Birth rates have declined globally from 32 per 1000 population in 1970 to 23 per 1000 population in 1996, but population growth continues at a rate of approximately 1.7% per year" (Foege, 1998, p. 1932). It has been shown that programs for family planning, child survival, and education of girls and women reduce the birth rate (Foege, 1998).

Accountability must be maintained. For example, "tobacco companies must be financially responsible for the adverse health effects of smoking worldwide.... The current annual global tobacco-related mortality of 3 million people will increase to an annual level of 10 million deaths by 2020" (Foege, 1998, p. 1932). Nurses and other health professionals need to be aware of and involved in seeking long-term solutions to societal health concerns. The following suggestions, while abstract and very difficult to implement, provide examples of important areas to pursue:

- Facilitate consumer involvement in the planning, policy-making, and operations of health systems at all levels. This is consistent with the empowerment approach advocated in Chapter 11, *Empowering Community Health*.

- Assure political commitment to making health, education, and human well-being higher priorities than military expansion in order to achieve security and peace.

- Strengthen ministries and departments of health to coordinate, integrate, and assure high-quality preventive and curative services, and provide trained health personnel to provide comprehensive health services and to administer those services effectively.

- Be alert of hazards from environmental tobacco, addictive drugs, occupational toxins, trauma, and violence, and take social action to minimize or eliminate these risks. Participate in the development of global surveillance systems to detect infectious disease outbreaks, chemical or bio-terrorist attack, or breakdowns in the safety of the global food supply.

- Provide maximum international collaboration for overall socioeconomic development to countries, sharing information to analyze risks that contribute to premature death and disability, and assessing cost-effective interventions to address the greatest health burdens.

The social environment is only one of the contexts that influence human health. The natural environment will be discussed in the next section.

Environmental Health Concerns

Nurses need to understand the influences on health of interactions between humans and their natural and social environments, social determinants of health—how social and environmental inequities contribute to health disparities (Schulz & Northridge, 2004, p. 455).

The literature (Grady et al., 1997; Green et al., 1996; Rogers & Cox, 1998; Spiegel & Yassi, 1997) suggests that environmental health refers to:

■ The whole of the physical aspects of our surroundings, including individual and natural or man-made environmental interactions that may affect health (human ecology).

■ The ecological balances essential to long-term human health.

■ The promotion of safe, healthful living conditions, and protection from environmental factors that may adversely affect human health.

■ The social, institutional, and cultural contexts of people-environment relations (social ecology).

One creative way of conceptualizing environment is through the geographic metaphor of "therapeutic landscape" (Gesler, 1992). Sense of place includes the meaning and significance that individuals and groups give to physical places, such as feelings of safety and security, and as settings for family life, employment, and aesthetic experience. In a positive way, the fresh air and pure water of the countryside, and magnificent scenery can be healing. In a negative context, "landscape" might incorporate nontherapeutic control relationships sometimes played out between clients and health care providers in physical settings such as hospitals and doctor's offices. As a blend of the place (physical setting) with its meaning to the client, landscape is related to, but not identical with, nature, scenery, environment, places, regions, areas, and geography (Gesler, 1992).

Dixon and Dixon (2002) propose an integrative model for environmental health, encompassing four broad domains and their interrelationships: physiological, vulnerability, epistemological, and health protection. The *physiological* domain includes a chemical or physical agent (potential cause of disease); exposure (contact with an agent); incorporation (accumulation within the body); and health effects (mortality and morbidity indicators such as disease diagnosis and symptom experience). The *vulnerability* domain includes individual characteristics (such as developmental, health, genetic, and gender-related) and community characteristics (such as sociodemographic and cultural). The *epistemological* domain concerns elements of personal thought (such as awareness of risks and challenges) and social knowledge (shared beliefs of what is true and who bears responsibility). The *health protection* domain includes concerns (appraisal of threat), sense of efficacy (confidence in ability to reduce health hazards), and actions (personal avoidance or changing the environment). The intent of the model is to promote thinking and research that encourages proactive changes in public policy ("upstream" thinking) to reduce environmental health hazards. Social and economic inequalities (fundamental factors) within the built environment, social context (intermediate factors) that influence stressors, health behaviors, and social relationships (proximate factors) ultimately result in individual and population health and well-being (Schulz & Northridge, 2004, p. 458).

Barriers to successful policy and environmental change interventions include:

■ Lack of trust in government.

■ Legal and bureaucratic distractions, particularly in the policy development arena, that demand more time, the involvement of outside partners, and legal expertise.

- "Turf issues" within the state and local official agencies, communities, nonprofit organizations, business groups, and health care institutions.

- Dependence on crisis management or reacting in situations rather than building advocacy over the longer term.

- Inability to handle sudden conflict. The fact that stakeholders often lack a shared vision and agenda does not help.

- Confusion over the differences among policy development, advocacy, politics, and lobbying.

- Organizational opposition. The tobacco industry and its allies, for example, opposed tobacco control programs, immediately.

- Benefits not immediate or evident. Many programs are under pressure to show results right away, whereas policy development and environmental change interventions take time and long-term commitment.

- Unfamiliarity with the concept of policy development and environmental change.

- Lack of legal capacity. (Hann et al., 2004, p. 380)

Environment can be viewed as a major determinant of disease, particularly in developing countries (Bradley, 1994). Underlying many current environmental health concerns is the perspective that the world's resources are "free and inexhaustible" (Helman, 1994, p. 381), and that humans are the most important of all the species and should therefore dominate nature. These views raise fundamental ethical questions such as the nature of our obligations to future generations and to other species on the planet (Smith, 1994). For example, environmental degradation from "the pressures of consumerism, population, increasing traffic density, technological hazards, land mines, and overexploitation of natural resources leads to droughts, soil erosion, famine, malnutrition, and related diseases" (Kaseje, 1995, p. 210). "Twenty percent of deaths in the United States can be attributed to such factors as pollution and toxic chemicals in the environment" (Bellack et al., 1996, p. 338).

TOXIC EXPOSURE

Toxic exposure is generally a result of human manipulations or an interaction with toxins in the environment. Environmental exposure occurs by way of inhalation through dust or fumes, ingestion of lead or pesticides from contaminated materials or foods, or skin absorption from direct contact with solvents (Rogers & Cox, 1998; Spiegel & Yassi, 1997). Examples of types of toxic exposure are presented in Box 9-1.

EXPLOITATION OF NATURAL RESOURCES

Non-renewable geochemical substances such as natural gas, oil, copper, lead, zinc, tin, gold, silver, mercury, and platinum metals will become physically scarce in the 21st century if we maintain current rates of use (Reijnders, 1993). In addition, renewable natural resources that are currently most exploited include soil, groundwater, and wood. To sustain renewable resources, their use should not exceed the current generation of the resource. "Sustainable development," a "steady-state" relation between society and the environment, is needed to protect natural resources (1993). However, sustainability appears improbable at the present

Box 9-1

Types of Toxic Exposure

- *Chemical hazards.* Synthetic fibers, plastics, solvents, fuels, detergents, pigments, metal alloys, pharmaceuticals, pesticides, and intermediate byproducts and waste products of these materials. Also included in this category is radon, a radioactive gas.

- *Physical agents.* Exposure to ultraviolet radiation, heat, cold, nuclear radiation, vibration, noise, and electromagnetic fields, acerbated by the depletion of the protective filtering effect of the ozone layer by chloroflourocarbons, which are widely used in refrigerants, air conditioning, and aerosol repellents (Rogers & Cox, 1998).

- *Car exhaust.* Air pollution from car exhaust fumes consists mainly of carbon monoxide, ozone, nitrous dioxide, and hydrocarbons.

- *Biological or infectious agents.* E.g., hepatitis or tuberculosis.

- *Toxic waste.* Industrial dumping and inappropriate disposal of medical, pathogenic, and radioactive wastes.

time as major changes in production and consumption, and restriction of the total world population to its present level would be required. Indeed, the true limits to growth are the capacity of the environment to deal with waste in all its forms and the "critical" resources, such as the ozone layer, the carbon cycle, and the global rain forests (Smith, 1994).

POLLUTION

Pollution may lead to the deterioration of an area's resource base. Examples of such resource-based deterioration include forest die-back due to acidification of soils and increased airborne ozone, which affects wood production and recreation; the threat to agriculture in low-lying areas due to the rise in sea level associated with the greenhouse effect; and the greenhouse effect itself—thinning of the ozone layer, rising levels of carbon dioxide, global warming, chlorofluorocarbons, and acid rain (Leaf, 1989; Reijnders, 1993).

Groundwater Pollution

Groundwater is the underground reserve of fresh water that supplies lakes and wells with drinkable water. "The importance of groundwater pollution derives from the importance of groundwater as a resource and ecological determinant, and the long-lasting effect of groundwater pollution, once it occurs" (Reijnders, 1993, p. 147). Intensively farmed and heavily industrialized areas are subject to pollution, particularly when the groundwater table is low (1993).

Depletion of the Ozone Layer

Another outcome of pollution is depletion of the atmospheric ozone layer. The ozone layer shields the earth from the damaging effects of the sun's ultraviolet radiation. Ozone is formed slowly from the action of sunlight on the rare molecules of oxygen in the stratosphere. Chloroflourocarbons, used in aerosols, refrigerants, and other industrial products; nitrous oxide, a byproduct of internal-combustion engines, industrial processes, and microbial activity; and carbon dioxide all absorb the longer infrared waves emitted from the earth, destroying ozone, trapping energy in the atmosphere, and warming the earth's surface. The term "greenhouse effect" refers to the effect on the balance between the energy the earth receives from solar radiation and the energy it loses by radiation from its surface back to space.

Since the Industrial Revolution, carbon dioxide, our society's single largest waste product and the predominant greenhouse gas, has been added to the atmosphere at an accelerating rate. The atmosphere today still contains half of all the carbon dioxide produced since the start of the Industrial Revolution (Leaf, 1989). Additionally, in the first half of the 21st century, carbon dioxide in the atmosphere is expected to double (Smith, 1994). "Once depleted, the ozone layer may require 8 to 10 years for reconstitution" (Leaf, 1989, p. 1579). Ozone depletion and climate change have major effects on health, including increases in vector-borne and water- and foodborne diseases, changes in food production, increase in stress from extreme heat or cold, skin cancer, cataracts, and immune suppression (Martens, 1998).

Climatic Change

Macro-effects of climatic change are heavily influenced by cycles of geochemicals such as carbon, nitrogen, sulfur, and water. These cycles strongly determine atmospheric concentrations of carbon dioxide, oxygen, and nitrogen compounds and precipitation (Reijnders, 1993). As concentrations of these gases build in the atmosphere, the earth's surface temperature slowly increases, creating global climate changes. Unfortunately, industrialized countries with the financial resources to do something about their tremendous production of waste gases, perceive little self-interest because global warming has limited effect on industry. Countries that rely on agricultural production (which will be greatly affected) have limited resources to invest (Smith, 1994).

Increases of 2° to 5° Centigrade in the next 50 to 100 years have been predicted, equaling the largest temperature change since the last ice age. The distribution and timing of climate change could have many outcomes, including:

- Creating drought and desert in areas that are now fertile but creating more arable areas in higher latitudes.

- Shifting patterns of tropical and monsoon rains that are so important to vegetation and agriculture in Africa, Asia, and South America.

- Greatly increasing malaria transmission, possibly "up to a hundredfold" (Bradley, 1994, p. 136).

- Melting the polar ice caps, inundating large population centers and much fertile land. "The expected rise may create 50 million environmental refugees worldwide, more than triple the number of all refugees today.... Displaced people and less arable land would compound the problem of feeding the world's increasing population... increased precipitation... intrusion of salt into surface water, increased flooding, runoffs contaminated with pesticides, salts, garbage, excreta, sewage, and eroded soil are all likely" (Leaf, 1989, pp. 1578-1579).

Examples of the possible health consequences of global climatic change include increased mortality from heat stress; decreased number of deaths from hypothermia and cold; increased morbidity and mortality from lung diseases such as bronchitis, bronchiectasis, asthma, and chronic obstructive pulmonary disease; increased incidence of all kinds of skin cancer among white populations; increased incidence of cataracts; depression of the immune system leading to an increase in infectious diseases; increased incidence of water- and air-borne diseases; spread of infectious diseases such as enteric infections, measles, pertussis, poliomyelitis, tuberculosis, leprosy; and malnutrition, hunger, and starvation (Leaf, 1989).

A number of suggestions have been made to reduce environmental pollution (Reijnders, 1993) including:

- Limit population size
- Limit pesticide and fertilizers through lower-input agriculture
- Prevent wastes associated with industrial production through good housekeeping, changes in production processes, and changes in inputs and internal recycling
- Improve energy efficiency. Switch away from nonrenewable primary energy
- Recycle organic wastes into fertilizers and/or composts
- Foster environmentally conscious buying behavior (green consumerism)

DEFORESTATION

Forests play a crucial role in reducing the "greenhouse effect" through the stabilization of global gases and in maintaining patterns of global rainfall. The destruction of forests can have a number of effects, including:

- Reduced rainfall in adjacent areas with irreversible soil erosion-causing crop failures and a fall in food production.
- Destruction of indigenous peoples through destruction of habitat and hunting grounds and violence.
- Species extinction. An estimated one-fourth of all species will become extinct within the next 50 years, more than 74 per day (Helman, 1994). "The global loss [of species] resulting from deforestation could be as much as 4000 to 6000 species a year, or some 10,000 times more than the naturally occurring rate of extinction that existed before human beings appeared" (Leaf, 1989, p. 1580).
- Infectious diseases "resulting from the destruction of the natural habitats and ecological niches of certain viruses or their vectors, and their release into human populations" (Helman, 1994, p. 379).
- Danger of mud-, rock-, and snowslides, as well as loss of topsoil, in mountainous regions.

The current loss of forested land due to human activity is higher than anything previously experienced (Smith, 1994). The expansion of the world's population, associated with the necessary production of food, is the main force driving deforestation, although factors such as logging, pollution, tourism, and bad productive practices are also involved (Reijnders, 1993).

NURSING IMPLICATIONS OF ENVIRONMENTAL HEALTH CONCERNS

Integrative health promotion emphasizes creating an environment that is conducive to healthy behaviors, health, and healing. As early as the mid-1800s, Florence Nightingale maintained that five essential environmental characteristics were needed to promote the health of individuals: pure air, pure water, efficient drainage, cleanliness, and light (Nightingale, 1859). Now, at the beginning of the 21st century, nurses appreciate Nightingale's focus on the importance of environmental factors in the promotion of health of individuals, communities, and society. At the individual and community levels, assessment may identify environmental conditions that are amenable to nursing interventions. Additionally, Bellack and colleagues (1996) indicate that nurses need to:

■ Acquire the knowledge and skills to recognize and treat environmentally induced disease.

■ Become advocates for environmental issues to protect clients' health.

■ Assess the environment for hazards and risks.

■ Work with employers and communities to reduce risk and prevent exposure to environmental hazards.

■ Promote healthy behaviors and lifestyles.

■ Identify resources for accomplishing population focused care related to environmental health.

■ Provide careful assessment, detection, and control of exposure sources.

A number of strategies have been proposed for accomplishing these goals. While all of these strategies are valuable, each nurse cannot do everything, and priorities have to be established. All nurses need to be cognizant and vigilant to environmental factors that influence health, and develop skill in environmental health history taking. Other strategies include (King & Harber, 1998; Rogers & Cox, 1998):

■ Identifying a potential irritant or toxic agent.

■ Identifying an exposure pathway and obtaining a risk assessment.

■ Strategizing with the client on how to eliminate or minimize exposure.

■ Administering appropriate screening and/or bio marker tests (e.g., blood lead or dichlorodiphenyldichloroethylene [DDE] levels).

■ Recommending treatment or further evaluation as appropriate.

■ Monitoring the client's health long-term, with follow-up as needed.

■ Reviewing the effect of the agent on the larger community (is this agent affecting others?).

■ Referring for support services as necessary.

■ Encouraging communication.

■ Creating networks where possible and educating clients about community action groups.

■ Lobbying for needed services and funding.

■ Identifying and encouraging successful coping strategies.

■ Encouraging general health promotion activities.

■ Working with interdisciplinary teams and public and private organizations to determine the impact of environmental health exposures.

■ Performing risk assessments.

■ Acting as a resource in providing data and materials about hazards and how to reduce exposures.

■ Educating other health care professionals.

■ Explaining basic environmental health principles, including exposure pathways, variability in susceptibility, toxicology of chemical of concern and steps to be taken, importance of dose in determining risk, and personal risk of specific future diseases.

■ Advocating on behalf of workers and others to alter hazardous conditions and prevent further health problems.

■ Identifying environmental health problems and developing a research plan.

■ Identifying linkages among workplace, home, community, and lifestyle.

The discussions of global, societal, and environmental health in this chapter have emphasized that everything is connected to everything else. The environment is predisposing, enabling, and reinforcing of health, in addition to being a determinant of disease. Although the main concern of biomedicine has been the treatment of individual risk factors, primary, preventive health promotion needs to be applied at all levels. Additionally, a focus on integrative health promotion demands consideration of moral and ethical issues for the just distribution of health and health care resources, locally, nationally, internationally, and globally.

Chapter Key Points

■ The ecocentric approach assumes that everything is connected to everything else and that there are links among environment, development, and human health.

■ Health professionals have traditionally been concerned almost exclusively with individual risk factors for diseases, ignoring unequal social, economic, and political structures that are the basic causes of health problems.

- The main variations in health status among countries result from environmental, socioeconomic, and cultural factors, with medical care of secondary importance.

- Underlying many of the current environmental health concerns is the view that the world's resources are inexhaustible and available for the taking.

- Environmental health concerns include toxic exposure, natural resources, pollution, deforestation, and climactic change.

- Societal health concerns include childhood health problems, infectious diseases, accidents, poor access to food, illiteracy, lack of clean water, migration, multinational business interests, poverty, overpopulation, and family planning.

- Empowerment involves assisting individuals and communities to articulate both their health problems and the solutions to address those problems, providing access to information, supporting indigenous community leadership, and assisting the community in overcoming bureaucratic obstacles to action.

References

Austin, W. (2001). Nursing ethics in an era of globilization. *Advances in Nursing Science, 24,* 1-18.

Beaglehole, R., & Bonita, R. (1998). Public health at the crossroads: Which way forward? *Lancet, 351,* 590-592.

Bellack, J. P., Musham, C., Hainer, A., Graber, D. R., & Holmes, D. (1996). Environmental health competencies: A survey of nurse practitioner programs. *American Association of Occupational Health Nurses, 44,* 337-344.

Benatar, S. R. (1998). Global disparities in health and human rights: A critical commentary. *American Journal of Public Health, 88,* 295-300.

Bradley, D. (1994). Health, environment, and tropical development. In B. Cartledge (Ed.), *Health and the environment* (pp. 126-149). Oxford, UK: Oxford University Press.

Coreil, J. (1997). Health behavior in developing countries. In D. S. Gochman (Ed.), *Handbook of health behavior* (Vol. 3, pp. 179-198). New York: Plenum Press.

Dixon, J. K., & Dixon, J. P. (2002). An integrative model for environmental health research. *Advances in Nursing Science, 24,* 43-57.

Foege, W. H. (1998). Global public health: Targeting inequities. *JAMA, 279,* 1931-1932.

Gesler, W. M. (1992). Therapeutic landscapes: Medical issues in light of the new cultural geography. *Social Science and Medicine, 34,* 735-746.

Grady, P. A., Harden, J. T., Moritz, P., & Amende, L. M. (1997). Incorporating environmental sciences and nursing research: An NINR initiative. *Nursing Outlook, 45,* 73-75.

Green, L. W., Richard, L., & Potvin, L. (1996). Ecological foundations of health promotion. *American Journal of Health Promotion, 10,* 270-281.

Hann, N. E., Kean, T. J., Matulionis, R. M., Russell, C. M., & Sterling, T. D. (2004). Policy and environmental change: New directions for public health. *Health Promotion Practice, 5,* 377-381.

Hegyvary, S. T. (2001). Editorial. *J Nurs Scholarsh, 33,* 304.

Helman, C. G. (1994). Medical anthropology and global health. In C. G. Helman (Ed.), *Culture, health and illness* (3rd ed., pp. 328-383). Oxford, UK: Butterworth-Heinemann Ltd.

Howson, C. P., Fineberg, H. V., & Bloom, B. R. (1998). The pursuit of global health: The relevance of engagement for developed countries. *Lancet, 351*, 586-590.

Israel, B. A., Checkoway, B., Schulz, A., & Zimmerman, M. (1994). Health education and community empowerment: Conceptualizing and measuring perceptions of individual, organizational, and community control. *Health Education Quarterly, 21*, 149-170.

Kaseje, D. (1995). The role of nursing in health care in the context of unjust social, economic, and political structures and systems. *Nursing and Health Care Perspectives on Community, 16*, 209-213.

King, C., & Harber, P. (1998). Community environmental health concerns and the nursing process. *American Association of Occupational Health Nurses, 46*, 20-27.

Kleffel, D. (1996). Environmental paradigms: Moving toward an ecocentric perspective. *Advances in Nursing Science, 18*(4), 1-10.

Lane, S. D., & Rubinstein, R. A. (1996). International health: Problems and programs in anthropological perspective. In C. F. Sargent, & T. M. Johnson (Eds.), *Medical anthropology. Contemporary theory and method* (Rev. ed., pp. 398-423). Westport, CT: Praeger.

Leaf, A. (1989). Potential health effects of global climatic and environmental changes. *New England Journal of Medicine, 321*, 1577-1583.

Lee, K. (1998). Shaping the future of global health cooperation: Where can we go from here? *Lancet, 351*, 899-902.

Leuning, C. J. (2001). Advancing a global perspective: The world as classroom. *Nursing Science Quarterly, 14*, 298-303

Martens, W. J. M. (1998). Health impacts of climate change and ozone depletion: An ecoepidemiologic modeling approach. *Environ Health Perspect, 106*(Suppl. 1), 241-245.

Murray, C. J. L., & Lopez, A. D. (1997). Mortality by cause for eight regions of the world: Global burden of disease study. *Lancet, 349*, 1269-1276.

Neighbors, H. W., Braithwaite, R. L., & Thompson, E. (1995). Health promotion and African-Americans: From personal empowerment to community action. *American Journal of Health Promotion, 9*, 281-287.

Nightingale, F. (1859). *Notes on nursing: What it is, and what it is not.* London: Harrison & Sons.

Reijnders, L. (1993). Health within an ecological perspective. In R. Lafaille, & S. Fulder (Eds.), *Towards a new science of health* (pp. 144-155). London: Routledge.

Robertson, A., & Minkler, M. (1994). New health promotion movement: A critical examination. *Health Education Quarterly, 21*, 295-312.

Roemer, M. I., & Roemer, R. (1990). Global health, national development, and the role of government. *Am J Public Health, 80*, 1188-1191.

Rogers, B., & Cox, A. R. (1998). Expanding horizons: Integrating environmental health in occupational health nursing. *American Association of Occupational Health Nurses Journal, 46*, 9-13.

Schultz, A., & Northridge, M. E. (2004). Social determinants of health: Implications for environmental health promotion. *Health Education and Behavior, 31*, 455-471.

Smith, D. (1994). How will it all end? In B. Cartledge, *Health and the environment* (pp. 207-218). Oxford, UK: Oxford University Press.

Spiegel, J., & Yassi, A. (1997). The use of health indicators in environmental assessment. *Journal of Medical Systems, 21*, 275-289.

Wait, G. (1998). Globalisation of international health. *Lancet, 351*, 434-437.

Wallerstein, N., & Bernstein, E. (1988). Empowerment education: Freire's ideas adapted to health education. *Health Education Quarterly, 15*, 379-394.

World Health Report. (1997). Conquering suffering, enriching humanity. *World Health Forum, 18*, 248-260.

Yach, D., Hawkes, C., Gould, C. L., & Hofman, K. J. (2004). The global burden of chronic diseases: Overcoming impediments to prevention and control. *Journal of the American Medical Association, 291*, 2616-2622.

THE PERSON WORLDVIEW

Section III, *The Person Worldview*, includes two chapters that emphasize healing approaches to the promotion of health. Chapter 10, *The Essence of Healing Helping Relationship*, discusses the elements of healing as a goal of nursing as contrasted with curing. A helping relationship that is characterized by presence (being rather than doing), mindfulness, respect, genuineness, active listening, empathy, and the therapeutic use of self are addressed. And, Chapter 11, *Empowering Community Health*, emphasizes community-level empowerment, collaboration, and capacity building to nurture and build on strengths and resources present in the community.

THE ESSENCE OF A HEALING HELPING RELATIONSHIP

Abstract

Healing is facilitated within a helping relationship that is characterized by such behaviors as presence (being with rather than doing for), mindfulness, respect, connected caring, genuineness, reciprocity, active listening, empathy, and communication. In this chapter, a helping relationship is viewed as one way to enhance a sense of well-being, lessen feelings of isolation and vulnerability, and facilitate health.

Learning Outcomes

By the end of the chapter the student will be able to:

- Differentiate between characteristics of prescriptive and healing helping relationships.

- Describe characteristics and outcomes of presence in a healing helping relationship.

- Discuss the use of challenge in a helping relationship.

- Discuss Patterson and Zderad's, Parse's, and Watson's use of presence in their nursing theories.

- Discuss behaviors associated with a healing helping relationship, such as presence, mindfulness, relating, respect, connected caring, genuineness, reciprocity, active listening, empathy, and communication.

Prescriptive Helping Relationship

Gadamer (1960) describes three kinds of interpersonal understanding. The first kind applies knowledge of human behavior in order to manipulate another person or serve one's own purpose(s). A second kind uses knowledge or understanding of another person's point of view in order to determine what the person needs. These two kinds of interpersonal understanding are demonstrated in a prescriptive helping relationship.

A medically oriented risk and illness prevention approach to health promotion is used by many nurses. This approach is characterized by "authoritarian, prescriptive, persuasive, and generalized information giving from 'expert' to 'ignorant' lay person" (Benson & Latter, 1998, p. 101). A prescriptive helping relationship is often characterized by dominating, generalized, reassuring, and directive interactions.

In a prescriptive helping relationship, the emphasis is on goal-directed nursing interactions aimed at problem resolution. An interaction is short and focuses on single dimensions of behavior such as verbal dialogue or actions (Morse et al., 1997). Relating and communicating are viewed as "something a nurse does using a set of defined communication skills" (Hartrick, 1997, p. 524). There is an emphasis on prescriptive information-giving about illness and detrimental individual lifestyle factors, with a lack of recognition of the broader social and environmental determinants of health (Benson & Latter, 1998).

Hartrick (1997, pp. 524-525) describes several constraints of a prescriptive helping relationship:

- The nurse's ability to experience and value human relationships is constrained by an emphasis on functions and productivity. The ability to be in a caring relationship requires far more than the refinement of behavioral communication skills. "Rather, it requires an appreciation of people's connectedness, the development of relational awareness and an interest in the movement of relationship, not just attention to self and others."

- Connection in a relationship is disrupted when the nurse concentrates attention and interest on her- or himself to the exclusion of the client. By focusing on performing (e.g., saying the "right thing"), the nurse may overlook or forget the relationship.

- Problem-resolution aims to achieve a conflict-free state of harmony. But, health and healing are promoted through the "development of an increasing openness to learning and growth, an increasing capacity to tolerate ambiguity and uncertainty, and an increasing experience of empowerment and choice."

- In addition, Newman (1999) noted that "the pathway of healing is one of exploration, not repair" (p. 229).

An emphasis on self-focused communication skills and on techniques to accomplish tasks is based on the mistaken belief that the nurse has to "do" something to solve client problems. Nurses, as well as other clinicians, tend to assume that it is the techniques they use which lead to change for patients. Indeed, nurses make so much investment in terms of time, money, and effort, in acquiring knowledge and skills, that it would be surprising if they were not highly committed to a belief in the effectiveness of their techniques. However, "it is the nontechnical factors which are central to healing" (Mitchell & Cormack, 1998, p. 77).

Gadamer's (1960) third kind of interpersonal understanding based on openness, mutuality, dialogue, and the possibility of change of both participants is consistent with a healing helping relationship that develops over time. Table 10-1 lists the selected characteristics of prescriptive and healing helping relationships differentiated by Hartrick (1997).

Table 10-1

Differentiating Characteristics of Prescriptive and Healing Helping Relationships

PRESCRIPTIVE	HEALING
Behavioral interpersonal practice	Relational caring practice
Subject-object separability	Relational inseparability
Objectivity	Intersubjectivity
I-It relationship (Buber, 1958)	I-Thou relationship (Buber, 1958)
Reciprocal relationship (Lyons, 1988)	Responsive relationship (Lyons, 1988)
Behavioral action/interaction	Human-to-human process
Method-centered doing	Relationship-centered being/knowing/doing
Problem identification and goal attainment	Understanding the meaning and complexity of human experience
Emphasizes increasing behavioural skillfulness of nurse	Emphasizes enhancing relational capacity of nurse
Communication skills: clarification, open-ended, questions, empathy, listening, attending, self-disclosure, confrontation, immediacy	Relational capacities: initiative, authenticity, responsiveness, mutuality and synchrony, honoring complexity and ambiguity, intentionality, re-imagining

Reprinted from Hartrick, G. (1997). Relational capacity: The foundation for interpersonal nursing practice. *J Adv Nurs, 26,* 525, with permission of Blackwell Science Ltd.

Healing Helping Relationship

When viewed from the perspective of a person as a composite (see the discussion of the disease perspective of health in Chapter 1), healing has been defined as the process of bringing together the parts of oneself (physical, mental, emotional, spiritual, and relational) at deeper levels of inner knowing. This leads to an integration and balance, with each part having equal importance and value (McKivergin, 2000) and, as "an inner process through which a person becomes whole" (Lerner, 1994, p. 13). When the reality of wholeness is viewed not as an ideal, but as a given (see the discussion of the person perspective of health in Chapter 1), the focus is on appreciating the wholeness of the pattern that arises from human-environment mutual process (Cowling, 2000).

Given that healing occurs within the client, the nurse healer's role is to facilitate another person's growth, assist with recovery from illness, or assist with transition to peaceful death (Dossey et al., 1995). The nurse assists and responds to the client, who is the central force in the healing process. "Nurses assume that their actions, as professionals, aim to facilitate wholeness in others through an interaction based on a mutuality of purpose" (Kritek, 1997, p. 14). Kritek (1997, p. 21) identified four fundamental elements of the healing encounter:

- Nurse and client interact within a given context

- The encounter is in response to a health experience

- The nurse works in a pattern of mutuality with the client

- Healing is facilitated in response to a client's elicitation of nursing involvement and expertise

Cowling (2000, p. 16) conceptualized healing "as the realization, knowledge, and appreciation of the inherent wholeness in life" that clarifies understanding and opportunities for action. He proposed a process of "pattern appreciation" that includes information gathering about the pattern of the whole and appreciating the transformative nature of a participatory engagement with people that "illuminates the possibilities." Newman (1999) identified mutuality, rhythm, and pattern in dynamic relatedness with one's environment as key features in a healing relationship. She stated that the development of a tolerance for uncertainty, and a mutually satisfying rhythm of relating with another person's interactive pattern are necessary for effective communication.

Lerner (1994) differentiated among universal, common, and unique conditions of healing. Examples of universal conditions are inner peace and a deep experience of love. Examples of common conditions are attention and care from friends and family, deeply enjoyed work, laughter, moving music, and great art. Lerner suggests that the unique conditions of healing are some of the most important. Thus, the nurse in a healing relationship needs to identify the unique conditions that are most meaningful for the individual client.

Benson and Latter (1998, p. 104) propose that the nurse should encourage "health promotion as an empowering, holistic, individualized approach applicable to any interaction as opposed to telling people what to do about unhealthy habits." Healers should try to cure sometimes, relieve often, and comfort always (Mitchell & Cormack, 1998). "Nurses offer the gift of walking with a person so that he or she is not alone at the crossroads of healing" (Mc-Kivergin, 1997, p. 24). A healing helping relationship is characterized by such principles as presence (being with rather than doing for), intention and purpose, empathy, guiding, creativity, imagery, and spirituality (Dossey et al., 1995; Keegan, 1994; Lerner, 1994).

BEHAVIORS ASSOCIATED WITH A HEALING HELPING RELATIONSHIP

Presence

Use of presence can be thought of as a particular way of using the self therapeutically (Minicucci, 1998). "*Presence* is of Latin and French derivation from the words *prae*, meaning in front, and *sens*, meaning being. Thus, the word presence has both spatial and temporal connotations. The same word in its verb form, *praesentare*, means to place before, to hold out, to offer, from which the nouns *gift* and *present* evolved" (Skeats, 1969, p. 409). Absence is the opposite of presence from *ab*, meaning away from, and *sens*, meaning being. Thus, from the nature of the word itself, "nursing presence can be construed as a state in which the nurse is in the same place, near or in front of a [client], and in the same moment, holding out to the [client] the gift of care" (Doona et al., 1997, p. 6).

Presence as a nursing phenomenon emerged in the 1960s as a coherent and consistent philosophical term based on the philosophy of Martin Buber and the existentialism of Gabriel Marcel and Martin Heidegger (Doona et al., 1997). Buber (1970) described I-It and I-Thou relationships, both of which he considered necessary for existence. The I-It relationship offers "familiar order, reliable experience, and continuity in space and time," while I-Thou relationships are "characterized by reciprocity or mutuality, spontaneity, acceptance, and confirmation of otherness or uniqueness, immediacy, wholeness, exclusiveness, [and] inclusion" (Cohn, 2001, p. 171).

For Heidegger (1987), presence means *being*. "Being then is the very personal, individual, unique attribute, quality, or spirit which makes one human" (Gilje, 1992, p. 55). "Being as a noun is commonly defined as *existence* and *actuality*. A synonym for being is *essence*.... To be present implies a quality and essence of being in the moment" (Dossey et al., 1995, pp. 67, 69). A major defining attribute of presence is the ability to psychologically or emotionally be with or attend to a person, place, or object. Valuing being and knowing are essential processes for understanding the concept and applying it to human experiences (Gilje, 1992).

Easter (2000) identified four distinct modes of presence. These are:

- *Physical presence*. Requires proximity or physical closeness; includes movement, touching, and being there.

- *Therapeutic presence*. "Used to provide support, hope, comfort, relaxation, and an increased ability to cope" (p. 366).

- *Holistic presence*. "It requires a nurse's mind, body, and spirit to connect with a [client's] mind, body, and spirit" (p. 369).

- *Spiritual presence*. Spirit-to-spirit communion.

Presence is an important part of several nursing theories, including those of Patterson and Zderad (1976), Parse (1990), and Watson (1985). Patterson and Zderad emphasize mutual outcomes. "Well-being and authenticity are benefits that both the [client] and the nurse experience.... Presence is the medium through which health in and between both the [client] and nurse is catalyzed. In this way, [clients] and nurses are equal partners in care" (Minicucci, 1998, pp. 10-11). Patterson and Zderad explicitly identify two components of presence: the physical (being there) and the psychological (being with). Table 10-2 differentiates "being there" and "being with."

Parse (1990, p. 139) suggests that "to approach a person as a nurturing gardener rather than a 'fix it' mechanic, believing that each person lives value priorities is to be truly present to the person as the person changes patterns of health.... It is a subject-to-subject interrelationship, a loving, true presence with the other to enhance the quality of life." In Parse's view, the true presence of the nurse is a way of "being with" in which a knowledgeable nurse is authentic, open, self-giving, and attentive to moment-to-moment changes in meaning within the relationship.

The concept of presence is mentioned rather than discussed throughout Watson's work. For example, she indicates that the development of her work was "influenced by Peplau's interpersonal domain and the notion of 'therapeutic use of self,' which later manifested... as presence, authentic caring relationship" (Watson, 1997, p. 49). However, it seems clear that presence is an essential and integral concept to Watson. This is evident when she discusses transpersonal caring, [which] "calls forth an authenticity of being and becoming, an ability to be present, to be reflective, to attend to mutuality of being and centering one's consciousness and intentionality toward caring, healing, wholeness, and health" (Watson, 1997, p. 51).

Presence has been described by a number of other nurses. For example, Doona and colleagues (1997, p. 3) describe nursing presence as "an intersubjective encounter between a nurse and a [client] in which the nurse encounters the [client] as a unique human being in a unique situation and chooses to 'spend' herself on his behalf." McKivergin (1997, p. 17) describes presence as "a multidimensional state of being available in a situation with the wholeness of one's individual being; relational style and quality of 'being with' rather than 'doing to'... and creates the space and opportunity for another to feel safe." Moch and Schaefer (1998, pp. 159-161) describe presence as "a process of being available with the whole of oneself and open to the experience of another through a reciprocal interpersonal encounter.... Presence implies an openness, a receptivity, readiness, or availability on the part of the nurse.... The union or total presencing that happens through the experience leads to healing, discovery, and finding meaning."

Romick (1997) frames presence within an encounter between a traveler and guide. Presence includes the guide's willingness to "be with another's reality," concentrate, fully attend, and let go of the outcome of the session. It includes intuitive inner knowing and "requires trust, empathy, acceptance, honesty, intention, and practice" (p. 473).

"The core element in presence is 'being there'... described as a gift of self... that is conveyed through open and giving behaviors of the nurse" (Osterman & Schwartz-Barcott, 1996, p. 24). Additionally, Fredriksson (1999) describes "being with" presence as a gift and an invitation, with the client choosing whether to accept or reject the gift. Osterman and Schwartz-Barcott (1996) describe four degrees of intensity of presence: presence, partial presence, full presence, and transcendent presence. Presence and partial presence involve being physically present with another

Table 10-2	**Differentiating "Being There" from "Being With"**	
	BEING THERE	BEING WITH
What is it?	A "state of being in one place and not elsewhere" in the context of another, and with attentive attitude focus on the other.	A gift of self that is conveyed through being available and at the disposal of the other person with all of self. An intersubjective encounter between a nurse and a patient in which the nurse encounters the patient as a unique human being in a unique situation and chooses to spend herself on the patient's behalf, while at the same time the patient invites the nurse into his experience.
Preconditions	To be physically close to a patient while using a quiet tone of voice, appropriate choice of words, eye contact and touch in ways that establish rapport and communicate empathy for the patient.	To be in touch with self and bring one's own humanness and acceptance of self to the encounter. To make room internally for the other person, being willing to be involved. To remain with the patient, enduring one's feelings of discomfort and awkwardness.
What is happening? (process)	Physically attending behavior, sensitivity to body language, use of touch in a judicious way to comfort or express concern, making eye contact and leaning forward toward the other. Listening, comfortable silence, and communication of understanding of the patient's experience.	A flow of feelings between two persons with different modes of being in a shared situation, in which the one caring is touched by the patient's feelings. Being there in the midst of a helpless situation rather than saying or doing the "right thing." Experience one's powerlessness in confronting, not knowing, not curing, and not healing.

continued

Table 10-2	*Differentiating "Being There" from "Being With" (continued)*	
	BEING THERE	BEING WITH
What does it lead to? (outcomes)	Assists coping. Diminishes intensity of feelings such as fear, powerlessness, anxiety, isolation, and distress. Support, comfort, sustained assistance, encouragement, and motivation. A sense of security and feeling reassured.	Alleviation of suffering. Growth through difficult experiences. Lessening of the sense of isolation, development of a sense of relationship and connectedness. Lessening of the sense of vulnerabilty, development of a sense of caring and being heard. Feelings and thoughts put into words. New ways of interpreting and understanding one's self-development, leading to new directions, solutions, decisions, and choices.

Reprinted from Frederiksson, L. (1999). Modes of relating in a caring conversation: A research synthesis on presence, touch, and listening. *J Adv Nurs, 30*, 1170, with permission of Blackwell Science Ltd.

person, while full and transcendent presence involve being physically and psychologically present. Additional characteristics of these four "ways of being there" are described in Table 10-3.

The nurse has to be present to her- or himself in order to "discover other presences." The nurse is invited to participate in the client's experience, and the nurse "gains affirmation of herself as a person and as a professional" instead of gaining satisfaction for caring for the client's needs (Doona et al., 1997, pp. 7-8).

Additional, selected descriptors of presence are discussed below:

1. "Nursing presence is an all-or-none phenomenon" (Doona et al., 1999, p. 57).

2. "Presence cannot be used or commanded because it is a choice that a nurse makes" (Doona et al., 1997, p. 11).

3. Presence cannot be made into a technique and cannot be taught, but can be cultivated.

4. Presence "does not depend on physical proximity" (McKivergin, 1997, p. 19). What is important is being there with the other person in a way the other person perceives as full of meaning, not the physical proximity of the nurse being in the same place and at the same time with a client.

Presence: *Characteristics of Four Ways of Being There*

Table 10-3

CHARACTERISTICS	PRESENCE	PARTIAL PRESENCE	FULL PRESENCE	TRANSCENDENT PRESENCE
Quality of being there	Physically present in context of another.	Physically present in context of another.	Physically present (there) (physical attending behavior—eye contact leaning toward). Psychologically present (with) (attentive listening behavior).	Physically present. Psychologically present (metaphysical beliefs). Holistic.
Focus of energy	Self-absorbed.	Objects or tasks in environment, relevant to the other individual but none of the energy is directed at the other. Mechanical/Technical reality.	Self/other (focusing on other influences response-reciprocal).	Centered (drawing from universal energy). Subject/Subject leads to oneness.
	Personal, subjective reality.		Present oriented (here and now) anchoring in present reality.	Transcending and oriented beyond here and now; sustaining while at the same time transforming reality.
Nature of interaction	No interaction, self-absorbed, intrapersonal encounter.	Interaction with part of other encounter.	Interactive; essential communication; boundaries—role constraints; professional relationship dyad caring.	Relationship; high degree of skilled communication; role free; human intimacy/love; humanistic caring, no boundaries; monad relationship.

continued

Table 10-3   *Presence: Characteristics of Four Ways of Being There (continued)*

CHARACTERISTICS	PRESENCE	PARTIAL PRESENCE	FULL PRESENCE	TRANSCENDENT PRESENCE
Positive outcomes	Reduce stress; reassurance that someone is there; may be quieting and restorative; facilitates creative thinking.	Reduce stress; solving a mechanical problem; reduces amount of stimuli in an encounter.	Solving of a human problem; relief of a here-and-now distress.	Transformations decreased loneliness; expansion of consciousness; spiritual peace, hope, and meaning in one's existence (love/connectedness); nice feeling generated in the environment; transpersonal (oneness).
Negative outcomes	No interpersonal engagement—missed communication; isolation, withdrawn, increased anxiety.	No interpersonal connectedness.	May be too much energy for recipient. Energy not always available for full presence; increased anxiety.	Fusion and possible loss of objective reality; danger of taking on recipient's problems.

Reprinted from Osterman, P., & Schwartz-Barcott, D. (1996). Presence: Four ways of being there. *Nursing Forum, 31,* 25. Used with permission.

5. The attitude shifts from "What can I do?" to "How can I be with the person in this moment?" The idea is to be with a client in a way that acknowledges a shared humanity.

6. "Being there" is "being with," an invitation that is accepted or rejected.

7. Presence is self-giving to another at the moment-at-hand, being available and at the disposal of the other.

8. Presence involves connecting with the client's experience and co-creating the outcome rather than imposing a preconceived agenda for the moment.

9. The process may be uncomfortable because remaining with the person exposes one's humanness and vulnerability (McKivergin, 1997).

10. Listening to the other is the context for informed judgment.

Barriers to Presence

The typical nursing work environment contains many barriers to presence. Many nurses cite a lack of time, high workload, tiredness, competing demands, distractions, and stress as factors that diminish nurse-client relationships. Other constraints include busyness and a goal-oriented task focus, feelings of inadequacy, a need to be in control, lack of openness, and concern about what other people will think. In addition, the client may not welcome presence, even though "the absence of nursing presence leaves [clients] feeling depersonalized and alone... the danger of nursing absence" (Doona et al., 1997, p. 5). Finally, there may be a clash of values between presence and the "professional" distance taught in many nursing schools.

Outcomes of Presence

In contrast to the depersonalization that characterizes many nurse-client relationships, McKivergin (1997) and Godkin (2001) suggest that for the client, presence can result in increased coping strength, even in the midst of unchanged circumstances; achievement of client goals; satisfaction with nursing care; healing and a sense of well-being; growth; a lessened sense of isolation with more connections; a decreased sense of vulnerability; and neutralization of the intimidating atmosphere of the health care system. For the nurse, presence can provide increased confidence in one's competence, job satisfaction, and joy.

A healing helping relationship includes other behaviors in addition to presence, including mindfulness, relating, respect, connected caring, genuineness, reciprocity, active listening, empathy, and communication. These behaviors are discussed in the next section.

Mindfulness

A healing helping relationship requires conscious attention (mindfulness). The nurse must focus and center her- or himself and detach from other distractions. Mindfulness involves the combination of slowing down and bringing one's full attention (thoughts, feelings, and bodily sensations) to the activity of the moment (Wells-Federman, 1996). See Chapter 15, *Reducing Energy Depletion: Relaxation and Stress Reduction*, for a discussion of mindfulness in relation to meditation and relaxation.

Centering

The centering process promotes openness and readiness for caring, both of which are essential to interpersonal presence (Moch & Schaefer, 1998). The concept of patterning energy is the basis for centering. Centering also is used in meditation, therapeutic touch, guided imagery, and self-hypnosis. "The experience of being centered is quiet, relaxed, peaceful, and insightful; a sense of well-being is established, whole and unitary, focused, compassionate, and timeless" (Dole, 1996, p. 34).

Centering is a powerful and easily achieved skill that can prevent fatigue, stress, depression, or anger when working with a client who displays these qualities. "Centering allows the practitioner to be separate from, yet open to, input from clients" (Clark, 1996, p. 21). The process of centering can be accomplished sitting or lying down, often with the eyes closed. The nurse chooses to acknowledge and then to release thoughts and tension. When breathing in, a calming thought is brought into and throughout the body. When breathing out, an awareness of tension is acknowledged and released naturally with the breath (Dole, 1996). One technique to facilitate centering is presented in Box 10-1.

Box 10-1

A Technique to Facilitate Centering

1. Sit in a comfortable chair with feet flat on the floor and hands resting quietly in your lap; close your eyes.
2. Check out your body for tension spots and relax these areas as you exhale.
3. Inhale easily, filling your body with relaxation.
4. Exhale, moving your breathing to your center, about the level of your navel.
5. Continue breathing in this manner until you feel calm, integrated, unified, and focused.
6. (Optional) Picture the body surrounded by a protective shield that allows positive energy in, but keeps negative energy out. The shield may be conceived as a color, light source, or spiritual sense.

Source: Clark, C. C. (1996). *Wellness practitioner* (2nd ed., pp. 21-22). New York: Springer.

Relating

Relating refers to establishing or demonstrating a connection (Soukhanov, 1992), which is essential to the establishment of a healing helping relationship. Relating in a healing helping relationship can be a connection with high intersubjectivity or a contact with limited intersubjectivity. "In a connection, the nurse is listening, using caring and connective touch and is present as 'being with' the [client]. In contrast, in a contact, the nurse is hearing, using task-orientated touch, and is present as 'being there' for the [client]" (Fredriksson, 1999, p. 1167).

Hartrick (1997) has identified relational capacities as taking initiative, being authentic and responsive, being open to mutuality and synchrony, honoring complexity and ambiguity, and relating intentionally. The focus for both the nurse and the client is on "being with" another person, sharing commonalties and differences of visions and goals, expanding the capacity to trust and experience uncertainty, and fostering the client's discovery of choice and power within his or her experience of health (Hartrick, 1997).

Respect

Respect is feeling or showing deferential regard or esteem (Soukhanov, 1992). Respect is demonstrated through acknowledgment (Smith, 1992). Respect is a nonpossessive affirmation that builds self-esteem and positive self-image. In a healing helping relationship, respect is demonstrated by equality, mutuality, and shared thinking about strengths and problems.

Connected Caring

Caring is "a nurturing way of relating to a valued other toward whom one feels a personal sense of commitment and responsibility.... The nurse cares without obligating the client to reciprocate" (Swanson, 1991, p. 165). According to Swanson (1991), the five categories or processes of caring are knowing, being with, doing for, enabling, and maintaining belief.

Caring has been described as overcoming the fear of crossing the boundaries to achieve connection, intimacy, and mutuality in a "sharing of humanness" (Gilje, 1992, p. 63). Connection indicates making contact, joining together, and linking through association with others to create a bond or special harmonious relationship with another person. Growth, integration, and healing are outcomes of connection and caring. Connecting takes courage and a willingness to take a risk (Sherwood, 1997).

The use of touch demonstrates and symbolizes connection with another in ways that can be both beneficial and harmful: to soothe, calm or comfort; to intervene directly or manipulate; to arouse, stimulate and seduce; or to hurt and damage. "The sensitive use of touch often depends on intuition rather than intellect.... When [clients] experience medical care as if their bodies were being dealt with independently of their minds, they complain of being treated impersonally, as unthinking objects" (Mitchell & Cormack, 1998, p. 65).

Genuineness (Authenticity)

In defining genuineness, which is used synonymously with authenticity, phrases such as "being actually and precisely what is claimed," acting in "good faith," and being "sincere" are used. "Being genuine means that you send the other person the real picture of you, not one distorted by being different than how you really think or feel" (Smith, 1992, p. 74). The genuine nurse in a healing helping relationship acts in ways that are unrehearsed and non-contrived, taking a risk by expressing negative thoughts, and confronting others when necessary.

Reciprocity

There is a fundamental difference between "understanding as an individual achievement and understanding as a mutual process or dialogue" (Widdershoven, 1999, p. 1163). Reciprocity is an interpersonal exchange that is symmetrical or equivalent in quality (Mendias, 1997). In addition, "therapeutic reciprocity is a mutual, collaborative, probabalistic, instructive, and empowering exchange of feelings, thoughts, and behaviors between nurse and client for the purpose of enhancing the human outcomes of the relationship for all parties concerned" (Marck, 1990, p. 57).

Both Peplau and Watson discuss mutuality as a reciprocal process (Mendias, 1997). Peplau's concept of mutuality has been described as legitimizing growth in both clients and nurses, while Watson describes a reciprocal transaction between nurses and patients (Mendias, 1997). Mutuality involves mutual exchange, gain, and responsibility; shared meaning for the participants; empowerment from shared control of the nurse-client relationship; and status and power balance between the client and the nurse.

Active Listening

Listening has been described as "an active process of searching for meaning" (Moch & Schaefer, 1998, p. 163). Active, or "empathetic," listening requires discipline and skilled interpersonal communication, which can be hard work (Ryden, 1998, p. 170). The nurse must really concentrate and focus to interpret verbal and nonverbal messages from the client, recognize themes and patterns, try to determine what is really being said and hear what is left unsaid, assist the client to communicate a message more clearly, and communicate an understanding of the client's verbal and nonverbal messages. Being able to really observe, listen, and interpret the meaning of a client message is essential to understanding (Ryden, 1998).

Klagsbrun (2001) discusses focusing as an essential part of active listening. As an alternative to analyzing, focusing is described as a way of getting in touch with vague, embodied awareness of a felt sense. By paying attention to a particular feeling and then noticing what is evoked inside the body, a felt sense forms. The nurse needs to stay "respectful, friendly, and welcoming toward whatever emerges" (2001, p. 120). Focusing is enhanced when the nurse "clears a space," by taking 5 minutes routinely to inventory and distance from stressors. Invoking and maintaining positive feelings also helps. Clients can use focusing to "get distance from [the] pain, can hear from it, or befriend it," allay apprehension, "promote acceptance and acknowledgment of the fearful and anxious place inside," gain a sense of mastery and control, and feel empowered (2001, p. 124).

Strategies to facilitate active listening are presented in Box 10-2.

Several authors (Clark, 1996, p. 21; McKay et al., 1995, pp. 16-19) suggest that by differentiating oneself from clients through the act of centering, many blocks to listening are removed. Selected blocks to listening are presented in Box 10-3.

Centering reduces blocks to listening by restoring internal quiet, thereby permitting the nurse to give attention and listen actively. Ryden (1998, p. 170) states that "active listening is the cognitive and communicative component of empathy."

Empathy

Empathy involves the ability to recognize and to some extent share the emotions and states of mind of another and to understand the meaning and significance of that person's

Box 10-2

Strategies to Facilitate Active Listening

- When giving external feedback, reflect the essence of what you have understood the client to say, ask for elaboration, encourage specificity and concreteness in place of vague global statements, and point out discrepancies in communication

- When interpreting the meaning of what is heard, critical thinking skills in addition to listening are required

- Use adeptness and sensitivity when communicating to the client what is understood

- Attempt to match the intensity of the feeling that has been communicated rather than overstating or minimizing

- Phrase interpretation in a tentative way rather than as a dogmatic assertion

- Allow the client's response to determine the direction of the subsequent interaction

Source: Ryden, M. B. (1998). Active listening. In M. Snyder, & R. Lindquist, *Complementary/alternative therapies in nursing* (3rd ed., pp. 173-174). New York: Springer.

behavior. Empathy is a feeling that is composed of thoughts and emotions related to understanding the client's situation (Baillie, 1996). Components of empathy have been described as moral compassion and concern for the welfare of others; emotive ability to subjectively perceive and share another person's psychological state or intrinsic feelings; cognitive intellectual ability to understand another's perspective; and behavioral ability to communicate empathetic understanding and concern. The actions resulting from empathy can be therapeutic (Morse et al., 1992).

The defining attributes of empathy include seeing the world as others see it, being nonjudgmental, understanding another's feelings, and communicating the understanding (Wiseman, 1996). Other characteristics include experiential knowledge, and the personal and human qualities of being able to trust, be honest and self-aware, and have reflective ability. Getting to know the patient promotes closeness and helps to develop rapport. Empathy is different from sympathy, "sympathy being more 'feeling sorry' for another person, while empathy requires more of an understanding of what the other person is experiencing" (Baillie, 1996, p. 1302).

Challenges point out discrepancies or contradictions that the client is unaware of or unwilling to change. "Discrepancies and contradictions are important because they are often signs of unresolved issues, ambivalence, or suppressed or repressed feelings" (Hill, 2004, p.

Box 10-3

Selected Blocks to Listening

- *Comparing.* Only partially listening because of trying to assess who is smarter, more competent, more emotionally healthy, or suffering more.

- *Mind reading.* Not paying attention to what is being communicated; trying to figure out what the client is really thinking and feeling, rather than listening closely to what is being said.

- *Rehearsing.* Not listening because of rehearsing what to say next.

- *Filtering.* Listening to only part of what is said.

- *Judging.* Not paying attention because the client's comments have already been labeled as stupid or unqualified.

- *Dreaming.* Not listening because the client says something that triggers a chain of private associations.

- *Identifying.* Taking what the client says and referring it back to one's own experience.

- *Advising.* Not listening for a full expression of the issue prior to suggesting what one should do.

- *Sparring.* Looking for ways to disagree, discount, or put down what the other person says.

- *Being right.* Unable to listen to criticism.

- *Derailing.* Changing the subject when bored or uncomfortable (e.g., joking).

- *Placating.* Agreeing with everything to be pleasant and nice.

---

227). Challenges are invitations to clients to become aware of their maladaptive issues, thoughts, feelings, and behaviors.

Our goal as helpers is not to break down or remove all of the defenses, but to give clients the option of choosing when and how often to use defenses. Another reason for using challenges is to help clients gain insight (p. 230).

A major task for helpers is presenting challenges in such a way that clients can hear them and feel supported rather than attacked. With challenges, helpers indicate that some aspect of a client's life is incongruent or problematic and imply that a client should change to feel, think, or act differently. Challenges should be done carefully, gently, respectfully, tentatively, thoughtfully, and with empathy. Challenges are most effective in the context of a caring and respectful therapeutic relationship.

Helpful hints to consider when using challenge in a relationship (Hill, 2004) are to:

- look for specific markers that indicate readiness for receiving challenges. Clients who are at precontemplation and contemplation stages of change may need a challenge to jolt them out of their complacency.

- use challenge as soon as possible after an example of the client's inconsistent behaviors.

- maintain a manner of puzzlement rather than hostility. Do not make judgments. A challenge should not be a criticism, but an encouragement for deeper examination.

- if you think your challenge was accurate but your client denies or dismisses it, you may need to back off until the client can handle the challenge or until you have more evidence for your observations.

- observe your client's reactions carefully. Listen attentively and observe the client's nonverbal behavior. Keep the lines of communication open.

- consider repeating challenges several times, in different ways, and applying them to different situations, so clients can hear the challenge and think about the issue in different ways.

- be warm and empathetic in challenging. Remember that you are offering your perception rather than providing the "truth."

- use nonabrasive words and state the challenge as a hunch rather than an accusation.

- not make judgments or interpretations.

- be curious and collaborative in working with clients.

- not be aggressive or blaming. Do not play a game of "gotcha" or try to score points by pointing out the client's inconsistencies. Be careful not to come across as trying to pin blame on the client.

- be alert to the client's culturally based reactions.

- use specific examples as evidence. A specific example is easier to respond to than a global characterization.

- give an example of something that just happened rather than a distant example that the client is not likely to remember.

- make sure the challenge is not for your needs (e.g., to appear insightful, to retaliate, or to elevate yourself in comparison with the client).

- not apologize before delivering the challenge or minimize its value.

- if the client is upset by the challenge or you feel you have blundered badly, apologize and ask how the client is feeling. Avoid apologizing too much or too often.

- leave enough time after a challenge to talk about it and to help the client learn from it. It takes time to process the challenge.

- follow challenges with reflections of feelings and open questions about feelings. When clients have come to a new awareness about their thoughts, behaviors, or feelings, you might go on to interpret or investigate the reason for them.

Communication

One aspect of a healing helping relationship that matters very much to clients is the nurse's ability and willingness to communicate effectively, both in terms of finding out what is important from the client's point of view and in conveying information and explanations back to the client. Knowledge and information can provide a feeling of control that helps to reduce anxiety and may have a direct association with the achievement of better outcomes. "Control comes through being able to do something oneself in order to manage the illness" (Mitchell & Cormack, 1998, p. 55). However, "the concept of empowerment becomes fundamentally flawed if positive outcomes are only identified as situations when the client makes the choice the nurse wanted them to make" (Benson & Latter, 1998, p. 106).

Mitchell & Cormack (1998, pp. 73-74) propose a number of concrete suggestions to enhance good communication in nursing practice:

1. Good communication takes place in the context of a respectful and caring therapeutic relationship. The tasks of the nurse are:

   - To negotiate an authentic relationship that may change over time and that is suited to the needs of the particular client

   - To listen carefully to what the client wants to communicate (both with words and with the body)

   - To offer support, encouragement, and realistic hope

   - To be sensitive to the client's emotional state and needs

2. Good communication requires the ability to take the other person's perspective into account. The nurse should try to clarify the client's beliefs, thoughts, and feelings about health and illness.

3. The nurse should also try to convey her perspective at a pace and level relevant to the client's understanding and desire to know. It is best to do this using the client's language, wherever possible, using words and metaphors that will be accessible.

4. Good communication includes trying to understand the person's experiences of the consequences of illness. Serious attention should be given to the client's account of their health history.

5. Clear, open, and respectful communication provides a framework for a shared understanding between client and nurse, which will change and develop over time.

The emphasis in this chapter has been on a healing helping relationship based on Gadamer's third kind of interpersonal understanding. It has been proposed that health is facilitated within a relationship that is characterized by such behaviors as presence, mindfulness, respect, genuineness, active listening, empathy, and communication. A healing helping relationship can be a mechanism for enhanced sense of well-being, growth, and the facilitation of health of both the nurse and the client.

Chapter Key Points

- Many nurses use a prescriptive approach to health promotion.

- The nurse healer's role is to facilitate another person's growth and wholeness, while being open to her own growth and change.

- Healing occurs within the person, and external interventions mobilize the client's inner healing resources.

- Through presence, "being there" and "being with," the nurse gives of him- or herself. The client has the choice to accept or reject the gift.

- Behaviors associated with a healing helping relationship include presence, mindfulness, relating, respect, connected caring, genuineness, reciprocity, active listening, empathy, and communication.

References

Baillie, L. (1996). A phenomenological study of the nature of empathy. *J Adv Nurs, 24,* 1300-1308.

Benson, A., & Latter, S. (1998). Implementing health promoting nursing: The integration of interpersonal skills and health promotion. *J Adv Nurs, 27,* 100-107.

Buber, M. (1970). *I and Thou* (W. Kaufman, Trans.). New York: Charles Scribner's Sons.

Clark, C. C. (1996). *Wellness practitioner* (2nd ed). New York: Springer.

Cohn, F. (2001). Existential medicine: Martin Buber and physician-patient relationships. *Journal of Continuing Education in the Health Professions, 21,* 170-181.

Cowling, W. R. (2000). Healing as appreciating wholeness. *Advances in Nursing Science, 22,* 16-32.

Dole, P. J. (1996). Centering: Reducing rape trauma syndrome anxiety during a gynecologic examination. *Journal of Psychosocial Nursing, 34,* 32-37.

Doona, M. E., Chase, S. K., & Haggerty, L. A. (1999). Nursing presence: As real as a milky way bar. *Journal of Holistic Nursing, 17,* 54-70.

Doona, M. E., Haggerty, L. A., & Chase, S. K., (1997). Nursing presence: An existential exploration of the concept. *Scholarly Inquiry for Nursing Practice: An International Journal, 11,* 3-16.

Dossey, B. M., Keegan, L., Guzzetta, C. E., & Kolkmeier, L. G. (1995). *Holistic nursing: A handbook for practice* (2nd ed.). Gaithersburg, MD: Aspen.

Easter, A. (2000). Construct analysis of four modes of being present. *Journal of Holistic Nursing, 18,* 362-377.

Fredriksson, L. (1999). Modes of relating in a caring conversation: A research synthesis on presence, touch, and listening. *Journal of Advanced Nursing, 30,* 1167-1176.

Gadamer, H. G. (1960). *Wahrheit and methods*. Tubingen, Germany: J. C. B. Mohr.

Gilje, F. (1992). Being there: An analysis of the concept of presence. In D. A. Gaut (Ed.), *The presence of caring in nursing* (pp. 53-67). New York: National League for Nursing.

Godkin, J. (2001). Healing presence. *Journal of Holistic Nursing, 19*, 5-21.

Hartrick, G. (1997). Relational capacity: The foundation for interpersonal nursing practice. *Journal of Advanced Nursing, 26*, 523-528.

Heidegger, M. (1987). *An introduction to metaphysics*. New Haven, CT: Yale University Press.

Hill, C. E. (2004). *Helping skills. Facilitating exploration, insight, and action* (2nd ed.). Washington, DC: Usical Association.

Keegan, L. (1994). *The nurse as healer*. Albany, NY: Delmar.

Klagsbrun, J. (2001). Listening and focusing: Holistic health care tools for nurses. *Nursing Clinics of North America, 36*, 115-129.

Kritek, P. B. (1997). Healing: A central nursing construct—Reflections on meaning. In P. B. Kritek (Ed.), *Reflections on healing. A central nursing construct* (pp. 11-27). New York: National League for Nursing.

Lerner, M. (1994). *Choices in healing*. Cambridge, MA: Massachusetts Institute of Technology.

Lyons, M. (1988). Two perspectives on self, relationships, and morality. In C. Gilligan (Ed.), *Mapping the moral domain: A contribution of women's thinking to psychological theory and education* (pp. 21-48). Cambridge, MA: Harvard University Press.

Marck, P. (1990). Therapeutic reciprocity: A caring phenomenon. *Advances in Nursing Science, 13*, 49-59.

McKay, M., Davis, M., & Fanning, P. (1995). *Messages: The communication book* (2nd ed.). Oakland, CA: New Harbinger.

McKivergin, M. (1997). The nurse as an instrument of healing. In B. M. Dossey (Ed.), *Core curriculum for holistic nursing* (pp. 17-25). Gaithersburg, MD: Aspen.

McKivergin, M. (2000). The nurse as an instrument of healing. In B. M. Dossey, L. Keegan, & C. E. Guzzetta (Eds.), *Holistic nursing: A handbook for practice* (3rd ed.). Gaithersburg, MD: Aspen.

Mendias, E. P. (1997). Reciprocity in the healing relationship between nurse and patient. In P. B. Kritek (Ed.), *Reflections on healing: A central nursing construct* (pp. 435-451). New York: National League for Nursing.

Minicucci, D. S. (1998). A review and synthesis of the literature: The use of presence in the nursing care of families. *Journal of the New York State Nurses Association, 29*, 9-15.

Mitchell, A., & Cormack, M. (1998). *The therapeutic relationship in complementary health care*. Edinburgh, UK: Churchill Livingstone.

Moch, S., & Schaefer, C. (1998). Presence. In M. Snyder, & R. Lindquist (Eds.), *Complementary/alternative therapies in nursing* (3rd ed., pp. 159-168). New York: Springer.

Morse, J. M., Anderson, G., Bottoroff, J. L., Yonge, O., O'Brien, B., Solberg, S. M., et al. (1992). Exploring empathy: A conceptual fit for nursing practice? *Image: Journal of Nursing Scholarship, 24*, 273-280.

Morse, J. M., Havens, G. A. D., & Wilson, S. (1997). The comforting interaction: Developing a model of nurse-patient relationship. *Scholarly Inquiry for Nursing Practice: An International Journal, 11*, 321-343.

Newman, M. A. (1999). The rhythm of relating in a paradigm of wholeness. *Image: Journal of Nursing Scholarship, 31*, 227-230.

Osterman, P., & Schwartz-Barcott, D. (1996). Presence: Four ways of being there. *Nursing Forum, 31*, 23-30.

Parse, R. R. (1990). Health: A personal commitment. *Nursing Science Quarterly, 3*, 136-140.

Patterson, J., & Zderad, L. (1976). *Humanistic nursing.* New York: Wiley.

Romick P. (1997). Psychosynthesis: A perspective for growth and healing of self. In P. B. Kritek (Ed.), *Reflections on healing: A central nursing construct* (pp. 435-451). New York: National League for Nursing.

Ryden, M. B. (1998). Active listening. In Snyder, M., & Lindquist, R. (Eds.), *Complementary/alternative therapies in nursing* (3rd ed., pp. 169-180). New York: Springer.

Sherwood, G. (1997). Patterns of caring: The healing connection of interpersonal harmony. *International Journal for Human Caring, 1*, 30-38.

Skeats, W. W. (1969). *A concise etymological dictionary of the English language.* New York: Capricorn.

Smith, S. (1992). Communications in nursing (2nd ed.). St. Louis: Mosby.

Soukhanov, A. H. (Ed.). (1992). *The American heritage dictionary of the English language* (3rd ed.). Boston: Houghton Mifflin.

Swanson, K. M. (1991). Empirical development of a middle range theory of caring. *Nurs Res, 40*, 161-166.

Watson, J. (1985). *Nursing: Human science and human care. A theory of nursing.* Norwalk, CT: Appleton-Century-Crofts.

Watson, J. (1997). The theory of human caring: Retrospective and prospective. *Nursing Science Quarterly, 10*, 49-52.

Wells-Federman, C. L. (1996). Awakening the nurse healer within. *Holistic Nursing Practice, 10*, 13-29.

Widdershoven, G. A. M. (1999). Care, cure and interpersonal understanding. *Journal of Advanced Nursing, 29*, 1163-1169.

Wiseman, T. (1996). A concept analysis of empathy. *Journal of Advanced Nursing, 23*, 1162-1167.

EMPOWERING COMMUNITY HEALTH

Abstract

Traditionally, health promotion activities have been directed at individual behavior change, and many interventions with the individual as the client may be community-based. In this chapter, however, the community is the client, and the emphasis is on community-level intervention to modify the social or power structure or allocation of resources of the community. It is proposed that the central processes for nursing facilitation of community-level change are empowerment, a process of increasing personal, interpersonal, or political power; interdisciplinary collaboration; and capacity building, the nurturing and building on strengths and resources already present in the community. Finally, principles for community organization and community-level health promotion are discussed.

Learning Outcomes

By the end of the chapter the student should be able to:

- Differentiate between community as place, social interaction, and political and social responsibility

- Differentiate between community-based and community-level nursing interventions

- Describe elements of community

- Describe characteristics of functionalist, conflict, and community-level social change theories

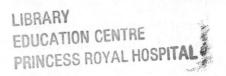

■ Discuss processes to empower individuals and communities

■ Differentiate between coordination, cooperation, and collaboration

■ Discuss individual, small group, and community levels of capacity building

■ Discuss strategies for community organizing to promote health

What Is Community?

Community has been defined as "a system of people with common values and institutions who identify with the system and share a locality, social structure, and personal relationships" (Hancock et al., 1997, p. 230). There are various approaches to community, including community as place, social interaction, and political/social responsibility (Patrick & Wickizer, 1995), as well as a holograph (Davis, 2000), each of which will be explored separately in the following sections.

COMMUNITY AS PLACE

Laffrey and Kulbok's (1999, p. 94) definition of community as "a designated area in which persons live, work, study, and play," is typical of community as place definitions. However, the field of human ecology, which draws analogies between plant ecology and the urban community, has expanded the geographic definition of community. The essential characteristics of community as defined by human ecology "are a population, territorially organized and more or less rooted in the soil it occupies, whose individual units live in a relationship of mutual interdependence" (Patrick & Wickizer, 1995, p. 49). From this perspective, both the localized population and the ecological boundaries of the community are influenced by the global economy, transportation, and mass communication (1995). Consequently, when defined primarily as place, community may be considered as "local places with distal influences" (1995, p. 68) such as the social and physical environment.

COMMUNITY AS SOCIAL INTERACTION

When community is viewed as social interaction, the emphasis is on a group of people sharing values and institutions. For example, Hancock and colleagues (1997, pp. 229–230) describe community as "a grouping of people who share a common purpose, interest or need, and who can express their relationship through communication face-to-face, as well as by other means, without difficulty." Israel, Checkoway, Schultz, and Zimmerman (1994, p. 151) more explicitly define community as "a locale or domain" (community as place) that is characterized by the following elements:

■ Membership, in the sense of identity and belonging

■ Common symbol systems, such as similar language, rituals, and ceremonies

■ Shared values, beliefs, and norms

■ Mutual influence, in which community members have influence and are influenced by each other

- Shared needs and a commitment to meeting them

- Shared emotional connection, in which members share common history, experiences, and mutual support

The community as social interaction perspective focuses on societal structures that can be considered community resources. Societal structures are functionally interdependent, relatively stable, enduring systems whose members share some consensus about societal goals, norms, and values (Thompson & Kinne, 1990). Patrick and Wickizer (1995) observe that household and family structure and the church are important sources of economic and social support. Households can be a source of resources and supports for dealing with social stress. Health is seen as "a resource of everyday life, not the objective of living" (Shields & Lindsey, 1998, p. 24)

COMMUNITY AS POLITICAL AND SOCIAL RESPONSIBILITY

The emphasis of health promotion in the community is changing lifestyle by changing socioeconomic-political structures in the local environment (Guldan, 1996). According to Patrick and Wickizer (1995), community involves a dynamic interaction in social relationships that creates a sense of solidarity, mutual obligation, and responsibility for social survival. However, Milio (1996, p. 38) suggests that "community in spirit and in a place are two sides of a coin," in which frequent and sustained contact between people creates a mutual identity and a sense of social responsibility for creating healthy surroundings. As a result of the surge in electronic communications in the last quarter of the twentieth century, "imagined communities" have resulted in social and physical distancing of people, "creating a narrower sense of place and social and local responsibility" (Milio, 1996, p. 38). There is concern that electronic communications may well reduce many elements of community, regardless of the definition.

HOLOGRAPHIC COMMUNITY

Davis (2000) moves beyond sociological or psychological definitions by describing community in terms of wholeness based on connection experienced through relationships. Community is defined as "a conscious connectedness based on shared values and moral integrity, where diversity within unity can be expressed, caring relationships experienced, learning environments that foster empowerment and development are evident, and individual and collective efforts are reflected and celebrated in mutual synergy toward greater levels of health for all" (2000, p. 296). Dimensions of this conception, each integral to the whole, are:

- *The consciousness of community* (awareness). An open connectedness to a greater world.

- *The heart of community* (values). Humanistic values based on human caring.

- *The soul of community* (service). Responsibility of serving others both personally and professionally.

- *The voice of community* (power). Operationalized as capacity, energy, and competence. "Principle-centered persons are change catalysts who influence without dominance and facilitate an empowerment process that creates synergistic solutions that are far better than individual efforts" (Davis, 2000, p. 297).

- *The body of community* (space, structure, relationships). The physical, social, economic, political, and relational structures of the environment.

- *The mind of community* (learning, development). Viewed as a transformative process to learn to solve problems and open the way for persons to empower themselves.

- *The spirit of community* (celebration, ritual). Common patterns that build bonds of intimacy and trust.

- *The vision of community* (health). Environments and expanding resources enable people to provide mutual support in functioning and developing to maximum potential.

The emphasis in this view of holographic community is on the centrality of moral leadership by nurses "to promote public policy, build healthy communities, and strengthen community action" (Davis, 2000, p. 299). The model is promoted as a way to recognize interconnectedness and interdependence in partnerships for community care, provide a vision for theory development, and guide decision making, health policy, and leadership skills such as mentoring, role modeling, advocacy, communication, priority setting, and creating values frameworks.

Elements of Community

Elements of community reflect all of the conceptions of community discussed in the previous section. Patrick and Wickizer (1995) have described several elements that are characteristic of community, including commitment, continuity, cohesion, and sense of community. Social interaction is important. Although some support such as informational, emotional, and instrumental support can be provided from a distance, vulnerable people require committed, direct, and continuous contact and continuity of leadership. Community cohesion, identity, and stability are affected by factors such as social mobility, intermarriage, changes in gender roles, the mixing of cultural traditions, and geographic mobility that contribute to a sense of loss of community. The sense of community includes a feeling of belonging and personal relatedness, the feeling that the person makes a difference to a group and that the group matters to them, the expectation that one's needs will be met through membership in the group, and a shared emotional connection and history. Additional elements of community that have been proposed include connectedness in social relationships (Patrick & Wickizer, 1995); participation in problem definition, planning, and resolution; maintenance of desired change (Thompson & Kinne, 1990); and a sense of responsibility or ownership over programs promoting change (Bracht, 1990).

What Is Social Change?

Change theories provides bases for understanding community health promotion. There are three major types of social change theories—functionalist theories, conflict theories, and community-level change theories. Characteristics of these major types of social change theories are summarized in Box 11-1.

Box 11-1

Characteristics of Major Social Change Theories

Functionalist theories:

- Emphasize patterns and processes that maintain a system.

- See social change as a gradual, adaptive process oriented toward system reform.

- Systems are based on cooperation and consensus, especially in the areas of societal goals, norms, and values.

- Norms are links that help hold the system together. When the system breaks down, external or environmental changes overwhelm the system, leading to new social norms and rules of conduct (Thompson & Kinne, 1990).

- Emphasize extrasystemic factors as impetus for change.

Conflict theories:

- See imbalance as a constant part of any system, resulting in ongoing adjustments.

- Social change occurs when one of several interests in a system gains ascendancy.

- Social norms help to maintain a system but in a coercive, rather than consensual sense, as those who control economic and political parts of a system establish norms and resist change.

- Emphasize internal explanations as impetus for change.

Community-level change theories:

- Deal with community organization and organizational relationships.

- Encourage local participation and ownership.

- Emphasize rational planning and problem solving.

- Encourage social action through mobilization and activation of disadvantaged groups who then demand redistribution of resources.

Thompson and Kinne (1990) have developed an integrated framework for social change. Consistent with a functionalist view, the system is initially stable, with most individuals and subsystems in agreement on societal goals, norms, and values. However, within the system are vested interests that act to preserve the status quo, and social movements that arise to conflict with vested interests. Change within the community may be planned either internally or externally. As the system interacts with the environment, external stimuli, in the form of laws, policies, and critical events, may influence norms and values within the system. External forces often use social planning or locality development theories to bring about change.

Additional theories can be used to support the major social change theories. For example, social network and interorganizational theories explain how connections are initiated and sustained at the subsystem level. Political and economic subsystems are frequently able to move a change in norms from the organizational level to the community level, after which the change is spread to other groups in the community through processes explained by diffusion, community development, and organizational development theories. Organizations that take on leadership roles become important as change agents. Individuals are subjected to changing norms and practices, with role models reinforcing new norms of behavior change. Social learning theory explains how individual change may occur in response to such role models. Eventually, due to organizational change and change in the interrelationships within subsystems, new norms and widespread individual change can occur.

Community-Level Interventions

Community health promotion is considered a collective rather than an individual approach to health, with the community involved in implementation and control of the process of the program (Hancock et al., 1997). Community ownership and program maintenance require early and sustained participation by community members and leaders (Bracht, 1990), although "community action does not relieve government of its responsibility to provide basic services for health to its citizens" (Kaseje, 1995, p. 211).

Community interventions may be community-based or targeted at the community-level. Community-based interventions are individual-directed attempts to modify or reallocate community social or power structures, whereas community-level interventions are organized to modify the entire community through community organization and activation (Patrick & Wickizer, 1995). Although most community nursing interventions in the past have been community-based, there is an urgent need for nurses to become involved in community-level interventions.

Community-level interventions involve active participation of the community at all stages of the intervention process (called community development in Australia, Canada, and the United Kingdom and community organizing in the Unite States) (Hancock et al., 1997). These are based on rejection both of professional dominance in decision making and emphasis on individual responsibility for health rather than on social, cultural, economic, and environmental determinants of health. This approach values the inclusion or involvement of historically marginalized individuals and groups, participation in and ownership of intervention programs by the community, and adaptation of strategies to local needs and resources (Judd et al., 2001).

The community-level approach to health promotion often includes multiple strategies, including "creating healthy public policy and supportive environments, fostering individual or group skills and capacities, strengthening community action and reorienting health services" (Judd et al., 2001, p. 370). It is assumed that permanent, large-scale behavior change is best achieved by developing positive role models for healthful behavior, while changing community expectations about health-related behavior. The community-level approach targets broad segments of the community or whole populations, emphasizing the role of social and environmental factors as key determinants of health.

EMPOWERMENT

Both conceptually and in practice, empowerment is the connecting link between health and community participation (Robertson & Minkler, 1994). In contrast to reactive approaches that are associated with a treatment or illness model, the concept of empowerment is positive and proactive (Israel et al., 1994). Community empowerment has been defined as "a social-action process in which individuals and groups act to gain mastery over their lives in the context of changing their social and political environment" (Wallerstein & Bernstein, 1994, p. 142), increasing their capacity to set priorities, control resources, and expand self-determination (Himmelman, 2001).

Personal, interpersonal, or political power is increased by empowerment (Robertson & Minkler, 1994). Given that power, "the capacity to produce intended results" (Himmelman, 2001, p. 278), makes it possible for individuals and communities to anticipate, influence, and participate with the environment, empowerment enables individuals and communities to take power and effectively transform their lives and their environment (Robertson & Minkler, 1994).

Dictionary definitions (Soukhanov, 1992) of empower include investing or giving power or authority to others, as well as enabling others, or giving others abilities in order that they may obtain power through their own efforts. However, if empowering means to give power to others, the empowering agent, such as the health professional, continues to control the terms of the interaction. As professionals often have more education, more access to sources of information, and use a different language to discuss health issues than either individual or community clients, "institutional embeddedness' confers a certain power on them" (Robertson & Minkler, 1994, p. 301). Consequently, clients remain relatively disempowered and continue to be the objects of professional actions (Labonte, 1994).

The lack of control over destiny that occurs with powerlessness promotes a susceptibility to disease for people who live in high demand or chronically marginalized situations and who lack adequate resources, supports, or abilities (Wallerstein, 1992). Relationships between governmental institutions and community groups can contribute to disempowerment. A more empowering relationship between professionals and clients and between institutions and community groups is needed for healthy social change (Labonte, 1994).

When power is taken rather than given, clients are able to set and achieve their own agendas (Robertson & Minkler, 1994). Power over clients in traditional hierarchical provider/client relationships tolerates others' views and tries to educate others to one's own terms, whereas power with clients respects others' views, trying to find common ground in a partnership between professionals and individuals or communities. (Labonte, 1994; Robertson & Minkler, 1994). However, Labonte (1994) suggests that one must have power in order to share it. Many nurses perceive a lack of professional autonomy, especially in acute care situations. "Disabling power-over tendencies within professional practice may simply reflect a projection of professional disempowerment" (p. 256). Figure 11-1 depicts the relationships in powerlessness and in empowerment.

Shields and Lindsey (1998) suggest that listening and critical reflection are important strategies that nurses can use to enhance empowerment of the community. Respect, trust, and

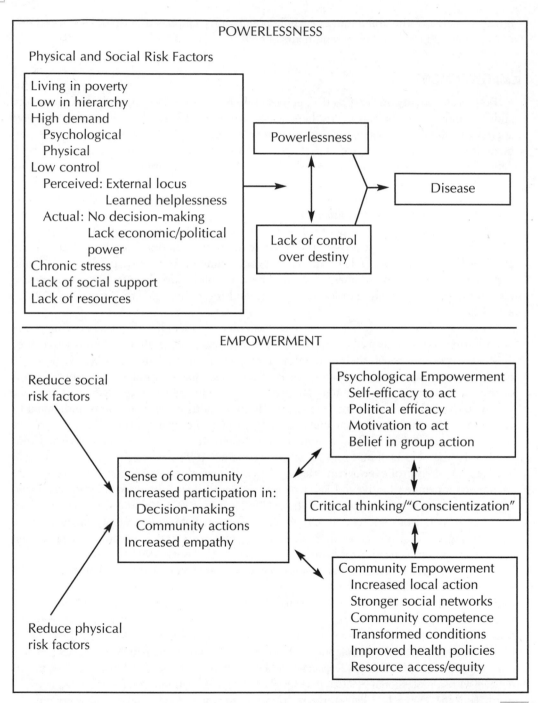

Figure 11-1. Relationships in powerlessness and empowerment (reprinted from Wallerstein, N. (1992). Powerlessness, empowerment, and health: Implications for health promotion programs, with permission of *American Journal of Health Promotion*, 6, 201).

a fundamental regard for people can be conveyed by listening, while critical reflection involves a conscious process of thinking about what is being heard. "The notion of voice, of having voice, and of giving voice to are central to community empowerment" (p. 30). Four components of listening and critical reflection have been proposed, including active engagement through participatory dialogue and critical questioning; identification of an emerging pattern in the dialogue; recognition of the capacity of the participants, with the nurse as a facilitator rather than the expert; and movement from dialogue to action.

Falk-Rafael (2001, p. 1) proposes that empowerment be considered as a process of evolving consciousness, "in which increasing awareness, knowledge, and skills interact with the clients' active participation to move toward actualizing potential." In this view, empowerment is an active, internal process of growth toward actualizing of one's potential. It occurs within the context of a nurturing and trusting nurse-client relationship, in which the nurse facilitates, rather than creates, empowerment in the community client. The process of becoming empowered evolves within the community, but nurses are also empowered in a reciprocal effect. Strategies to foster empowerment include collaborating with other health care professionals and using positional power, building capacity to help community members to identify the communities' health goals and resources, and using political processes to advocate for the community.

Collaboration

Collaboration is defined as "exchanging information, altering activities, sharing resources, and a willingness to enhance the capacity of another for mutual benefit and a common purpose; it requires the highest levels of trust, considerable amounts of time, and an extensive sharing of turf" (Himmelman, 2001, p. 278). "The distinguishing feature of collaborative partnerships for community health is broad community engagement in creating and sustaining conditions that promote and maintain behaviors associated with widespread health and well-being" (Roussos & Fawcett, 2000, pp. 369-370).

Collaboration incorporates but goes beyond cooperation and coordination. Cooperation is defined as "exchanging information, altering activities, and sharing resources for mutual benefit and a common purpose. It requires significant amounts of time, high levels of trust, and a significant sharing of turf" (Himmelman, 2001, p. 277-278). In contrast, coordination is defined as "exchanging information for mutual benefit and altering activities for a common purpose" (Himmelman, 2001, p. 277). It requires time and trust but does not necessitate sharing professional territory. The most direct form of coordination is mutual adjustment, in which two or more people simply adapt to each other, usually by informal communication, as their work progresses. A second mechanism is direct supervision, in which a hierarchy of authority is created by focusing responsibility for coordinating the work on someone who does not actually do the work, such as a supervisor or manager (Glouberman & Mintzberg, 2001). Additionally, coordination can also be achieved through standardization of work procedures, results or consequences, education or training, or socialization to establish common values, beliefs, and expectations. Glouberman and Mintzberg (2001) suggest that coordination of professional work through bridge building and mutual adjustment is preferable to the almost automatic standardization of skills and knowledge that is emphasized in the current health care system. What is needed is a culture that values attitudes of understanding, commitment, mutual respect, a sense of belonging, purpose and trust, encourages identification with collective need, and facilitates flexible communication among peers.

Laffrey and Kulbok (1999) emphasize the need for nurses to work in partnership with other team members to achieve comprehensive and holistic community care. Helman (1994) describes four different types of community health workers (CHWs) who are found primarily in indigenous cultures:

1. *Workers from the community*. They advise the community on preventive strategies; give advice on child care, healthy nutrition, immunizations, and hygiene; as well as providing some limited curative and first-aid services. They include "barefoot doctors" in China, family welfare educators in Botswana, the village health development workers in Indonesia, the village health volunteers in Thailand, and the community health agents in Egypt. They usually have a short course of training (a few weeks to a few months) and a small amount of equipment such as basic drugs, dressings, disinfectants, thermometer, and scales and charts. However, "the combination of inadequate diagnostic and treatment skills, infrequent supervision, and shortage of drugs undermine the acceptance of CHWs by their communities" (p. 370).

2. *Community health groups*. Are often organized to share information about health issues such as family planning or breast feeding and give help to their members. Many are women's groups.

3. *Traditional healers*. Examples include folk healers, a shaman, or "bone-setter." They are usually trained in an apprenticeship, and often claim to have some contact with the spirit world that is believed to aid in healing.

4. *Community leaders*. People of influence due to family position or job title and responsibility in the community. For example, a tribal head would be able to exert the authority of position and the influence of lineage.

In the United States, the emphasis of collaboration is on professional providers. "The purpose of interprofessional collaboration is to bring a broader scope of expertise to the efforts to improve the quality of care outcomes" (Schmitt, 2001, p. 53). It is assumed that a collaborative effort is needed for cost efficiencies, quality improvement, and comprehensive continuity of care. However, in a comprehensive review of research relating collaboration to improved quality of care, Schmitt (2001) described a number of conceptual and methodological challenges. Collaboration is a multidimensional construct that is not simply present or absent but is present to varying degrees. However, in many studies it is not clear whether the interest is in collaboration as a global concept or in specific components such as collegiality, interaction, coordination or communication. The measurement of outcomes has also been hindered by lack of conceptual clarity, and by the limited number of psychometrically evaluated instruments. Few studies have assessed longitudinal intervention effects. Schmitt (2001, p. 63) concludes, "if there is an important place for interprofessional collaboration in health care delivery then it is a high priority task to get on with the research, difficult as that is, that demonstrates what mix of collaborators, for what purposes, for whom, with what outcomes, and at what cost matters."

A number of benefits of interprofessional collaboration have been identified, including increased networking, information sharing, and resource access; attaining desired outcomes; enjoying working in the partnership; receiving personal recognition; and enhancement of skills. Costs include the time devoted; possible lack of direction, appreciation, recognition, or skills; being pressured for additional commitment; and loss of autonomy. A complete focus on interdisciplinary collaboration can result in loss of the identity of nursing (Disch, 2001). The degree of reciprosity and mutuality in the relationship between autonomous disciplines is critical (el Ansari & Phillips, 2001).

Long (2001) stresses incremental approaches to achieving interdisciplinary collaboration, defining interdisciplinary as activities that involve just two disciplines. Suggestions include focusing on small steps and moderate successes, taking advantage of committed leadership, and acknowledging the give and take, trust, and goodwill that are needed across professional boundaries. However, she acknowledges that professional orientation (identity and stature of one's own profession) and workplace structure (accreditation, licensure, national rankings, and practice reimbursement) tend to work against the success of interdisciplinary activities and toward the achievements, activities, or accomplishments of single disciplines.

Capacity Building

Capacity building as a process "is conceived of as the nurturing of and building upon the strengths, resources, and problem-solving abilities already present in individuals and communities" (Robertson & Minkler, 1994, p. 303) in order to "enhance the capacity of a system to prolong and multiply health effects" (Judd et al., 2001, p. 368). As an outcome, community capacity is "the characteristics of communities that affect their ability to identify, mobilize, and address social and public health problems" (Goodman, 1998, p. 259). In Freudenberg, Israel and colleagues (1994) suggest that the health professional identify and work within contexts that already show some sense of community. If community does not exist, then the initial task is to try to strengthen communality or recognize that the individual, family, or social network may be more appropriate as the unit of practice. Capacity building can occur at the individual, small group, or community level, affecting member, relational, organizational, and/or programmatic capacity.

Individual Level of Capacity Building

Individual or psychological empowerment refers to an individual's ability to make decisions and have control over his or her personal life. Psychological empowerment at the individual level combines personal efficacy and competence, a sense of mastery and control, and a process of participation to influence institutions and decisions. Additionally, empowerment incorporates an analytical understanding of the social and political context, and the cultivation of both individual and collective resources and skills for social action (Israel et al., 1994), contributing to the empowerment of the community.

According to Booker and colleagues (1997) and Foster-Fishman and colleagues (2001), characteristics of individual collaborative capacity and empowerment include:

- Valuing health enhancing outcomes

- Holding positive attitudes about the need for and value of collaboration

- Making decisions by consensus

- Sharing of information and power

- Demonstrating mutual respect and support

- Participating in supportive and noncontrolling relationships

- Having skills to cooperate with and respect others, resolve conflict, communicate, and understand member diversity

- Possessing perceived self-efficacy (a positive social identity)

- Having future life goals and perspective

- Feeling a sense of coherence in life

- Identifying with others and seeing problems in common

- Feeling capable of helping others

- Understanding member roles and responsibilities to build an effective coalition infrastructure

An internal feeling of increased efficacy and competence can provide a basis for willingness to take public action. Acceptance of individual responsibility for health is an important first step toward personal empowerment (Neighbors et al., 1995). Neighbors and colleagues (1995), in discussing self-help specifically among African Americans, stress that individual enterprise, mutual aid, and community action exist as fundamental strengths and critical survival strategies in the black community. However, even well-intentioned paternalistic efforts inadvertently reinforce dependency, an external locus of control, and a feeling of "collective despair and frustration that are major risk factors in poverty, substance abuse, violence, and other public health problems." (p. 285).

Small Group Level of Capacity Building

Capacity building can be enhanced with the support of a group. In interacting with others, people gain control, capacity, coherence, connectedness, and critical thinking. Both nurturing groups and groups that challenge the status quo are needed (Labonte, 1994). In addition, in group building with ethnic minorities, the health professional must be aware of the need for cultural competence, knowledge about a particular ethnic group, and cultural sensitivity (Neighbors et al., 1995).

The creation of positive internal relationships is crucial to the success of community coalitions. The working climate needs to be cohesive, trusting, and capable of resolving conflict. It is helpful if members can identify and unite around a shared vision. And, an inclusive culture needs to be created where group members share decision-making power. All members need to be provided with up-to-date information to keep everyone informed and prevent problems from escalating. Additionally, groups need to develop external relationships with community organizations to increase visibility, access to resources, and the likelihood of adoption of proposed policies. To increase the chances that group efforts will lead to long- term system change, relationships also need to be developed with key community leaders and policy makers. Goups need to interact with other community groups who are addressing similar issues, to identify new innovations and best practice solutions (Foster-Fishman et al., 2001). For progress to continue over time, the group must be able to maintain its focus on manageable projects and be able to reposition assets, competencies, and resources, colloquially known as patching, when needs and priorities change. When individuals are personally empowered, they will come together to form effective community organizations (Neighbors et al., 1995). This is the macro level of capacity building.

Community (Macro) Level of Capacity Building

Among many influences, community empowerment in public health has been affected by community and social psychology; the mandate for community participation in the World Health Organization and Ottawa Health Promotion Charters; the liberating and popular educational philosophy of Brazilian educator Paulo Freire; and the critical theory, feminist, and post-modernist schools (Wallerstein & Bernstein, 1994).

Best and colleagues (2003) have proposed an integrative framework to facilitate the translation of theory into effective community-level health promotion strategy. The components of the framework are the social ecology model, the PRECEDE-PROCEED model, and the Life Course Health Development model, integrated by tenets of systems theory. The empowerment orientation weighs process heavily, the behavior orientation weighs outcome, and the organization orientation weighs structure.

Social ecology models suggest that efforts to promote well-being should be based on an understanding of the relationships among diverse environmental and personal factors rather than on analyses that focus exclusively on environmental, biological, or behavioral factors. In turn, health promotion planning models give increased attention to policy and organizational changes needed to support people in their efforts to gain greater control over their health. Additionally, developmental models emphasize multiple determinants operating in a nested genetic, biological, behavioral, social, and economic context (Best et al., 2003). A systems thinking perspective suggests that more comprehensive, participatory, and collaborative approaches to health promotion are potentially more effective than narrowly targeted and less collaborative approaches.

Community organization describes the process of organizing people around problems or issues that are larger than group members' own immediate concerns (Labonte, 1994). Robertson & Minkler (1994) suggest helpful strategies to increase community problem-solving abilities, or "community competence" including:

- Assisting individuals and communities to articulate both health problems and their solutions

- Providing access to information

- Supporting indigenous community leadership

- Assisting the community in overcoming bureaucratic obstacles to action

However, community ownership is often prevented when service providers drive the coalition. The grassroots community must be involved in defining the issues, solutions, and strategies, and must know that it will be given tools and resources to control the implementation of programs and strategies (Kaye, 2001).

The relevant dimensions of community capacity can be distinguished, made operational, measured, and then used to compare communities or to design and evaluate interventions to improve capacity. Some relevant dimensions of community capacity include leadership, participation, skills, resources, social and organizational networks, sense of community, understanding of community history, community power, values, and critical reflection (Freudenberg, 2004).

Organizational capacity requires leaders with strong skills, relationships, and vision. "Effective leaders create an internal work environment that is simultaneously empowering, efficient, and task oriented, fostering member satisfaction and commitment and coalition effectiveness" (Foster-Fishman et al., 2001, pp. 253-254). Other leadership tasks include setting clear guidelines through formalized processes and procedures, promoting the focus necessary to achieve targeted goals, developing an internal communication system to promote information sharing and problem discussion and resolution, providing for human and financial resources, and "a continuous learning orientation, consistently seeking and responding to feedback and evaluation data, adapting to shifting contextual conditions, dialoguing about problems, and seeking external information and expertise" (Foster-Fishman et al., 2001, p. 255).

Kaye (2001) notes that a community organizer acts as a strategy coach, meeting facilitator, and an identifier and developer of community leadership. Specific suggestions for the nurse who functions as a community organizer to reach out to the community include:

- Setting up town meetings to reach out to the organized community, or meetings in someone's home, apartment, or the local coffee shop where people are usually invited by word of mouth (Kaye, 2001).

- Going door-to-door with face-to-face contact breaking down barriers and suspicions (Kaye, 2001).

- Doing street outreach such as handing out flyers at the factory gate, going out to the basketball court, or hanging out on a certain street corner with someone credible to the community (Kaye, 2001).

- Setting up a table in front of a busy supermarket, train station, or anywhere else that people pass by (Kaye, 2001).

- Attending local community meetings (Kaye, 2001).

- Holding meetings in the evening (after people get out of work), and providing childcare (Kaye, 2001).

- Having materials and meeting agendas translated into languages other than English if necessary, and providing translators at meetings (Kaye, 2001).

- Having regular orientation meetings each month for new members (Kaye, 2001).

- Building social time and interaction with people in power into meeting agendas (Kaye, 2001).

- Beginning and ending meetings with an expression of faith or spirituality as a way to make people feel welcome and connected (Kaye, 2001).

- The nurse is a facilitator who, "like a midwife, helps people give birth to their own ideas and initiatives and provides leadership when crisis opens up opportunity for change" (Kaseje, 1995, p. 213).

- Working wonders through quick and easy interventions creates dependency. Time is needed for the processes of dialogue and "truly empowered participation" (Kaseje, 1995, p. 212).

Much work in community empowerment is based on the writings of the health educator Paulo Freire (1973) and his concept of conscientization. Empowerment education, as developed from Freire's writings by Wallerstein and Bernstein (1988), brings people together in groups to identify the social and historical roots of health problems and to develop strategies to overcome obstacles in achieving goals.

Freire's Concept of Conscientization

"Conscientization involves the development of a sense of identification with a group, of shared fate with that group, and of self and collective efficacy" (Israel et al., 1994, p. 153). Freire proposes a dialogue approach in which everyone participates as equals and co-learners to create social knowledge and foster critical thinking. While health education assumes that individuals can make health decisions with enough information, skills, and reinforcement, Freire emphasizes collective knowledge from shared experience rather than knowledge from experts giving information. Accordingly, the nurse enters into a dialogue with the community group, contributing information once themes have been proposed for mutual reflection. The emphasis is on listening to each other, developing effective strategies for action, and subsequent reflection to facilitate learning (Wallerstein & Bernstein, 1988).

As a social action process, a community empowerment model "conceives of power as an expanding commodity," (Israel et al., 1994, p. 154) and emphasizes participation, caring, connectedness and responsibility to others, sharing, critical thinking, and personal and social capacity building (Wallerstein & Bernstein, 1994). In order to promote empowering education, Wallerstein and Bernstein (1988, pp. 382-383) propose a three-stage, problem posing methodology:

1. Listening to understand the felt issues or themes of the community. Listening is conducted in equal partnership with community members to identify problems and determine priorities. It is a continual process.

2. Participatory dialogue about the investigated issues using a problem-posing methodology. The dialogue is structured in order to reflect the community reality back to discussion participants.

3. Action, or the positive changes that people envision during their dialogue. The envisioned action changes can lead to a deeper cycle of reflection.

Community Empowerment

Community empowerment seeks to enhance a community's ability to identify, mobilize, and address the issues that it faces to improve the overall health of the community. Central to the concept of community empowerment is community capacity, defined as "the cultivation and use of transferable knowledge, skills, systems, and resources that affect community- and individual-level changes consistent with public health-related goals and objectives" (Yoo et al., 2004, p. 256).

In a study of 668 participants from five community partnerships in South Africa, it was found that: (a) involvement, commitment, and sense of ownership were associated with high benefits and low costs; (b) benefits, commitment, and ownership might be more sensitive monitors of involvement than costs and satisfaction; and (c) an increase in involvement was initially associated with decreased costs and increased satisfaction up to a point beyond which costs increased and satisfaction decreased despite increasing benefits. It was established that for favorable cost-benefit ratios, benefits needed to be at least 60% more than costs (Ansari & Phillips, 2004).

Social Capital

Social capital is a concept that originated within the discipline of sociology, with the idea of capital drawn from economics. Bourdieu (1986, p. 248) initially defined social capital as "the aggregate of the actual or potential resources which are linked to possession of a durable network of more or less institutionalized relationships of mutual acquaintance or recognition—or in other words to membership of a group." In simpler terms, Portes (1998, p. 6) defined social capital as "the ability of actors to secure benefits by virtue of membership in social networks." The central idea of social capital is that membership in a social group confers obligations and benefits on individuals. Whereas economic capital is durable and tangible, and builds up a stock of value that can be converted into money, the stock of social capital is in network relationships with no individual ownership (Hawe & Shiell, 2000).

Social capital can be the source of benefits such as social control, family support, and benefits through extrafamilial networks (Portes, 1998). However, there also are potential negative consequences. Strong ties enable members of a group to bar others from access, for potential economic advantage. For example, Korean immigrants have a growing control of the produce business in several East coast cities, Jewish merchants have a traditional monopoly over the New York diamond trade, and Cubans dominate numerous sectors of the Miami economy (Portes, 1998). In addition, the social network can demand conformity and constrain individual freedom. In order to create a unified entity, differences and divisions can be suppressed, "at times to the point of homogenization of the community members" (Drevdahl, 2002, p. 10). In situations where there has been a common experience of adversity and opposition to mainstream society, there can be "downward leveling norms," hindering individual advancement unless the person leaves the group (Portes, 1998, p. 17).

Hawe and Shiell (2000) express concern that the social capital literature emphasizes relational rather than political and material aspects, potentially diluting social health initiatives already underway under the labels of empowerment, capacity building, and community health promotion. Social capital also has been criticized for not advancing social justice (Drevdahl et al., 2001). Drevdahl and colleagues (2001, p. 23) indicate that access to "more substantial sources of social capital" leads to domination, rather than promoting an equitable "bearing of burdens and reaping of benefits in society." The authors emphasize that nurses must expose and change the "overpowering dominance of market philosophies and policies," and the ways in which they generate health inequalities. "Ultimately, it is the development of social policies directed at decreasing material and social disparities that will have any meaningful effect on reducing or eliminating health disparities, rather than promoting social capital, cohesion, or trust in communities" (2001, p. 28). Given that "supportive relational ties are not a sufficient antidote to material deprivation and learned helplessness" (Hawe & Shiell, 2000, p. 879), political action and advocacy to change material, social, and health disparities and inequities are essential.

Political Action and Advocacy

Advocacy means taking a position on an issue and initiating actions in a deliberate attempt to influence private and public policy choices (Labonte, 1994). Nurses have a reputation for being trustworthy, building consensus, and getting along with people. Nurses also can use their breadth of knowledge and experience with health care issues to advance the desired agenda. According to Neighbors and colleagues (1995) and Feldman and Lewenson (2000), recommendations to facilitate advocacy and political action include:

- Begin with an analysis of perceived needs of the target group rather than the needs and expectations of the program planners.

- Focus explicitly on neighborhood issues and community resources.

- Start at the grassroots family and neighborhood level with community service.

- Be part of the solution.

- Use a nonjudgmental, self-confident approach. Polish problem-solving, team building, networking, and coalition building skills.

- Praise health messages within the context of self-help, self-reliance, community control, empowerment, and self-pride. Messages should be firm and culturally sensitive.

- Incorporate specific skill-oriented training.

- Use members of a target group who have expertise concerning their culture and health problems, and more important, know what solutions are likely to work in their communities.

- Build relationships with community leaders and local and state political representatives.

Barriers to Community Empowerment

Despite the numerous advantages inherent in community empowerment, Israel and colleagues (1994) suggest that there are also a number of barriers. For example, there are situations where past experiences and beliefs result in community members feeling that they do not have influence within the system. Some community members may feel powerless and therefore remain quiet and uninvolved in an empowerment intervention.

The differences in, for example, social class, race, and ethnicity that often exist between community members and nurses or health educators may impede trust, communication, and collaborative work. Swanson and colleagues (2001) propose that people must first know themselves before forming cross-cultural partnerships. To reduce inherent conflicts and misunderstandings, they propose a number of characteristics that partners need, including understanding; common goals; commitment; persistence; a sense of humor; trust; an open and flexible approach to others; being willing to change personal attitudes, beliefs, behaviors, and values; being willing to set assumptions aside and withhold judgment; learning appropriate foreign languages; curiosity; tolerance and appreciation for differences; acceptance of ambiguity; low goal and task orientation; and the ability to understand another's reality.

Capacity can be undermined as well as created. Some external social processes that may damage community capacity include urban renewal, crime and fear of crime, war, extreme poverty, recession or other economic dislocation, job loss, racism, competition for limited resources, and other types of intergroup conflict. Additionally, certain types of experiences may dissipate rather than build capacity, and diminish the capacity to act in the future. These may include unresolved racial, ethnic, gender, or other conflicts within a community coalition; repression that succeeds in demobilizing an initiative; an inability to engage policy makers in serious discussions; or the long delays that opponents of change can sometimes impose (Freudenberg, 2004).

In addition, some health educators, their employers, and community members have short timeframe expectations that are inconsistent with the sustained effort and long-time commitment of financial and personal resources that are required by the community empowerment approach. For example, funds may be contributed by a foundation or charitable organization but require a report with measurable outcomes at the end of a year. Other barriers to community empowerment include the following:

■ Dealing with role-related tensions and differences arising around the issues of values and interests, resources and skills, control, political realities, rewards and costs.

■ Encountering risks and potential resistance when challenging the status quo.

■ Measuring change in community empowerment. For example, the collection and analysis of extensive amounts of data to be used for action as well as evaluation purposes may be perceived as slowing down the process.

Principles for Community Organization

Community organization is a process planned primarily by community representatives, consistent with local values. Individuals, groups, or organizations from within the community use their own social structures and internal or external resources to accomplish community goals and attain and then sustain community improvements and/or new opportunities (Bracht & Kingsbury, 1990).

Community activation or stimulation begins with the creation or presence of an issue. The community must identify the condition or situation as a priority for community action, identify and activate community groups and individuals to deal with the issue, institute a process for change, and establish structures to implement and maintain program solutions. One important outcome of this ongoing process of community and citizen involvement is community ownership, with an organizer or change agent potentially facilitating the process. The change agent must be socially acceptable and trusted by the group (Bracht & Kingsbury, 1990).

The key areas of community analysis are the assessment of community capacity to support a project, identification of potential barriers that exist, and determination of community readiness for involvement. Community analysis is the process of assessing and defining needs, opportunities, and resources involved in initiating community health action programs. A community analysis results in a "dynamic community profile," done not on the community but with the community (Haglund et al., 1990 p. 91).

There are several different types of approaches to community analysis (Haglund et al., 1990). The medical science approach focuses on absence of disease, health improvements through use of science and technology, and lack of direct citizen involvement, relying on diagnosis by experts. The health planning approach emphasizes technical needs assessment, with a focus on improvements in delivering medical and preventive services. The community development approach views health within the broader context of social and economic improvement and views citizen empowerment and "bottom-up" decision-making as vital. Community is considered both a context and the vehicle for change. Bracht and Kingsbury (1990, pp. 73-86), propose a community health promotion model with five stages of organizing. These key elements of community analysis are identified in Box 11-2.

Box 11-2

Key Elements of Community Analysis

Stage 1: Define the community. Determining the geographic focus and/or community boundaries of the project.

- Collecting data. A "community profile" should include information on community resources, history, readiness for action, needs, who can get things done, and who may be opposed to health promotion efforts.

  1. Compile a comprehensive profile of community health, demographics, resources, history, and readiness for action. (For example, population by age, sex, and racial or ethnic heritage; family structure, marital status, housing conditions, education levels, immigration, divorce rates, crime rates, quality-of-life; employment business conditions, welfare and social security beneficiary rates).

  2. Compile a profile of health risks including behavioral risks such as dietary habits; use of drugs, alcohol, and tobacco; and patterns of physical activity; social risks such as long-term unemployment, isolation, poor education, and social support mechanisms; and environmental risks such as quality of the physical water, soil, air, climate, and housing.

  3. Compile a profile of health and wellness outcomes such as distribution of illness and well-being in the community through age-specific death rates, unnecessary deaths, morbidity and mortality rates.

- Assessing community capacities that support change.

- Assessing community barriers that hinder or create resistance to change. People may resist changes not clearly understood, that threaten vested interests and security, or that do not fit with cultural values of the community.

continued

Box 11-2 CONTINUED

- Assessing readiness for change. How urgent is the problem? How receptive are top decision makers?
- Synthesizing data and setting priorities. It is desirable to use a consensus decision-making process involving key community leaders.

Stage 2: Design and initiation. Establishing a structure to elicit and/or coordinate broad citizen support and involvement. The key elements include:

- Establishing a core planning group and selecting a local organizer or coordinator.
- Choosing a dynamic organizational structure. Examples include an advisory board, coalition, lead agency, informal network, or grass-roots or advocacy movement for program planning, community development, social action, advocacy, or consciousness raising (Shields & Lindsey, 1998).
- Identifying, selecting, and recruiting organization members. They should represent all major community institutions and groups including commercial, volunteer, political, minority, religious, recreational, medical, public health, and media, and can speak and make decisions for the people they represent. Ideally, those people would be positive thinkers, enthusiastic, enjoy a challenge, and believe in the project.
- Identifying influential and leadership persons.
- Defining the organization's mission and goals. Develop a mission statement.
- Clarifying roles and responsibilities of board members, staff, and volunteers.
- Providing training and recognition.

Stage 3: Implementation. Mobilizing and involving professionals and citizens in the planning of a sequential set of activities to accomplish their mission. Plans should be adapted to local constraints and values and make maximum use of available resources and existing institutions.

- Generating broad citizen participation.
- Developing a sequential work plan.
- Using comprehensive, integrated strategies. More than "one-shot" interventions are needed.
- Integrating community values into the programs, materials, and messages.

continued

Box 11-2 CONTINUED

Stage 4: Program maintenance and consolidation. Having gained experience and success with the programs and dealt successfully with problems, community members and staff are developing a solid foundation in the community, and the programs are gaining acceptance. The key elements of this stage include:

- Integrating intervention activities into community networks.
- Establishing a positive organizational culture.
- Establishing an ongoing recruitment plan.
- Disseminating results.

Stage 5: Dissemination and reassessment. Reassessment occurs continually throughout the various stages, but the key elements of this stage include:

- Updating the community analysis.
- Assessing the effectiveness of interventions and programs.
- Charting future directions and modifications.
- Summarizing and disseminating results.

Source: Adapted from Bracht, N., & Kingsbury, L. (1990). Community organization principles in health promotion. In N. Bracht (Ed.), *Health promotion at the community level* (pp. 66-88). Newbury Park, CA: Sage.

This kind of a model can provide an organizational and structural framework for community health promotion activities. Additionally, Stokols (1996) suggests a number of strategies that nurses can use to promote community health, including:

1. Exploring the links between facets of well-being and diverse geographic, architectural, technological, organizational, and sociocultural environmental conditions.

2. Combining active (behavioral) and passive (environmental) interventions, given the dynamic interaction of intrapersonal and environmental factors on individual and community well-being.

3. Enhancing the fit between people and their surroundings, giving participants control over their surroundings with flexibility and freedom to initiate goal-directed efforts to modify the environment in accord with their preferences and plans.

4. Focusing health promotion interventions on high-impact behavioral and organizational leverage points. Leverage points are personal health behaviors that directly affect a person's well-being (such as only selecting menu items that are labeled "heart-healthy") or others' well-being (such as only "heart-healthy" foods being included on a menu).

5. Concentrating on leverage points that have the most influence for the individual or the organization.

6. Addressing interdependencies between multiple settings and life domains such as residential, educational, occupational, recreational, religious, and health care environments, which have a cumulative and combined influence on well-being.

7. Integrating multidisciplinary perspectives in the design of health promotion programs and using multiple and longitudinal methods to gauge the methodologic rigor and theoretical adequacy of a research or intervention program.

8. Gauging the societal value and practical significance of a research or intervention program with such data as epidemiologic prevalence of particular health problems, economic costs and sustainability of programs designed to alleviate those problems, the number of people who are likely to benefit from or be adversely affected by the intervention program, possible occurrence of undesirable side effects from the program, and public opinion about community health priorities.

Empowerment cannot be bestowed on a community. Communities need to participate in an equal partnership with health professionals in setting the health agenda, in defining their health problems, and developing the solutions to address those problems (Robertson & Minkler, 1994). The role of the professional changes from that of an expert who defines the community's needs and provides the solutions through professionally oriented strategies to that of a consultant who provides technical and informational support to the community, and builds community capacity to address health needs. The community and the professionals are equal partners in setting the health agenda for the community (Robertson & Minkler, 1994).

Although there are obvious advantages to community health promotion, Guldan (1996) outlines a number of obstacles in our current health care delivery system, including the fact that current medical training does not yet produce health-promoting physicians. Current nursing education does not yet produce sufficient health-promoting nurses either. There is a need for more primary care physicians and nurses alongside other community-based workers. The system needs to move toward a community-based health system based on health promotion and disease prevention.

In addition, the market shapes demand toward wants rather than health needs. Industrial interests can act as a barrier to health promotion through globally pervasive and aggressive advertising. Sound, current information promoting health does not reach relatively unconnected and less educated community members quickly enough to promote a turnaround in attitudes. For example, few programs have been designed for and partnered with their target audiences in informal "centers of health" such as shopping malls and hairdressers. Therefore, misinformation is often prevalent. Other obstacles to community health promotion include the long time period necessary for change and for the results of community health promotion to become evident, the significant financial commitment necessary for long-term intensive work and the complexity of effective engaging and coordinating many people.

In order to promote community health, nurses need political savvy. Kaseje (1995) suggests that nurses have to learn how to identify partners and opponents in the political process, do thorough research, present a cohesive front, carefully work out action plans, and present their position clearly but not aggressively in order to have the greatest influence at various levels of policy formulation and implementation.

Community-level health promotion is not a panacea. Some communities may be unable or unwilling to support the process; there is a high personal cost to those involved in community mobilization; and the process can emphasize conflict between professional and community health goals. However, the many advantages of community-level action are sufficient reasons to encourage nursing's involvement and leadership in community-level health promotion. These include the ability to reach inaccessible populations through the use of informal community networks; the ability to maximize social pressure through social support, modeling, and peer pressure strategies; and the ability to use local knowledge, expertise, and resources to address community-wide health-related issues (Hancock et al., 1997).

The emphasis in this chapter has been on empowering strategies, such as collaboration, capacity building, and political action/advocacy that nurses can use for community-level organization to promote social and political change toward health. The nurse is viewed as a consultant who provides the moral leadership to strengthen action and promote public policy to build healthy communities. However, in this "information age," perhaps an even greater challenge is fostering a sense of community built on shared values, relatedness, a feeling of belonging, and trust, that is necessary for community ownership of change.

Chapter Key Points

- Community can be described with the emphasis on place, people with shared institutions and values, social interaction, distribution of power, or a social system.

- Characteristics of community include commitment, continuity, cohesion, sense of community, membership, influence, shared emotional connection, and the expectation that one's needs will be met through membership in the group.

- Community-based interventions are directed at individual health behaviors, with the individual as the client.

- This chapter has emphasized community-level interventions to modify the entire community through community empowerment, interdisciplinary collaboration, and capacity building.

- Empowerment and capacity building can be directed at individuals, small groups, or the community level.

- Examples of barriers to community empowerment include perceived powerlessness by community members, lack of trust, communication, collaboration, and role-related tensions and differences.

- Community health promotion includes analysis of community capacity, potential barriers, and readiness; establishment of a structure to elicit and/or coordinate broad citizen support and involvement; development of an implementation plan; maintenance and consolidation of the program; and dissemination and reassessment of results.

- Nurses need to develop political savvy in order to influence community health promotion.

References

Ansari, W. L., & Phillips, C. J. (2004). The costs and benefits to participants in community partnerships: A paradox? *Health Promotion Practice, 5,* 35-48.

Best, A., Stokols, D., Green, L., Leischow, S., Holmes, B., & Buchholz, K. (2003). An integrative framework for community partnering to translate theory into effective health promotion strategy. *American Journal of Health Promotion, 18,* 168-176.

Booker, V. K., Robinson, J. G., Kay, B. J., Najera, L. G., & Stewart, G. (1997). Changes in empowerment: Effects of participation in a lay health promotion program. *Health Education & Behavior, 24,* 452-464.

Bourdieu, P. (1986). The forms of capital. In Richardson, J. G. (Ed.), *Handbook of theory and research for the sociology of education* (pp. 248-258). New York: Macmillan.

Bracht, N. (1990). Introduction. In N. Bracht (Ed.), *Health promotion at the community level* (pp. 19-21). Newbury Park, CA: Sage.

Bracht, N., & Kingsbury, L. (1990). Community organization principles in health promotion. In N. Bracht (Ed.), *Health promotion at the community level* (pp. 66-88). Newbury Park, CA: Sage.

Davis, R. (2000). Holographic community: Reconceptualizing the meaning of community in an era of health care reform. *Nurs Outlook, 48,* 294-301.

Disch, J. (2001). Strengthening nursing and interdisciplinary collaboration. *J Prof Nurs, 17,* 275.

Drevdahl, D. J. (2002). Home and border: The contradictions of community. *Advances in Nursing Science, 24,* 8-20.

Drevdahl, D., Kneipp, S. M., Canales, M. K., & Dorcy, K. S. (2001). Reinvesting in social justice: A capital idea for public health nursing? *Advances in Nursing Science, 24,* 19-31.

el Ansari, W., & Phillips, C. J. (2001). Interprofessional collaboration: A stakeholder approach to evaluation of voluntary participation in community partnerships. *Journal of Interprofessional Care, 15,* 351-368.

Falk-Rafael, A. R. (2001). Empowerment as a process of evolving consciousness: A model of empowered caring. *Advances in Nursing Science, 24*(1), 1-16.

Feldman, H. R., & Lewenson, S. B. (2000). *Nurses in the political arena: The public face of nursing.* New York: Springer.

Foster-Fishman, P. G., Berkowitz, S. L., Lounsbury, D. W., Jacobson, S., & Allen, N.A. (2001). Building collaborative capacity in community coalitions: A review and integrative framework. *Am J Community Psychol, 29,* 241-261.

Freire, P. (1973). *Pedagogy of the oppressed.* New York: Continuum.

Freudenberg, N. (2004). Community capacity for environmental health promotion: Determinants and implications for practice. *Health Education and Behavior, 31,* 472-490.

Glouberman, S., & Mintzberg, H. (2001). Managing the care of health and the cure of disease-Part II: Integration. *Health Care Manag Rev, 26,* 70-84.

Guldan, G. S. (1996). Obstacles to community health promotion. *Soc Sci Med, 43,* 689-695.

Haglund, B., Weisbrod, R. R., & Bracht, N. (1990). Assessing the community. In N. Bracht (Ed.), *Health promotion at the community level* (pp. 91-108). Newbury Park, CA: Sage.

Hancock, L., Sanson-Fisher, R. W., Redman, S., Burton, R., Burton, L., Butler, J., et al. (1997). Community action for health promotion: A review of methods and outcomes 1990-1995. *Am J Prev Med, 13*, 229-239.

Hawe, P., & Sheill, A. (2000). Social capital and health promotion: A review. *Soc Sci Med, 51*, 871-885.

Helman, C. G. (1994). *Culture, health, and illness* (3rd ed.). Oxford, UK: Butterworth-Heinemann.

Himmelman, A. T., (2001). On coalitions and the transformation of power relations: Collaborative betterment and collaborative empowerment. *American Journal of Community Psychology, 29*, 277-284.

Israel, B. A., Checkoway, B., Schulz, A., & Zimmerman, M. (1994). Health education and community empowerment: Conceptualizing and measuring perceptions of individual, organizational, and community control. *Health Educ Q, 21*, 149-170.

Judd, J., Frankish, C. J., & Moulton, G. (2001). Setting standards in the evaluation of community-based health promotion programmes—A unifying approach. *Health Promotion International, 16*, 367-380.

Kaseje, D. (1995). The role of nursing in health care in the context of unjust social, economic, and political structures and systems. *Nursing and Health Care Perspectives on Community, 16*, 209-213.

Kaye, G. (2001). Grassroots involvement. *American Journal of Community Psychology, 29*, 269-275.

Labonte, R. (1994). Health promotion and empowerment: Reflections on professional practice. *Health Educ Q, 21*, 253-268.

Laffrey, S. C., & Kulbok, P. A. (1999). An integrative model for holistic community health nursing. *Journal of Holistic Nursing, 17*, 88-103.

Long, K. A. (2001). A reality-oriented approach to interdisciplinary work. *J Prof Nurs, 17*, 278-282.

Milio, N. (1996). *Engines of empowerment.* Chicago, IL: Health Administration Press.

Neighbors, H. W., Braithwaite, R. L., & Thompson, E. (1995). Health promotion and African-Americans: From personal empowerment to community action. *American Journal of Health Promotion, 9*, 281-287.

Patrick, D. L., & Wickizer, T. M. (1995). Community and health. In B. C. Amick, S, Levine, A. R. Tarlov, & D. C. Walsh (Eds.), *Society and health* (pp. 46-71). Oxford, UK: Oxford University Press.

Portes, A. (1998). Social capital: Its origins and applications in modern sociology. *Annual Review of Sociology, 24*, 1-24.

Robertson, A., & Minkler, M. (1994). New health promotion movement: A critical examination. *Health Educ Q, 21*, 295-312.

Roussos, S. T., & Fawcett, S. B. (2000). A review of collaborative partnerships as a strategy for improving community health. *Annu Rev Public Health, 21*, 369-402.

Schmitt, M. H. (2001). Collaboration improves the quality of care: Methodological challenges and evidence from US health care research. *Journal of Interprofessional Care, 15*, 47-66.

Sheilds, L. E., & Lindsey, A. E. (1998). Community health promotion nursing practice. *Advances in Nursing Science, 20*, 23-36.

Soukhanov, A. H. (Ed.). (1992). *The American heritage dictionary of the English language* (3rd ed). Boston: Houghton Mifflin.

Stokols, D. (1996). Translating social ecological theory into guidelines for community health promotion. *American Journal of Health Promotion, 10*, 282-298.

Swanson, E., Goody, C. M., Frolova, E. V., Kuznetsova, O., Plavinski, S., & Nelson, G. (2001). An application of an effective interdisciplinary health-focused cross-cultural collaboration. *J Prof Nurs, 17*, 33-39.

Thompson, B., & Kinne, S. (1990). Social change theory. In N. Bracht (Ed.), *Health promotion at the community level* (pp. 45-65). Newbury Park, CA: Sage.

Wallerstein, N. (1992). Powerlessness, empowerment, and health: Implications for health promotion programs. *American Journal of Health Promotion, 6*, 197-205.

Wallerstein, N., & Bernstein, E. (1988). Empowerment education: Freire's ideas adapted to health education. *Health Educ Q, 15*, 379-394.

Wallerstein, N., & Bernstein, E. (1994). Introduction to community empowerment, participatory education, and health. *Health Educ Q, 21*, 141-148.

Yao, S., Weed, N.E., Lempa, M.L., Mbondo, U., Shada, R.E., & Goodman, R.M. (2004), Collaborative community empowerment: An illustration of a six-step process. *Health Promotion Practice, 5*, 256-265.

IV

INTEGRATIVE NURSING
INTERVENTIONS TO PROMOTE
HEALTH AND HEALING

Section IV, *Integrative Nursing Interventions to Promote Health and Healing*, provides a comprehensive introduction to non-invasive therapeutic modalities that are appropriate as nursing interventions (with proper supervised training and credentialing) and/or to be taught to clients for self-use in promoting health and healing. Chapter 12, *Relinquishing Bound Energy: Herbal Therapy and Aromatherapy* presents clinical applications for a number of selected herbs and essential oils. Chapter 13, *Re-establishing Energy Flow: Physical Activity and Exercise*, proposes a number of strategies to empower clients to adopt a more active lifestyle. The chapter also introduces the Chinese energy exercises of tai chi and qigong, which use breathing, mental concentration, and physical postures to facilitate the flow of energy throughout the body. In Chapter 14, *Releasing Blocked Energy: Touch and Bodywork Techniques*, massage therapies, acupressure, and various postural/movement reeducation therapies are presented. Chapter 15, *Reducing Energy Depletion: Relaxation and Stress Reduction*, describes modalities such as different forms of meditation, breathing, yoga, biofeedback, and guided imagery that are designed to reduce stress responses through relaxation. Chapter 16, *Regenerating Energy: Nutrition*, explores Western dietary guidelines and goals, essential dietary nutrients, phytonutrients, antioxidants, nutritional medicine supplements, and basic diets to affect disease processes and promote health. And, Chapter 17, *Restoring Energy Field Harmony: Energy Patterning*, explores Reiki and prayer as examples of modalities that are based on channeling of a spiritual energy that has innate intelligence or logic, while music, color therapy, polarity therapy, and Therapeutic Touch pattern the vibrations of the environmental energy field for healing purposes.

RELINQUISHING BOUND ENERGY

Herbal Therapy and Aromatherapy

Abstract

Because herbal therapy and aromatherapy are based on the use of components of natural plants, they both are presented in this chapter. Clinical applications for a number of selected herbs and essential oils that have been well studied and appear to be both effective and low in side effects are presented. Parameters for dosage and administration are also included. However, the nurse is urged to pursue thorough educational preparation prior to the use of herbs and essential oils in practice. In addition, there is a professional obligation to restrict the use of herbs and essential oils to the promotion of health and well-being, and to refer clients to an appropriate medical practitioner for the treatment of disease.

Learning Outcomes

By the end of this chapter the student will be able to:

- Describe examples of forms of delivery of herbal preparations
- Identify selected herbs and essential oils that have been well studied and appear to be both effective and low in side effects
- Describe the clinical applications of selected herbs and essential oils
- Identify selected drug/herbal interactions
- Discuss ways of using aromatherapy for self-care

■ Discuss the professional obligation to restrict the use of herbs and essential oils to the promotion of health and well-being, and to refer clients to an appropriate medical practitioner for the treatment of disease

Herbal Therapy

Herbal therapy is an established and growing modality used in health care. According to the World Health Organization (WHO), "approximately 75% of the global population—most of the developing world—depends on botanical medicines for their basic health care needs" (Barrett et al., 1999, p. 41). In the United States, approximately 60 million American adults, or 30 % of the nation's adult population, were estimated to have used herbs or herbal preparations in 1996 (Integrative Medicine Communications, 1998).

There are a number of reasons why Americans are interested in the use of herbs, including (Berman & Larson, 1994; Jonas & Ernst, 1999):

■ Availability of traditional European and North American herbs, Chinese, Japanese, and Ayurvedic herbals, herbs from Central and South America and Mexico, and Native American herbal medicines.

■ Pharmaceutical drugs are seen increasingly as overprescribed, expensive, and even dangerous. Herbal remedies are seen as less expensive and less toxic.

■ Therapies labeled as natural are perceived as safer.

■ Exposure to exotic foreign foods prepared with non-European culinary herbs has led to exploration of medicinal herbs from those countries.

■ People are increasingly willing to "self-doctor" by investigating and using herbs and herbal preparations as adjuncts to other treatments, especially for chronic illnesses such as arthritis, diabetes, cancer, and AIDS.

An herb is a plant whose stem does not produce woody persistent tissue and generally dies back at the end of each growing season (Soukhanov, 1992). Herbs occur naturally in a number of forms, including flowering plants, shrubs, or trees, or a moss, lichen, fern, algae, seaweed, or fungus. The entire plant may be used for an herb, or specifically the flowers, fruits, leaves, twigs, bark, roots, rhizomes, seeds, or exudates (such as tapped and purified maple syrup), or a combination of parts. Additionally, nonplants are used as healing agents in many herbal traditions, including animal parts (organs, bone, tissue), insects, animal and insect secretions, worm castings, shells, rocks, metals, minerals, and gemstones (Meserole, 1996).

Both herbs and standard pharmaceuticals are absorbed into the blood stream in the same way. Barrett et al. (1999, p. 40) suggest that "regulation, preparation, and degree of chemical refinement form the primary boundaries that divide botanical medicines from their more conventional prescription and over-the-counter counterparts." However, as a rule, herbal preparations are less toxic than their synthetically produced counterparts and offer less risk of side effects. In addition, the mechanism of action of an herb is often to correct the underlying cause of a health problem, in contrast to the use of a synthetic drug to alleviate a symptom (Murray, 1995).

Herbal therapy is an integral part of Chinese medicine. The goal of therapy is to find and treat the integrally related underlying causes of a problem, and not just treat isolated, specific manifestations and symptoms. As a result, the whole plant or crude extract is often much more effective than isolated chemical constituents, and a formula made up of combinations of herbs is often prescribed for individualized needs. Herbal therapies are not very effective when they are used as pharmaceutical substitutes, although they are often labeled and marketed to treat individual symptoms. Herbs tend to work best preventively or therapeutically as slow-acting, gradual, healing agents. They must be taken consistently, in the correct form and dose. "Additionally, the herbal practitioner's familiarity with each medicinal plant or herbal formula usually is much greater than the medical doctor's familiarity with each individual pharmaceutical, and this permits the herbalist to precisely select a particular plant or formula for each [client]" (Meserole, 1996, p. 117).

The importance of the individualized use of a whole plant is stressed by Ballentine (1999), who suggests that each whole plant possesses a "pattern of function." Congruence between the pattern of the plant and that of a particular individual creates an energy field "resonance" that can be used therapeutically. When a congruent plant is introduced into a person whose symptoms reflect a pattern of disorder, something "clicks," and a pattern of reorganization occurs at the energy level. The pattern of energy flow then has an impact on the physical body and how it functions.

Messerole (1996) describes common aspects of herbalism as follows:

- Optimization of health and wellness

- Emphasis on the whole person and the community

- Enhancement of the quality of life

- Promotion of simple self-treatment and preventive self-care

LEVELS OF HERBALISTS

No training is legally required to recommend herbal remedies in the United States and Canada. Herbal education varies greatly. There are weekend workshops, correspondence courses, and schools of herbal medicine. Although the American Herbalists Guild, the only professional group of herbalists in the United States, bestows the title "Herbalist AHG" upon herbalists who have passed a peer-review process, there is no official recognition or licensing of herbalists in the United States (Dog, 1999; Prescriber's Letter, 1998).

There also is no recognized standard training program for herbal therapy. However, in the United States and Europe, a number of professionals have been trained in the use of herbs, including officially trained medical herbalists, clinical herbalists, registered nurses, licensed naturopathic doctors specializing in botanical medicine, licensed acupuncturists with training in Chinese herbal medicine, licensed Aryurvedic doctors, Native American herbalists and shamans, and Latin American curanderos. "A professional herbalist undertakes formalized training or a long apprenticeship in plant and medical studies, or alternatively in plant and spiritual or healing studies. This knowledge includes extensive familiarity—often a relationship—with specific plants, which involves their identification, habitat, harvesting criteria, preparation, storage, therapeutic indications, contraindications, and dosing" (Meserole, 1996, p. 113).

In contrast, a lay herbalist has a broad knowledge of plants useful for health problems, but does not have extensive training in medical and spiritual diagnosis and management. Evaluation of medicinal plant quality, strength, uses, and doses are included in the lay herbalist's domain. Additionally, "plant gatherers, growers, and medicine makers… are to the practicing herbalist what the contemporary pharmacist is to the clinical physician" (Meserole, 1996, p. 114).

Herbs and botanical remedies, when prescribed to treat illness, are part of medical practice by the physician and, where authorized, the licensed professional nurse. The unauthorized practice of medicine is a legal misdemeanor. The use of herbs as part of a plan to promote client well-being, quality of life, and health falls within the jurisdiction of professional nurses who have formal training and experience within courses offered by a respected institution that include exposure to a number of different systems of herbology.

SYSTEMS OF HERBOLOGY

A number of health care systems use herbology, including traditional Chinese medicine, Ayurveda, Western medicine, and Native American medicine. Important elements of herbology in each of these systems are described below (Burton Goldberg Group, 1995; Pizzorno, 1997), and are summarized in Table 12-1.

Table 12-1

Elements of Herbology in Selected Health Care Systems

	PURPOSE	ADMINISTRATION	CLASSIFICATION
Traditional Chinese Medicine	Restoration of harmony	Given in balanced formulas rather than singly	According to energies and flavors
Ayurveda	Balance	Formula is based on regulation of doshas	According to the humor (vata, pitta, or kapha) whose qualities they promote
Western Medicine	Biochemical "magic bullets"	Individual herbs	Active biochemical constituents
Native American Medicine	Energy unites all living beings	Therapeutic effect cannot be reduced to sum of qualities or chemical constituents	According to spiritual and therapeutic energies

Traditional Chinese Medicine

In Chapter 3, the major concepts that interact to affect health in traditional Chinese medicine (TCM) were identified as qi, yin/yang, energy phases, organ networks, and body climates. Herbal therapies are classified according to their energetic qualities and administered for their action on energy disorders, disturbed internal energy, blockage of the meridians or corresponding organ dysfunction, or seasonable physical demands. The chief ingredient of the herbal formula treats the principal pattern of the underlying problem, while the other ingredients assist, enhance, and integrate actions.

- Restoration of harmony is integral to TCM.

- Since the goal is balancing the body, medicines are typically given in balanced formulas rather than singly.

- Each taste is said to have a particular medicinal action: bitter-tasting herbs (goldenseal, dandelion, and milk thistle) drain and dry, clear, and detoxify; sweet herbs (Panax ginseng and licorice) tonify and may reduce pain, warm, sooth, build and nourish; acrid herbs (cinnamon and ginger) disperse and expel cold; salty herbs (oyster shell) nourish the kidneys and cool; sour herbs (rosehips and hawthorn berries) nourish the yin and astringe, preventing unwanted loss of body fluids or qi; bland herbs may have a diuretic effect.

- The taste can also indicate the organ to which it has a natural affinity.

- Different temperatures are ascribed to herbs—hot, warm, neutral, cool, and cold.

Ayurveda

As discussed in Chapter 3, in Ayurveda the functional aspect of the body is governed by three metabolic principles, the doshas. The doshas are forces of energy, patterns, and movements, not substances and structures. Ether and air together constitute vata (the energy of movement); fire and water, pitta (the energy of digestion or metabolism); and water and earth, kapha (the energy that forms the body's structure and holds the cells together). "Balanced vata creates energy and creativity; pitta, when balanced, creates perfect digestion and contentment; and balanced kapha provides strength, stamina, immunity, and even temperament" (Larson-Presswalla, 1994, p. 22). In every person, the doshas that make up one's nature (prakriti) differ in emphases and combinations.

Application of herbal therapy in Ayurveda is based on taste, as taste is indicative of the properties of the herb. There are six taste essences: sweet, sour, salty, pungent, bitter, and astringent:

- Sweet (such as licorice or comfrey root) are nutritive and anti-inflammatory.

- Sour (such as rosehips or hawthorn berries) encourage salivation, increase digestive secretions, and induce sweating.

- Salty tasting herbs cause heat and so increase pitta (fire).

- Pungent (such as peppers or garlic) counteract congestion and stagnation, and stimulate the nervous system and digestion.

- Bitter (such as goldenseal or barberry) clear, dry, detoxify, and cleanse.

- Astringent (such as alum, witch hazel, or bayberry) contract, dry, and clear, and are cooling and decrease pitta.

For vata imbalance, therapeutic herbs are demulcent, nutritive tonics with a sweet taste and warm energy. Herbs that are drying, diuretic, bitter, or astringent—qualities similar to vata—aggravate vata imbalance (Pizzorno, 1997). Therapeutic herbs that help a pitta person are drying and cooling with bitter, astringent, and sweet flavors. On the other hand, herbs that exacerbate a person's pitta are warming and moistening with pungent, sour, or salty flavors (1997). Kapha types should take therapeutic herbs that are drying, warm and eliminative with spicy, bitter, and astringent flavors. Herbs that are moist, demulcent, nutritive, tonic, sweet, and salty aggravate kapha people (1997).

Western Medicine

- Medicines are viewed as biochemical "magic bullets."

- The philosophy of science-based herbalism is that the primary action produced by herbal medicines is the result of pharmacological (chemical) actions.

- In contrast to the other healing systems, science-based herbalism typically prescribes herbs individually.

Native American Medicine

- Native American medicine promotes respect for an energy that unites all living beings. Therefore, an herb's therapeutic properties cannot be reduced to the sum of its qualities or chemical constituents (Pizzorno, 1997).

REGULATION

Medicinal herbs are regulated as dietary supplements under the Dietary Supplement Health and Education Act (DSHEA) of 1994. Dietary supplements under this law are considered safe unless proven unsafe by the Food and Drug Administration (FDA). The DSHEA prohibits labels on dietary supplements from making medical claims. Labels are restricted to making "structure and function" claims, which are somewhat general statements about how the product affects people (Prescriber's Letter, 1998). Herbal products may be produced without the assurance of compliance standards for Good Manufacturing Practice (although such standards are being developed), and they are marketed without prior approval of their efficacy and safety by the FDA (deSmet, 2002).

The European Economic Community (EEC), recognizing the need to standardize approval of herbal medicines, developed a series of guidelines, *The Quality of Herbal Remedies*. The guidelines outline standards for quality, quantity, and production of herbal remedies and provide labeling requirements that member countries must meet. The EEC guidelines are based on the principles of the WHO's *Guidelines for the Assessment of Herbal Medicines* (1991). According to these guidelines, a substance's historical use is a valid way to document safety and efficacy in the absence of contradictory scientific evidence (Berman & Larson, 1994).

In Germany, the German Federal Institute for Drugs and Medical Devices established an expert committee on herbal remedies. This committee became known as the Commission E. The German Commission E prepared a total of 391 monographs on medicinal plants in use up to 1995. The monographs do not contain references. Many of the materials that the monographs are based on are unpublished studies provided by German herb manufacturers. The monographs were developed to inform the consumer, not for scientific debate (Prescriber's Letter, 1998). The European Commission (which governs the European Union) has recently developed a draft directive on the licensing of traditional herbal preparations.

In Europe, herbal remedies fall into three categories. The most rigorously controlled are prescription drugs, which include injectable forms of phytomedicines (from plant sources) and those used to treat life-threatening diseases. A second category is over the counter (OTC) phytomedicines, which are similar to American OTC drugs. The third category are traditional herbal remedies, products that typically have not undergone extensive clinical testing but are judged safe on the basis of generations of use without serious incident (Berman & Larson, 1994).

In more developed Asian countries such as Japan, China, and India, "patent" herbal remedies are composed of dried and powdered whole herbs or herb extracts in liquid or tablet form. In China, traditional herbal remedies are still the backbone of medicine. However, in 1984, the People's Republic of China implemented the Drug Administration Law, which said that traditional herbal preparations were generally considered "old drugs" and, except for new uses, were exempt from testing for efficacy or side effects. The Chinese Ministry of Public Health now oversees the administration of new herbal products (Berman & Larson, 1994).

In Japan, almost half (42.7 %) of Western-trained medical practitioners prescribe kampo (traditional Japanese) medicines, and the Japanese national health insurance pays for these medicines. In 1988, the Japanese herbal medicine industry established regulations to manufacture and control the quality of extract products in kampo medicine. Those regulations comply with the Japanese government's Regulations for Manufacturing Control and Quality Control of Drugs (Berman & Larson, 1994).

ACTIONS OF HERBS

There are a number of possible actions of herbs. Table 12-2 describes selected herbal actions.

HERBAL PREPARATIONS

The predominant form of delivery of herbal medicines varies among different herbal traditions. Tinctures are widely used in Britain and the United States; tablets of standardized extracts of certain herbs (e.g., Ginko biloba) are popular in Germany and the United States; decoctions are common in Tibetan, Chinese, and African traditions; therapeutic oils are used topically and internally in Ayurvedic treatments; and teas, smokes, and compresses are used in the Native American tradition.

Oral Herbal Forms

Whole Herbs

Whole herbs are plants or plant parts that are dried and then either cut or powered. Some plants are best used fresh, but are seldom marketed fresh since they are highly perishable.

Table 12-2	**Selected Actions of Herbs**

ACTION	DESCRIPTION
Adaptogenic	Increase resistance and resilience to stress, enabling the body to adapt around the problem and avoid collapse. Adaptogens by supporting the adrenal glands.
Alterative	Gradually restore proper functioning of the body, increasing health and vitality.
Anthelminitic	Destroy or expel intestinal worms.
Anti-inflammatory	Soothe inflammations or reduce the inflammatory response of the tissue directly. They work in a number of different ways, but rarely inhibit the natural inflammatory reaction as such.
Antimicrobial	Help the body destroy or resist pathogenic microorganisms. Herbs help the body strengthen its own resistance to infective organisms and resist illness.
Antispasmodic	Ease cramps in smooth and skeletal muscles. They alleviate muscular tension and can ease psychological tension as well.
Astringent	Have a binding action on mucous membranes, skin, and other tissue. They have the effect of reducing irritation and inflammation, and creating a barrier against infection that is helpful to wounds and burns.
Bitter	The taste triggers a sensory response in the central nervous system, which stimulates appetite and the flow of digestive juices, aid the liver's detoxification work, increase bile flow, and motivate gut self-repair mechanisms.
Carminative	Plants that are rich in aromatic volatile oils stimulate the digestive system to work properly and with ease. They soothe the gut wall, reduce inflammation, and ease gripping pains and help with the removal of gas from the digestive tract.
Demulcent	Rich in mucilage and soothe and protect irritated or inflamed tissue. They reduce irritation down the whole length of the bowel, reduce sensitivity to potentially corrosive gastric acids, help prevent diarrhea, and reduce the muscle spasms that cause colic.
Diuretic	Increase production and elimination of urine. They help the body eliminate waste and support the whole process of inner cleansing.

continued

Table
12-2

Selected Actions of Herbs (continued)

ACTION	DESCRIPTION
Emmenagogue	Stimulate menstrual flow and activity. With most herbs, however, the term is used in the wider sense for a remedy that affects the female reproductive system.
Expectorant	Stimulate removal of mucus from the lungs. Stimulating expectorants "irritate" the bronchioles causing expulsion of material. Relaxing expectorants soothe bronchial spasm and loosen mucous secretions, helping in dry, irritating coughs.
Hepatic	Aid the liver. They tone and strengthen the liver and in some cases increase the flow of bile.
Hypotensive	Lower abnormally elevated blood pressure.
Laxative	Promote bowel movements. They are divided into those that work by providing bulk, those that stimulate the production of bile in the liver and its release from the gallbladder, and those that directly trigger peristalsis.
Nervine	Help the nervous system. Tonics strengthen and restore the nervous system. Relaxants ease anxiety and tension. Stimulants directly stimulate nerve activity.
Stimulating	Quicken and invigorate the physiological and metabolic activity of the body.
Tonic	Nurture and enliven. They are used frequently in traditional Chinese medicine and Ayurvedic medicine, often as a preventative measure.

Teas (Infusion)

Either loose or in teabag form, dried, whole, or chopped herbs can be prepared as infusions (steeped as tea) or decoctions (simmered over low heat). Flowers, leaves, and powdered herbs are infused (chamomile or peppermint); while fruits, seeds, barks, and roots require decocting (rose hips, cinnamon bark, licorice root). When steeped in boiled water for a few minutes, the fragrant, aromatic flavor and medicinal properties are released. Teas are used to prepare the more delicate parts of the plants, such as leaves and flowers. Most teas are consumed as alternatives to caffeinated tea or coffee, with meals for the flavor, or for their mild medicinal effects. Suggestions for preparation:

■ Always use a glass or enamel container, as this will best preserve the integrity of the medicine. Stainless steel may be used also, but aluminum must be avoided because it can contaminate the formulas. Chemicals can be absorbed from plastic containers. Use distilled water, as it will pull the medicinal properties of the plant into solution.

- General proportions are 1 tablespoon dried herb per cup of water (1 part herb to 16 parts water). If you are using fresh herbs, use 3 tablespoons per cup water.

- For general use, the tea is taken warm; however, to produce a sweat, drink it hot.

Decoctions

A decoction is a stronger, more potent tea than an infusion. The purpose of a decoction is to pull the mineral salts and bitter principles of the plant. Many of the volatile oils and vitamins will escape with this process. This method is generally used for the harder parts of the plant, such as roots, bark, and seeds, but it is also used to reduce or boil down any herbs to make a stronger preparation, such as cough syrup. Suggestions for preparation:

- Proportions are generally 1 ounce dried herbs per 1.5 pints of water (can vary, consult directions).

- Put the herbs into the distilled water, bring the water to boil, and then turn down to a simmer. Simmer for 10 minutes, turn off the heat, let sit for 5 more minutes, strain, and drink.

Capsules and Tablets

These offer convenience and the bonus of not having to taste the herbs. Herbs are available either powdered or freeze-dried, in bulk, tablets, troches, pastes, or capsules.

Extracts and Tinctures

These provide a high concentration of drug in low weight and space. Many fresh and dried herbs can be tinctured as preserved medicines in alcohol; some plants are suited to extracts (vinegar extracts) and others are active and well preserved as syrups, glycerites (in vegetable glycerine), or miels (in honey). They are quickly assimilated. Alcohol is used as a solvent and as a preservative to maintain shelf life. Tinctures usually contain more alcohol than extracts. Fluid and solid extracts are strong concentrates, four to six times the crude herb strength, and fresh plant juices that are preserved in approximately 25% alcohol (as in the fresh plant echinacea succus).

If an extract or tincture contains known active principles, the strength is commonly expressed in terms of the content of these active principles. Otherwise, the strength is expressed in terms of their concentration. For example, tinctures are typically made at a 1:5 concentration. This means one part herb (in grams) is soaked in five parts liquid (in milliliters of volume), or that there are five times the amount of solvent (alcohol or water) in a tincture as there is herbal material. Expressing the strength of an extract by the concentration method does not accurately measure potency because there may be great variation among manufacturing techniques and raw materials (Murray, 1995).

"The term standardized extract (or guaranteed potency extract) refers to an extract guaranteed to contain a 'standardized' level of active compounds. Stating the content of active compounds rather than the concentration ratio allows for more accurate dosages to be made" (Murray, 1995, p. 17). One minum of the extract represents one grain of the crude drug.

The solvent (menstruum) is usually a combination of food grade grain alcohol and distilled water. Fresh plants require different proportions. A general rule for dried plant tinctures is 50% alcohol and 50% water, which is the equivalent of 100 proof vodka. General proportional rules for dried herb tinctures are 8 oz herb per quart of menstruum. To prepare a tincture using maceration, finely cut, blended or powdered herbs are put in a jar in the quantity specified by the formula, covered with the appropriate menstruum, and closed tightly. Each day for a minimum of 14 days, the mixture is shaken. The more the tincture is agitated, the better chance the menstruum has to work through the herb. The mixture should be poured through a strainer into a bowl, then placed into a cheesecloth which has been draped over a strainer sitting in a bowl to catch drips. The cheesecloth can be gathered up into a ball, with the remaining menstruum squeezed out. The menstruum should then be filtered through a coffee or milk filter or a double layer gauze diaper to remove any remaining particles. The remaining tincture can be transferred to small-mouthed bottles and stored in a dark cool place.

Elixirs

Similar to tinctures, elixirs are made quite sweet using honey or sucanet. They are often made with brandy and are normally used as tonics.

Nonoral Herbal Forms

Nonoral delivery forms include rectal administration of herbal suppositories or enemas; application to the skin of creams, ointments, gels, liniments, oils, distilled waters, washes, baths, poultices, or compresses; or inhalation of steams, smokes, or aromatics (volatile oils).

- *Salves, balms, and ointments.* Made with vegetable oil or petroleum jelly. Semi-solid, designed to be applied to the skin. Best to use dried herbs, as fresh herbs contain moisture that could lead to spoilage of the formula.

- *Liniments.* Tinctures used externally only. They are the only preparations that use isopropyl alcohol, but vodka can be used instead. Alcohol is quickly absorbed and carries the medicine into the tissues. Sprains, strains, and sore muscles all respond quickly to liniment therapy. Preparation is the same as with a regular tincture.

- *Essential oils.* Concentrated, with one or two drops often constituting adequate dosage. They should be diluted in fatty oils or water before topical application (see the section on Aromatherapy later in this chapter).

USES FOR HERBAL THERAPIES

Herbal remedies can be used for a wide range of minor ailments that are amenable to self-medication, including stomach upset, the common cold, flus, minor aches and pains, constipation and diarrhea, coughs, headaches, menstrual cramps, digestive disturbances, sore muscles, skin rashes, sunburn, dandruff, and insomnia. Other conditions that respond well to herbal medicine include digestive disorders such as peptic ulcers, colitis, and irritable bowel syndrome; rheumatic and arthritic conditions; chronic skin problems such as eczema and psoriasis; problems of the menstrual cycle and especially premenstrual syndrome; anxiety and tension-related stress; bronchitis and other respiratory conditions; hypertension; and allergies (Burton Goldberg Group, 1995).

SPECIFIC HERBAL THERAPIES

Below are descriptions of 10 herbs that have possible self-care health promotion applications, as described by Landis (1997). They are widely used, and, in most cases, have demonstrated effectiveness in at least some scientific clinical studies. For each herb, the common name is followed by the species name in parentheses.

Astragalus (Membranaceus)

The astragalus root is a traditional Chinese herb from the pea family. Dried, sliced astragalus root looks like rough yellow tongue depressors. Astragalus has the following uses:

1. Immune enhancer. As a long-term tonic, it assists healing and recovery in chronic infection or illness:

   - Stimulates phagocytosis
   - Increases macrophage activity
   - Increases number of stem cells
   - Increases spleen activity
   - Increases release of antibodies
   - Boosts the production of hormonal messenger molecules that signal for virus destruction

2. Reduces the side effects of steroid therapy and counteracts the immunosuppressive effects of toxic cancer therapies such as chemotherapy and radiation.

3. Antiviral. Decreases incidence of colds.

4. Tonic. Builds energy:

   - Reduces sweating
   - Increases appetite
   - Cools fever
   - Diuretic
   - Digestive tonic

Astragalus is sold in capsules and tinctures. In Asia, it is used in a fresh broth or soup. Use 4 to 8 mL per day of the 1:2 liquid extract or tincture (1:5): 2 to 6 mL (1: 1.5 teaspoons) three times a day for a cold (Mills & Bone, 2000). There is no toxicity, but note, it is advisable in acute infections. Astragalus is considered mild and safe.

Chamomile (Matricaria Recutita)

Chamomile flower is used in many cultures for its pleasant-tasting tea, consumed as an after-dinner beverage to help digestion. Its uses include:

1. Digestive aid, antispasmodic

2. Inflammatory diseases of the digestive tract

   - Mouthwash for minor mouth irritation or gum infections
   - Irritable bowel syndrome and infant's colic

Chamomile tea is made by pouring boiling water over a tablespoon of the flower heads and steeping for 10 to 15 minutes; this is drunk three to four times daily. An allergic reaction involving urticaria or bronchoconstriction can occur, though extremely rarely, in a person who is hypersensitive to daisy or ragweed-type plants.

Echinacea (E. Purpurea)

Echinacea (purple coneflower) species are perennial herbs native to midwestern North America, from Saskatchewan to Texas.

Although the root is believed to possess the greatest immune enhancing properties, most studies have used fresh-pressed juice from the aerial portion of E. purpurea. Standardized preparations are guaranteed to contain a minimum of 2.4% beta-1,2-fructofuranosides. "Standardizing the product for these compounds guarantees that the plant was harvested in the blossom stage, the product was carefully prepared and suffered no enzymatic or microbiological degradation, and that the product is stabilized" (Murray, 1995, p. 104).

Echinacea is used to treat:

1. Common cold. May be able to moderate the severity and duration of symptoms, but no benefit for prevention of upper respiratory infection has been demonstrated (Barrett, Kiefer, & Rabago, 1999).

2. Infections:

   - Promotes tissue regeneration and reduces inflammation (helps alleviate rheumatoid arthritis)

   - Nonspecific antiviral effect

   - Mild direct antibacterial activity

3. Low immune status:

   - Elevates serum white blood cell counts when they are low

   - Promotes nonspecific T cell activation

   - Increases number of circulating neutrophils

4. Cancer:

   - Increases the activity of natural killer cells

   - Stimulates macrophages to greater cytotoxic activity against tumor cells

As a general immune stimulant during infection, the herb should be given three times daily. The dose of juice of aerial portion of E. purpurea, stabilized in 22% ethanol (standardized), is 2 to 3 mL (0.5 to 0.75 teaspoon). The usual dose for the root extract is 900 mg 2 to 4 times a day, while the tincture (1:5) dose is 3 to 4 mL (0.75 to 1 teaspoon) (Dog, 1999).

"Powdered echinacea administered orally in the form of capsules would probably be relatively inactive" (Tyler, 1993, p. 116). However, "there is no evidence to suggest that long-term usage will have an adverse effect on immune function" (Mills & Bone, 2000, p. 355).

The usual recommendation for long-term use is 8 weeks on followed by 1 week off. In patients with impaired immune function, long-term administration can provide long-term benefit. Echinacea is not toxic when used at the recommended doses, but should not be used by patients with infectious or autoimmune diseases such as multiple sclerosis, tuberculosis, Lupus, AIDS, and HIV infection. It also may interfere with immunosuppressive therapy.

Garlic (Allium Sativum)

Garlic, a member of the lily family, is a perennial plant that is cultivated worldwide. The bulb, either fresh or dehydrated, is used as a medicinal herb and assists with:

1. Cancer prevention; inhibits formation of nitrosamines.

2. Diabetes; hypoglycemia.

3. Protects against heart disease and strokes:

   ■ Lowers blood pressure

   ■ Lowers cholesterol and hyperlipidemia

   ■ Intervenes in the process of atherosclerosis at many steps

   ■ Antioxidant

4. Infection:

   ■ Broad-spectrum antimicrobial activity against many genera of bacteria, virus, worms, and fungi

   ■ Anti-inflammatory

5. Garlic possesses diuretic, diaphoretic, emmenagogue, and expectorant action. It is also a carminative, antispasmodic, and digestant, making it useful in cases of flatulence, nausea, vomiting, colic, and indigestion" (Murray, 1995, p. 125). A meta-analysis suggested that across all 13 randomized clinical trials meeting the inclusion criteria, the effect on total cholesterol was statistically significant but too small to be clinically relevant. The most rigorous randomized clinical trials did not show a statistically significant effect (Ernst & Pittler, 2002).

Stability, quality control, and standardization of the content of several active ingredients is variable from product to product, making treatment effects unpredictable (Dog, 1999). Therefore, "preparations standardized for alliin content provide the greatest assurance of quality... Make sure that the level of alliin and the total allicin potential is clearly stated and that the product is stable. The commercial product should provide a daily dose of at least 10 mg of alliin or a total alliin potential of 4,000 micrograms" (Murray, 1995, pp. 128-129), an amount equal to approximately 1 clove (4 grams) of fresh garlic. Garlic is nontoxic at the dosages commonly used for most people. In large amounts, however, it can cause irritation to the digestive tract. To avoid the taste or offensive odor of garlic, the best formulations are enteric coated tablets or capsules of dried garlic or garlic powder. Garlic may potentially interact with anticoagulants such as warfarin.

Ginkgo Biloba

Ginkgo biloba is a deciduous tree that lives as long as 1,000 years. Ginkgo bears a foul-smelling, inedible fruit and an edible, ivory-colored inner seed that is sold in marketplaces in the orient. Extracts from the leaves of the ginko tree are used medicinally for the following purposes:

1. Vascular insufficiency:

    ■ Reduces symptoms of cerebral insufficiency, including impaired mental function (senility) in the elderly

    ■ Anti-aggregatory effect on platelets

2. Memory enhancing:

    ■ Increases cerebral blood flow with oxygen and glucose utilization

    ■ Increases the rate at which information is transmitted at the nerve cell level

    ■ Delays mental deterioration in the early stages of Alzheimer's disease equivalent to a 6-month delay in the progression of the disease

3. Retinopathy. Addresses the underlying factors in senile macular degeneration.

4. Peripheral vascular disorders. Improves limb blood flow and walking tolerance.

5. Impotence. Erectile dysfunction due to lack of blood flow.

6. Ginkgo biloba extract (GBE) "may be of benefit in cases of angina, congestive heart failure, and in acute respiratory distress syndrome. Its action on inhibiting platelet activating factor may also make it useful in the treatment of conditions other than allergies, including various types of shock, thrombosis, graft protection during organ transplantation, multiple sclerosis, and burns" (Murray, 1995, p. 158).

Ginkgo biloba has been shown in several systematic reviews to be effective for the symptomatic treatment of dementia and intermittent claudication (Ernst & Pittler, 2002). Most of the clinical research has used a standardized extract, containing 24% ginkgo heterosides (flavone glycosides) at a dosage of 40 mg three times a day. GBE should be taken consistently for at least 12 weeks in order to be effective. Although most people report benefits within 2 to 3 weeks, some may take longer to respond. GBE is extremely safe and side effects are uncommon but may include mild gastrointestinal disturbances, headache, dizziness, and vertigo. In contrast, contact with or ingestion of the fruit pulp has produced severe allergic reactions like poison ivy, oak, or sumac group.

Panax Ginseng

Ginseng is a widely cultivated plant, especially in Korea, but also in Russia, China, and Japan. Old, wild, well-formed roots are the most valued, while rootlets of cultivated plants are considered the lowest grade. "For largely economic purposes, most ginseng in the American marketplace is derived from the lowest grade root, diluted with excipients, blended with adulterants, or totally devoid of active ingredients, that is ginsenosides. High-quality roots and extracts are available, however. These preparations consist of the main root of plants between 4 to 6 years of age, or extracts that have been standardized for ginsenoside content and ratio to ensure optimum pharmacological effect" (Murray, 1995, p. 266). In China, ginseng is used to restore the yang quality and as a tonic for its revitalizing properties, especially after a long illness. The genus name Panax is derived from the Latin word panacea meaning "cure all." It is used to treat:

1. Fatigue and recovery from illness.

2. Stress. Adaptogen:

   ■ Spares glycogen utilization in exercising muscle

   ■ Promotes secretion of ACTH

3. Diabetes, hypoglycemia.

Products should be standardized by their ginsenoside content. The standard dose for high-quality ginseng root is in the range of 4 to 6 grams daily. It is best to begin at lower doses and increase gradually. "The Russian approach for long-term administration is to use ginseng cyclically for a period of 15 to 20 days, followed by a 2-week interval without any ginseng" (Murray, 1995, p. 276). "Many clinical trials have been conducted using a dose of 200 mg of a standardized extract" (Mills & Bone, 2000, p. 419). Studies with standardized extracts have demonstrated the absence of side effects, but women may experience breast tenderness that can be reversed by lowering the dose or stopping the treatment. However, a systematic review found no convincing evidence for efficacy in any indication, and another systematic review of all nine randomized clinical trials available was inconclusive. Many of the studies had poor methodological quality (Ernst & Pittler, 2002). Interactions are possible with warfarin, insulin, and phenelzine.

Siberian Ginseng (Eleutherococcus Senticosus)

Siberian ginseng grows abundantly in parts of the Soviet Far East, Korea, China, and Japan, north of latitude 38. The root is the most widely used medicinal part, and assists with:

1. Stress and fatigue. Ability to "normalize" irrespective of the direction of pathology. However, in a prospective, double-blind, placebo-controlled, randomized clinical trial with 83 healthy young adults, ginseng supplementation had no effect on positive affect, negative affect, or total mood disturbance at the clinically recommended level or twice that level (Cardinal & Engels, 2001):

   ■ Inhibit the alarm phase of the stress reaction

   ■ Protective and medicinal action in animals exposed to both single and prolonged x-ray radiation

   ■ Chronic fatigue syndrome

2. Atherosclerosis.

3. Impaired kidney function.

"The standard dosage of the 33% ethanol extract (fluid extract) used in the majority of studies ranged from 2.0 to 4.0 mL, one to three times a day, for periods up to 60 consecutive days. In multiple dosing regimens, there is usually a 2- to 3-week interval between courses. The dose to be administered three times a day of fluid extract (1:1) is 2.0 to 4.0 mL" (Murray, 1995, p. 319). "Adult doses used in most studies were in the range of 1 to 4 g daily, which corresponds to 2 to 8 mL/day of a 1:2 extract" (Mills & Bone, 2000, p. 535). Siberian ginseng extracts are virtually nontoxic, but side effects are often reported at dosages of 4.5 to 6 mL three times daily. These include insomnia, irritability, melancholy, and anxiety. Individuals with rheumatic heart disease have reported pericardial pain, headaches, palpitations, and elevations in blood pressure.

Green Tea (Camellia Sinensis)

Both green tea and black tea are derived from the tea plant. The parts used are the leaf bud and the two adjacent young leaves together with the stem, broken between the second and third leaf. Older leaves are considered inferior in quality. Green tea is produced by lightly steaming the fresh-cut leaf, while the leaves are allowed to oxidize to produce black tea. Green tea is produced and consumed primarily in China, Japan, and a few countries in North Africa and the Middle East. One cup of green tea usually contains about 300 to 400 mg of polyphenols and between 50 and 100 mg of caffeine. Green tea is used to assist with:

1. Antioxidant supplementation

2. Cancer prevention

   - Blocks the formation of cancer-causing compounds such as nitrosamines suppresses the activation of carcinogens and detoxifies or traps cancer-causing agents.

   - "The forms of cancer that appear to be best prevented by green tea are cancers of the gastrointestinal tract, including cancers of the stomach, small intestine, pancreas, and colon; lung cancer; and estrogen-related cancers including most breast cancers" (Murray, 1995, p. 194).

The normal amount of green tea consumed by Japanese and other green tea-drinking cultures is about 3 cups daily or about 3 grams of soluable components, providing roughly 240 to 320 mg of polyphenols. For a green tea extract standardized for 80% total polyphenol and 55 percent epigallocatechin gallate content, this means a daily dose of 300 to 400 mg. Green tea is not associated with any significant side effects or toxicity. Overconsumption may produce a stimulant effect (nervousness, anxiety, insomnia, irritability, etc.) as with any caffeine-containing beverage; however, for some reason green tea usually does not produce those symptoms even in those who are usually quite sensitive to caffeine.

St. John's Wort (Hypericum Perforatum)

St. John's wort is a shrubby perennial plant with numerous bright yellow flowers. It is native to many parts of the world, including Europe and the United States. It grows especially well in northern California and southern Oregon. The major compounds of interest in St. John's wort leaves and flowers are hypericin and pseudohypericin. In Europe, St. John's wort has a long history of use, particularly as a folk remedy in the treatment of wounds, kidney and lung ailments, and depression. Clinical trials have shown St. John's wort extract to be more effective than placebo and equally effective as standard synthetic antidepressants (Dog, 1999). Its clinical applications include the treatment of:

1. Depression. Inhibits monoamine oxidase (MAO) types A and B, which leads to an increase in nerve impulse transmitters that maintain normal mood and emotional stability. "The results of 26 double-blind controlled studies with the standardized St. John's wort extract (0.3% hypericin) indicate that at a dosage of 300 mg three times daily it is as effective in relieving symptoms of depression as standard antidepressants but is much better tolerated with fewer side effects" (Murray, 1995, p. 298).

2. Sleep disorders.

3. Viral infections. Inhibits herpes simplex virus types 1 and 2, influenza types A and B, and Epstein-Barr virus. The greatest promise may be in treatment of AIDS.

4. Healing of wounds. As a lotion it will speed the healing of wounds and bruises, varicose veins, and mild burns. The oil is especially useful for healing sunburn.

A typical regimen is "hypericum tablets (1.5 g standardized to contain 0.9 mg TH): 2 to 3 tablets per day" (Mills & Bone, 2000, p. 543). Can also be taken as tea prepared from 1 to 2 teaspoonfuls of the herb steeped for 10 minutes; 1 to 2 cups of the tea are drunk daily for 4 to 6 weeks.

Advantages of St. John's wort compared with antidepressant drugs include (Coss & Cott, 2002):

- Side effects are generally mild and infrequent

- Nonhabituating and nonaddictive, and has no withdrawal symptoms upon discontinuing use

- Does not interfere with REM sleep; most often it enhances sleep and dreaming

- Shows no adverse effects when mixed with alcohol or most drugs

- Far less likely to cause drowsiness or agitation

- Not a single reported death from an overdose

St. John's wort is unlikely to be toxic to humans when used at recommended medicinal doses. Side effects reported for St. John's wort are generally mild, including gastrointestinal symptoms and fatigue (Coss & Cott, 2002). "Because of the possibility of photosensitivity, some herbalists recommend that individuals, especially those with fair skin, avoid exposure to strong sunlight and other sources of ultraviolet light when using the herb. Those taking the herb should also avoid foods and medications that are known to interact negatively with MAO-inhibiting drugs. Tyramine-containing foods (cheeses, beer, wine, pickled herring, yeast, etc.) and drugs such as L-dopa and 5-hydroxytryptophan should be avoided. St. John's wort should also be taken with food, as it may cause mild gastric upset in sensitive individuals" (Murray, 1995, p. 300).

Valerian

Valerian is a perennial plant native to North America and Europe. The rootstock is the portion used medicinally for:

1. Insomnia. Binds to the same brain receptors as Valium and other benzodiazepine drugs without side effects such as impaired mental function, morning hangover, and depend-

ency. However, "larger, better controlled, and more representative clinical trials are needed before clear recommendations can be made" (Barrett et al., 1999, p. 47).

2. Stress and anxiety.

As a mild sedative, valerian may be taken 30 to 45 minutes before retiring as 2 to 6 mL of 1:2 liquid extract per day, 5 to 15 mL of 1:5 tincture per day (Mills & Bone, 2000), or Valerian extract (0.8% valeric acid): 150 to 300 mg.

For best results, eliminate dietary factors such as caffeine and alcohol, which disrupt sleep. Valerian is generally regarded as safe and is approved for food use by the FDA. It does not have a synergy with alcohol. Approximately 5% to 10% of users have reported paradoxical stimulant effects.

There are a number of tonic, energizing, and endurance herbs that can be used to promote general well-being based on many years of anecdotal experience particularly in The People's Republic of China. Table 12-3 lists some of the most common herbs used for these purposes.

Table 12-3

Selected Tonic, Energizing, and Endurance Herbs

TONIC HERBS	ENERGIZING HERBS	STAMINA AND ENDURANCE HERBS
Astragalus membranaceus	**Short-term energizers:**	Panax (Asian) ginseng
Echinacea	Guarana seed	Eleuthero
Triphala (Ayurvedic)	Kola nut	Triphala
Turmeric root	Yohimbe	
Ginseng	Yerba mate	
Eleuthero	Ma huang	
Dong quai	**Medium-term energizers:**	
Licorice root	Licorice root	
	Cubeb berry	
	Garlic, onion, and ginger	
	Long-term energizers:	
	Fo-ti root	
	Astragalus root	
	Eleuthero root	
	Saw palmetto berry	
	Triphala	
	Black cohosh root	
	Prickly ash bark	
	Muira puama root	
	Sarsaparilla root	
	Bladderwack	

Unfortunately, a number of herbs may have dangerous interactions with conventional drugs when they are taken together. Table 12-4 indicates some examples of selected drug and herbal interactions.

Table
12-4

Selected Herbal Medicine Interactions with Prescribed Drugs

HERBAL MEDICINE	HERB AND DRUG INTERACTIONS
St. John's wort (Hypericum perforatum)	Lowers blood concentrations of cyclosporin, amitriptyline, digoxin, indinavir, warfarin, phenprocoumon, and theophylline.
	Causes intermenstrual bleeding when used with oral contraceptives (ethinylestradiol/desogestrel).
	Causes delirium when used with loperamide.
	Causes mild seratonin syndrome when used with selective serotonin-reuptake inhibitors (sertaline, paroxetine, nefazodone).
	Should not be used with monoamine oxidase inhibitors (MAOI antidepressants), narcotics, reserpine, and photosensitizing drugs.
	Discontinue use at least 5 days prior to surgery. Should not take postoperatively if oral anticoagulation is needed.
	May inhibit iron absorption, undermining the benefits of prescribed anemia drugs.
Ginkgo biloba	Causes bleeding when combined with warfarin.
	Raises blood pressure when used with a thiazide diuretic.
	Causes coma when used with trazodone.
	Should discontinue at least 36 hours prior to surgery (inhibits platelet-activating factor).
Ginseng (Panax ginseng)	Lowers blood concentrations of alcohol and warfarin.
	May induce headaches, tremulousness, or manic episodes if used with phenelzine sulfate (antidepressant).
	Should discontinue use at least 7 days prior to surgery.
Garlic (Alluim sativum)	Changes pharmacokinetic variables of paracetamol.
	Decreases blood concentrations of warfarin.
	Produces hypoglycemia when taken with chlorpropamide.
Kava (Piper methysticum)	Increases "off" periods in Parkinson's patients taking levadopa.
	Can cause a semicomatose state with alprazolam.
	Potentiates the sedative effects of anesthetics.

continued

| Table 12-4 | ***Selected Herbal Medicine Interactions with Prescribed Drugs (continued)*** |

HERBAL MEDICINE	HERB AND DRUG INTERACTIONS
Echinacea (E. angustifolia; E. purpurea; E. pallida)	May interfere with immunosuppressive drugs. Use with caution in patients with allergic reactions (e.g., asthma, atopy, or allergic rhinitis) Potential concern for hepatotoxicity.
Ginger	Can cause adverse reactions with acid-inhibiting, anticoagulant, antiplatelet, cardiac, and diabetes drugs
Melatonin	Can interfere with central nervous system depressants, verapamil, and immunosuppressive drugs.
Green tea	Can cause hypertension with MAOIs. Can have adverse reactions with chlorpromazine, cimetidine, clozapine, disulfiram, theophylline, and verapamil.

Sources: Adapted from Ang-Lee, M. K., Moss, J., & Yuan, C. (2001). Herbal medicines and perioperative care. *JAMA, 286*, 208-216; Coleman, S. (2001, July 30). Proceed with caution. *Advance for nurses*, 23-24; Eastman, P. (1999). Drugs that fight can hurt you. *American Association of Retired Persons Review, 40*, 14-16; Izzo, A. A., & Ernst, E. (2001). Interactions between herbal medicines and prescribed drugs: A systematic review. *Drugs, 61*, 2163-75.

KEY CONCERNS

There are a number of concerns with the use of herbal remedies. One concern is that developing countries have minimal regulation and oversight, even though herbal medicines are the staple of medical treatment, with visits to Western-trained doctors or prescription pharmacists reserved for life-threatening or hard-to-treat disorders. Healers rely mainly on indigenous "crude drugs." These are unprocessed herbs, plants or plant parts, dried and used in whole or cut form. Herbs are prepared as teas (sometimes as pills or capsules) for internal use and as salves and poultices for external use (Berman & Larson, 1994).

Another concern is the lack of support by the U. S. federal government. Because herbs have not been "discovered," they cannot be patented. Consequently, drug companies are not motivated to invest money in testing or promotion of herbs. "The collection and preparation of herbal medicine cannot be as easily controlled as the manufacture of synthetic drugs, making its profits less dependable" (Burton Goldberg Group, 1995, p. 253). The federal government has not intervened to promote quality control of herbs.

There is a limited supply of educated botanists, and traditional healers are elderly and have few disciples. In addition, the academic infrastructure for study of ethnomedical systems has eroded. Today, only a handful of active full-time ethnobotanists are trained to catalog information on the medicinal properties of plants, and in the mid-1990s only 12 American pharmacy schools offered courses on botanical medicine (D'Epiro, 1997).

Also of concern is the lack of a holistic approach to studying the efficacy of herbals as phytomedicines (whole plant medicines) rather than individual chemicals. Most herb products contain a combination of several ingredients because they come from plants. It is possible that "plant composition alone offers an incomplete explanation of the full scope of the properties and actions of food and healing plants.... Many herbalists hold that healing energy is inherent to plants; it is primarily this energy, rather than nutritive or chemical constituents, which promotes healing" (Meserole, 1996, p. 116).

Americans have been conditioned to rely on synthetic, commercial drugs to provide quick relief, regardless of side effects (Burton Goldberg Group, 1995). Despite the lack of research models to test herbal preparations that may contain many active ingredients and the fact that, in many cases, experts have not yet determined which pharmacologically active ingredient or combination of ingredients is causing the pharmacologic activity, the emphasis of many herbal manufacturers is to isolate single active ingredients that can be packaged and sold separately (Prescriber's Letter, 1998).

Herbal products can interact with either prescription or nonprescription drugs. However, providers often do not ask, and "[clients] frequently don't tell their health care providers that they use herbs. Maybe [clients] forget, or they just don't consider herbs as drugs. They might think herbs are not powerful enough or important enough to bring up" (Prescriber's Letter, 1998, p. 1). Selected herb and drug interactions were discussed earlier in this chapter.

"Natural" doesn't necessarily mean safe. Some herbs have toxic effects. However, "true attributable adverse effect rates appear to be in the range of 3%" (Jonas & Ernst, 1999, p. 104). Unfortunately, herbal products often lack consistency. Many factors influence the content of herbal medicine products such as soil, weather, other environmental conditions, time of harvest, storage, and manufacturing procedures (Prescriber's Letter, 1998). Thus, issues of quality control are of concern.

Herbs are not required to demonstrate bioequivalence. A standardized extract merely means that the manufacturer asserts that one specific ingredient is present in a certain concentration and that subsequent lots of the herbal product contain the same concentration of the standardized component. But, the other ingredients could be higher or lower depending on many other factors. Two brands of a standardized herb extract may not be identical (Prescriber's Letter, 1998) and can vary in efficacy and results, even at the same doses (D'Epiro, 1997). Mislabeling and misrepresentation occur. Without quality control, there is no guarantee that the herb contained in the bottle is the same as what is stated on the label (Murray, 1995). Quality assurance is needed to ensure: (a) that the product has the expected effects, (b) the quality of available product information, and (c) product safety (deSmet, 2002).

Despite these concerns, companies supplying standardized extracts currently offer the greatest degree of quality control, hence these products typically offer the highest quality. The European Economic Council (EEC) has proposed guidelines for acceptable levels of impurities such as parasites (bacterial counts), pesticides, residual solvents and heavy metals, and product stability. Most standardized extracts are currently made in Europe under these strict guidelines (Murray, 1995). Extracts made in the United States. do not have to meet these guidelines.

Incorrect, inaccurate, or inappropriate diagnosis can result in the application of effective therapies for the incorrect condition. Misapplication usually occurs because of inadequate training, knowledge, skills, or experience of the clinician (Jonas & Ernst, 1999). Additionally, treating with herbs with unproven therapeutic potential may delay or replace a more effective form of conventional medication therapy. These concerns highlight the need for practitioners to obtain thorough educational preparation before prescribing herbal therapies.

Given these many concerns, there are many challenges for the future including the conservation of biodiversity and plant habitat; training professional and other herbalists; exchanging information with traditional healers; providing health care professionals with a familiarity with plant medicines; educating the public in the appropriate use of herbs for self-care; ensuring the funding of medicinal plant research that focuses on public health, clinical therapeutics, and wellness, and not just drug development; and preserving public access to inexpensive, tonic, and therapeutic herbs through economic, environmental, market, legislative, and health policy (Meserole, 1996).

Aromatherapy

Aromatherapy is the therapeutic use of the odor or fragrance of essential oils extracted from plants (Stevensen, 1996). Essential oils are volatile, organic components extracted from fragrant plants by steam distillation or expression (Buckle, 2001). Essential oils may be extracted from the roots, bark, stalks, flowers, or leaves of the plant. Chemical changes occur, changing the composition of the oil, immediately after the flower is cut.

Essential oils are highly volatile and dissolve in pure alcohol, fats, and oils but not in water. Because they are sensitive to heat and light, they are preferably kept in dark glass bottles that should be stored to prevent contamination from other sources. Plastic bottles should never be used to store essential oils because the oils will interact with the plastic. The oils will evaporate readily if left exposed to the air. Most essential oils have a limited lifespan of approximately 2 years, and citrus oils such as lemon, orange, and lime do not keep that long (Glickstein, 1996; James, 1998). Essential oils should not be bought or used unless the smell is pleasing.

Clinical aromatherapy includes both environmental and personal (esthetic) applications to calm, balance, and rejuvenate. The purposes of esthetic aromatherapy include pleasure and healing, whereas commercial aromatherapy relies almost exclusively on use of environmental fragrances in work, purchasing, and sales settings (Holmes, 1995). In clinical aromatherapy, the concern is for 100% purity of oil extracted from a specific plant genus, species, and chemotype, with nothing added, removed, or reconstructed. Good or high quality oils are crucial to the success of clinical treatments.

CLINICAL APPLICATIONS

The basis of the action of aromatherapy is thought to be the same as that of modern pharmacology, using smaller doses. The chemical constituents are absorbed into the body, affecting particular physiologic processes. In addition, the emotional and psychological benefits of aromatherapy are important. By affecting the limbic system, the part of the brain involved in memory and emotion, the inhaled oils exert their effects through learned responses as well as inherent pharmacological properties (Horowitz, 1999).

The chemical makeup of essential oils gives them a number of desirable pharmacological properties ranging from antibacterial, antiviral, and antispasmodic, to uses as diuretics, vasodilators, and vasoconstrictors. Essential oils act on the adrenals, ovaries, and the thyroid and can energize or pacify, detoxify, and facilitate the digestive process. The therapeutic properties of the oils also make them effective for interacting with the various branches of the nervous system and modifying immune response, moods, and emotions (Burton Goldberg Group, 1995).

Aromatherapy aims first to enhance and balance the individual constitution and thereby prevent the development of disease. Second, it aims to treat actual sickness when it arises. Clinical aromatherapy involves numerous treatment modalities, some more preventive, others more curative. Aromatherapy can easily be incorporated within a nursing plan for the promotion of well-being and health. In addition, reasons to administer aromatherapy in conventional biomedical settings include:

- Relaxation, stress, and anxiety relief
- Headache (e.g., migraine) and chronic pain relief
- Reduction of insomnia and restlessness
- Reduction of anxiety, depression, and fatigue
- Self-image enhancement
- Stimulating immune function (e.g., against the Epstein-Barr virus)
- Infection fighting
- Wound healing
- Burn treatment
- Addiction treatment
- Reduction of compulsive eating
- Relief of menopausal symptoms
- Constipation
- Topical treatment of herpes simplex (shingles) and numerous skin disorders
- Ability to relieve muscle spasm
- Anxiety and nausea of chemotherapy
- Anti-inflammatory effects in treating arthritis

There are few well-designed studies investigating the effects of aromatherapy in humans, although several in vitro and animal studies have been conducted. Although "little is known about possible interactions with conventional medications or treatments, it is presumed that because the dosages of essential oils absorbed in the body generally are small, and because there has been no reported incidence of difficulties, that essential oils administered in physiologic doses are safe given the contraindications" (Stevensen, 1996, p. 145). It is clear that more scientific evidence is needed concerning basic mechanisms of action and efficacy of particular oils in particular populations.

Methods of Administering Essential Oils

A number of routes of administration can be used to administer essential oils. Some of the most common routes of administration are:

1. Through a diffusor. Diffusors disperse microparticles of the essential oil into the air. They can be used to achieve beneficial results in respiratory conditions, or to simply change the air with the mood-lifting or calming qualities of the fragrance. Simple inhalation of the oils is a method used for respiratory conditions, insomnia, and mood elevation and enhancement, or simply for making an environment more pleasant.

   - Electric. 5 to 6 drops added to water in the diffuser.

   - Candle generated. 8 to 10 drops added to water in dish.

   - Inhalation. Put 4 to 5 drops of essential oil in a bowl of very hot water. (Eyes should be closed to avoid a stinging sensation from the steam and essential oils. The client's head can be covered with a towel, while the client inhales for 5 minutes. The nurse should stay with the client and remove the bowl if the client starts expectorating). This method has a rapid effect. Another technique is to place 1 to 5 drops on a tissue to be inhaled slowly for 5 to 10 minutes.

2. External applications. Oils are readily absorbed through the skin. Therefore, they may be administered via baths, massages, hot and cold compresses, or a simple topical application of diluted oils. Because the essential oils are the same as those used for their aroma, external applications are discussed briefly here:

   - Essential oils in a hot bath can stimulate the skin, induce relaxation, eliminate toxins, and energize the body. Add 6 to 8 drops to the bath. The oils can be mixed with milk before adding to facilitate dispersion. Gently pat the skin dry afterward to leave a fine layer of oils on the skin for further absorption.

   - In massage (gentle rubbing touch rather than vigorous rubbing), the oils can be worked into the skin and depending on the oil and massage technique, can either calm or stimulate an individual. Rubbing or heating increases the rate of absorption of essential oils through the skin. In general, essential oils should not be applied directly to the skin, but should be mixed in a carrier oil. Clark (1996, p. 238) describes possible carrier oils: apricot kernel oil soothes and smooths dry or inflamed skin and is high in vitamin A; canola oil promotes skin health and resists rancidity; olive oil is beneficial to skin and hair but because of its strong odor, works better with stronger smelling oils such as basil, rosemary, and tea tree; peanut oil can be used on any skin type and is absorbed readily; and wheat germ oil nourishes dry or cracked skin and soothes eczema and psoriasis, may prevent stretch marks, and helps reduce scarring.

- Caution is appropriate when working with clients who have very sensitive skin or respiratory disorders such as asthma. For massage, the ratio should be half the number of essential oil drops to milliliters of base oil.

- When used in compresses, essential oils soothe minor aches and pains, reduce swelling, and treat sprains. Place 3 to 4 drops of essential oil in a bowl of water (can be diluted in cold-pressed vegetable oil, a cream, a gel, or water). Agitate water gently to disperse oil, then soak a small cotton or toweling cloth in bowl, ensuring that the cloth has absorbed the oil. Gently squeeze the cloth of excess water and apply to skin. Floral waters can be sprayed into the air or on skin that is too sensitive to touch.

- Buckle (2000) describes a gentle and soothing stroking process she has called the "M" (for manual) technique, which can be used with aromatherapy. The technique is done in a distinctive pattern (sequence, number, and pressure) of strokes, which is never modified, and is completely reproducible for use in research. Each stroke, within each movement, is repeated three times, with a pressure of 3 on a scale from 1 to 10. The "M" technique takes as little as 5 minutes for a client's hand, or 15 minutes for both feet. The back also may be stroked in a sequence lasting no more than 11 minutes. See the additional information at the end of the chapter to obtain more information about this technique.

3. Internal application. For certain conditions (such as organ dysfunction/disorder), it can be advantageous to take oils internally. However, "when essential oils are taken internally, the therapy is generally thought to be part of herbal medicine, not aromatherapy" (Buckle, 1999, p. 42). It is essential to receive proper medical guidance for internal use of oils, as they can cause a toxic reaction if ingested.

SPECIFIC ESSENTIAL OILS AND THEIR APPLICATIONS

Presented below are commonly used essential oils for clinical or self-care aromatherapy (Burton Goldberg Group, 1995).

Eucalyptus (Eucalyptus Radiata)

Eucalyptus is a classic antiviral (can help deal with herpes and shingles) and expectorant agent. It is antifungal, antiparasitic, a mosquito repellent and larvicide, and can inhibit granulation. It is also a muscle relaxant that may be useful in postoperative physiotherapy. It is best used through a diffusor or topically as a chest rub.

Everlast (Helichrysum Italicum)

When used in dilutions of 2% or lower, everlast can be used for tissue-regenerating on scars. Applied topically, it is a powerful anti-inflammatory agent and can prevent hemorrhaging and swelling after sports injuries or bruising. Because of its ketone content, this oil should only be used topically and in concentrations not exceeding 2%.

Geranium (Pelargonium Xasperum)

This fragrant oil has both antifungal and antiviral properties. It is gentle on the skin and gives body to the fragrance of many essential oil compositions.

Lavender (Lavandula Angustifolia)

Lavender is considered the classic oil of aromatherapy. It can be used undiluted on burns, small injuries, and insect bites. A high ester content gives it a calming, almost sedative quality. Two to 5 drops of the essential oil should be diluted in 5 mL of aloe vera gel to produce a 2% to 5% solution for use as a cell rejuvenator (Buckle, 2001). As an antiseptic it can be used as a gargle or mouth wash, with 1 to 3 drops added to a glass full of warm water (Buckle, 2001). For its analgesic action in earache, 1 drop of lavender should first be diluted with 2 drops of vegetable oil (e.g., sweet almond oil) and then the mixture should be placed on a cotton ball and placed in the child's ear (Buckle, 2001). As an antispasmodic, 1 to 5 drops should be added to a fixed carrier oil or hand cream and rubbed gently on the affected area (Buckle, 2001). Lavender is known for its calming effects, and inhaling 1 to 5 drops of lavender from a facial tissue for about 10 minutes can enhance well-being (Buckle, 2001; Robins, 1999). It is also used topically for pain relief "that also seems to enhance the effect of orthodox pain medication" (Buckle, 2001, p. 61).

Mandarin (Citrus Reticulata)

Mandarin's calming properties and universally pleasing fragrance make this oil a top choice to release anxiety. It has also been found to improve immune function (Buckle, 2001). It is typically dispersed in a room with a diffusor.

Niaouli (Melaleuca Quinquenervia Viridflora)

Niaouli calms respiratory allergies, is a vitalizing, balancing agent for overactive and oily skin, and helps with hemorrhoids (in the nonacute stage).

Palmarosa (Cymbopogon Martinii)

Palmarosa's pleasant fragrance and excellent antiseptic/antiviral activity have uses in skin care and in the treatment of herpes.

Peppermint (Meentha Piperita)

A drop of this oil on the tongue provides excellent relief for nausea and travel sickness. It is also effective for irritable bowel syndrome. However, it has up to 30% of ketones, which in high doses are known to be neurotoxic (Campbell et al., 2001).

Roman Chamomile (Anthemis Nobilis)

Recommended to calm an upset mind or body, a drop of Roman chamomile rubbed on the solar plexus can bring rapid relief of mental or physical stress.

Rosemary (Rosmarinus Officinalis)

Rosemary activates the metabolism in the outer layer of the skin and improves cell regeneration.

Spikenard (Nardostachys Jatamansi)

Spikenard is aimed as much toward benefiting the psyche as the skin.

Tea Tree (Melaleuca Alternifolia)

A nonirritating antiseptic, tea tree has antibacterial, antiviral, and antifungal properties. Applied topically, it is useful in healing pus-filled wounds and for treating many types of mild or chronic infections. Tea tree can be used in a hand wash, room spray, and body wash. One percent to 3% can be used as a mouthwash for mouth infections (Buckle, 2001).

Contraindications to the use of aromatherapy agents include the following (d'Angelo, 2002):

1. Epilepsy: eucalyptus, lavender, rosemary, basil, fennel, and sage

2. Hypertension: thyme, rosemary, pine, and sage

3. Asthma: rosemary and camphor

4. Pregnancy: lemon balm, cinnamon, basil, and thyme

CAUTIONS IN USING ESSENTIAL OILS

"An essential oil has cautions and/or contraindications associated with it for essentially three possible reasons: the intrinsic toxicity level of the oil itself, irritation to the skin and mucosa, and spontaneous idiosyncratic reactions" (Holmes, 1995, p. 181). The practitioner must consider a number of factors, including:

- Which oils to select

- The exact dosage required

- The correct dilution of the oils and in what medium

- The cautions and contraindications associated with each oil

- The duration of the treatment

Although essential oils are considered generally safe (Stevensen, 2001), there are potential side effects such as neurotoxic and abortive qualities, dermal toxicity, photosensitivity, allergic reactions, problems with internal usage, and liver sensitivity. Specific untoward effects include:

- Essential oils derived from thuja, wormwood, mugwort, tansy, hyssop, and sage can cause a toxic reaction if taken internally. Their toxicity is much lower when applied externally.

- Essential oils with a high phenol (disinfectant) content, such as oregano and savory, should not be taken internally for a period exceeding 10 to 21 days because of negative effects on liver metabolism.

- Clove and cinnamon should be used with caution, as they are known allergens.

- Overexposure to oils absorbed via diffuser can result in headaches, fatigue, or allergic reactions such as streaming eyes and skin problems.

In general, essential oils should not be ingested (Robins, 1999). Balanced formulas rather than single formulations should be used. However, herbals and essential oils can interact with prescription and nonprescription drugs, and can have toxic effects. Lack of standardization, bioequivalence, and limited quality control are also of concern. Education and experience are needed in order to learn how to find and treat the root causes of a problem (not just manifestations and symptoms). All nurses (as well as other clinicians) should have thorough preparation before using herbs and essential oils in practice.

SELF-CARE WITH AROMATHERAPY

Aromatherapy can be used for a number of self-care purposes. When used as part of daily hygiene, gentle antiviral essential oils, such as eucalyptus radiata, ravensera aromatica, and niaouli can be spread over the skin before, during, or after the morning shower. This practice strengthens the body's resistance to sickness during the cold or flu season (Burton Goldberg Group, 1995). The essential oils of black spruce and peppermint are effective stimulants that work by strengthening the adrenal cortex. Or, for relaxation, essential oils like citronella and eucalyptus citriodora can be diffused in the air or rubbed on the wrists, solar plexus and temples for quick and effective relaxation. Mandarin is favored by children, and its calming qualities can slow down highly active children. Lavender oil added to the bath or sprayed on the bed sheets reduces tension and enhances relaxation (Buckle, 2001).

Essential oils can also be used to relieve symptoms. For digestive and stress-related discomfort, a drop of anise seed oil taken with a spoon of honey (or by itself) helps to reduce gastrointestinal cramping (Burton Goldberg Group, 1995). Tarragon stimulates digestion and calms the digestive tract. Peppermint is the classic oil for alleviating nausea and travel sickness. It is also beneficial for an irritated colon (1995). Everlast relieves pain after injuries, and prevents hemorrhaging and swelling. For mosquito and other insect bites, lavender is unsurpassed in treating itching or stinging (1995). Lavender oil is restorative on burnt skin (Buckle, 2001). The antihistamines peppermint, anise, and ginger open tightened air passages (Keville, 1998). Anise and fennel will reduce coughing (1998).

In a randomized study of 51 patients with cancer pain, 1% chamomile nobile was administered to one group via full body massage once a week for 3 weeks. The other two groups had either massage without aromatherapy, or neither. When after massage measurements were compared with before massage, the aromatherapy with massage group had a significant decrease in anxiety, tension, and pain compared with the other groups. The authors suggest that since outcomes were measured 1 week after the treatment, aromatherapy using Roman chamomile can have a lasting effect on pain (Wilkinson, 1995).

NURSING ISSUES

Aromatherapy should be used as only a part of a comprehensive program to enhance well-being and health. The intent is to balance the body in order to optimize health and wellness and not wait for signs of illness. Care should be individualized. Given the belief that energy works at different levels, essential oils work differently in each person. Therefore, the choice of oil or oils must be individualized for each client.

Clients need to be involved in their own healing. A thorough history is needed as clients may not think to tell the nurse that they are using essential oils. Historical use is a valid way to document safety and efficacy in the absence of scientific evidence to the contrary, but aromas should not be released indiscriminately. "A smell that is unasked for and that has unpleasant associations can feel like an invasion of personal space" (Avis, 1999, p. 117). The impact of an aroma decreases over time as the olfactory neurons become accustomed to it, but people become more aware of a smell each time it is used and, as time passes, are able to detect smaller amounts. This suggests that constantly bombarding people with an aroma without altering the concentration is both counter-productive and increases the risk of an adverse reaction (Avis, 1999).

Aromatherapy is a growing therapeutic modality. As of 2002, aromatherapy has been accepted as part of nursing practice by the state boards of nursing in Massachusetts, Maryland, Nevada, New Mexico, New York, Arizona, North Carolina, Oregon, and California, and other states are considering authorizing its use by nurses (Buckle, 2001).

The emphasis in this chapter has been on the use of herbal therapies and aromatherapies to promote health and well-being, not to treat disease. Given the lack of regulation, oversight and standardization of potency, control of quality of herbal preparations and essential oils, and the possibility of negative interactions with pharmaceutical drugs, the nurse who uses these therapies needs to have thorough education preparation and supervised experience in order to practice competently. There is a need for well-designed research to study the holistic effects of phytomedicines and foster individualized therapies that involve clients in their own healing.

Chapter Key Points

- Selected herbs and essential oils have been well studied and appear to be both effective and low in side effects.

- The nurse is urged to pursue thorough educational preparation as a basis for the use of herbs and essential oils in practice.

- There is a professional obligation to restrict the use of herbs and essential oils to the promotion of health and well-being, and to refer clients to an appropriate medical practitioner for the treatment of disease.

- Extracts, which are made with petrochemical solvents, and synthetic chemicals frequently used in perfumes, may cause allergic or sensitizing reactions and should not be used for aromatherapy.

References

Ang-Lee, M. K., Moss, J., & Yuan, C. (2001). Herbal medicines and perioperative care. *Journal of the American Medical Assoication, 286,* 208-216.

Avis, A. (1999). When is an aromatherapist not an aromatherapist? *Complementary Therapies in Medicine, 7,* 116-118.

Ballentine, R. (1999). *Radical Healing.* New York: Harmony Books.

Barrett, B., Kiefer, D., & Rabago, D. (1999). Assessing the risks and benefits of herbal medicine: An overview of scientific evidence. *Alternative Therapies in Health and Medicine, 5,* 40-49.

Berman, B. M., & Larson, D. B. (Eds). (1994). *Alternative medicine: Expanding medical horizons.* Washington, DC: U.S. Government Printing Office.

Buckle, J. (1999). Use of aromatherapy as a complementary treatment for chronic pain. *Alternative Therapies, 5,* 42- 51.

Buckle, J. (2000, February/March).The "M" technique. *Massage and Bodywork,* 52-64.

Buckle, J. (2001). The role of aromatherapy in nursing care. *Nursing Clinics of North America, 36,* 57-74.

Burton Goldberg Group. (1995). *Alternative medicine: The definitive guide.* Fife, WA: Future Medicine Publishing.

Campbell, L., Pollard, A., & Boeton, C. (2001). The development of clinical practice guidelines for the use of aromatherapy in a cancer setting. *Australian Journal of Holistic Nursing, 8,* 14-22.

Cardinal, B. J., & Engels, H. J. (2001). Ginseng does not enhance psychological well-being in health, young adults: Results of a double-blind, placebo-controlled, randomized clinical trial. *Journal of the American Dietetic Association, 101,* 655-660.

Clark, C. C. (1996). *Wellness practitioner: Concepts, research and strategies* (2nd ed.). New York: Springer.

Coleman, S. (2001, July 30). Proceed with caution. *Advance for Nurses,* 23-24

Coss, H., & Cott, J. (2002). Herbal medicine. In S. Shannon (Ed.), *The handbook of complementary and alternative therapies in mental health* (pp. 377-400). San Diego: Academic Press

d'Angelo, R. (2002). Aromatherapy. In S. Shannon. (Ed.), *Handbook of complementary and alternative therapies in mental health* (pp. 72-92). San Diego: Academic Press.

D'Epiro, N. W. (Ed.). (1997, October 15). Herbal medicine: What works, what's safe. *Patient Care,* 49-77.

DeSmet, P. A. G. M. (2002). Herbal remedies. *New England Journal of Medicine, 347,* 2046-2054.

Dog, T. L. (1999). Phytomedicine. In W. B. Jonas, & J. S. Levin (Eds.), *Essentials of complementary and alternative medicine* (pp. 355-368). Philadelphia: Lippincott Williams & Wilkins.

Eastman, P. (1999). Drugs that fight can hurt you. *American Association of Retired Persons Review, 40,* 14-16.

Ernst, E., & Pihler, M.H. (2002). Herbal medicine. *Medical Clinics of North America, 86,* 149-161.

Glickstein, J. K. (1996). Motivation in geriatric rehabilitation. *Focus on Geriatric Care and Rehabilitation, 9,* 1-8.

Holmes, P. (1995, April/May). Aromatherapy: Applications for clinical practice. *Alternative and Complementary Therapies,* 177-182.

Horowitz, S. (1999). Aromatherapy: Modern applications of essential oils. *Alternative and Complimentary Therapies, 5,* 199-203.

Integrative Medicine Consult. (1998). *A primer: Integrative medicine.* Boston: Integrative Medicine Communications.

Izzo, A. A., & Ernst, E. (2001). Interactions between herbal medicines and prescribed drugs: A systematic review. *Drugs, 61,* 2163-2175.

James, K. (1998). In M. Snyder & R. Lindquist, *Complementary/Alternative therapies in nursing.* New York: Springer.

Jonas, W. B., & Ernst, E. (1999). Evaluating the safety of complementary and alternative products and practices. In W. B. Jonas & J. S. Levin (Eds.), *Essentials of complementary and alternative medicine* (pp. 89-107). Philadelphia: Lippincott Williams & Wilkins.

Keville, K. (1998). Breathe easy with aromatherapy. *Great Life,* 18-20.

Landis, R. (1997). *Herbal defense.* New York: Warner.

Larson-Presswalla, J. (1994). Insights into eastern health care: Some transcultural nursing. *Perspectives: Journal of Transcultural Nursing, 5,* 21-24.

Meserole, L. (1996). Western herbalism. In M. S. Micozzi (Ed.), *Fundamentals of complementary and alternative medicine*. New York: Churchill Livingstone.

Mills, S., & Bone, K. (2000). *Principles and practice of phytotherapy*. Edinburgh, Scotland: Churchill Livingstone.

Murray, M. T. (1995). *The healing power of herbs* (2nd ed.). Rocklin, CA: Prima.

Pizzorno, L. (1997, July). Tracing the roots of American herbalism. *Delicious*, 30-34.

Prescriber's Letter. (1998). *Continuing education therapeutic use of herbs*. Stockton, CA.

Robins, J. L. W. (1999). The science and art of aromatherapy. *Journal of Holistic Nursing, 17*, 5-17.

Soukanov, A. H. (Ed.). (1992). *The American heritage dictionary* (3rd ed.). Boston: Houghton Mifflin.

Stevensen, C. J. (2001). Aromatherapy. In M. S. Micozzi (Ed.), *Fundamentals of complementary and alternative medicine* (2nd ed., pp. 146-158). New York: Churchill Livingstone.

Tyler, V. E. (1993). *The honest herbal. A sensible guide to the use of herbs and related remedies* (3rd ed.). Binghamton, NY: Pharmaceutical Products.

Wilkinson, S. (1995). Aromatherapy and massage in palliative care. *International Journal of Palliative Nursing, 1*(1), 21-30.

World Health Organization. (1991). *Guidelines for the assessment of herbal medicines: Programme on traditional medicines*. Geneva, Switzerland: Author.

Additional Information

ASSOCIATIONS AND CREDENTIALING

Chinese Herbal Medicine

National Commission for the Certification of Acupuncture and Oriental Medicine
1421 16th Street N. W. Suite 501
Washington, D. C. 20036
www.nccaom.org

This is the accrediting body of schools. The student must graduate from an accredited school before sitting for the state board exam or national certification commission exam. In some states, NCCAOM certification is the only educational, training, or examination criteria for licensure. Other jurisdictions have set additional eligibility criteria. Training in Chinese herbal medicine is part of the total training in acupuncture and oriental medicine. The programs range in length from 2 to 4 years depending on the state requirements and degree level.

Aromatherapy

National Association for Holistic Aromatherapy
PO Box 17622
Boulder, CO 80308
Tel: (888) ASK-NAHA
www.naha.org

At the moment, there is no recognized national certification examination. There is no governing body at present, but the steering committee for Educational Standards in Aromatherapy in the United States is currently setting up the Aromatherapy Registration Board, which as a nonprofit entity will be responsible for administering a national exam and providing the public with a list of registered practitioners.

Jane Buckle is director of R. J. Buckle Associates LLC, an educational consulting firm in complementary therapies. Her website is www.rjbuckle.com.

RE-ESTABLISHING ENERGY FLOW

Physical Activity and Exercise

13

Abstract

Movement of energy is essential for a person's well-being. Physical activity or physical exercise (disease perspective) and energy exercise (person perspective) are different approaches to the movement of energy. Although activity and exercise have many benefits, most adults are, however, sedentary. Therefore, a number of strategies are proposed to encourage clients to adopt a more active lifestyle. In addition, the Chinese energy exercises of tai chi and qigong are introduced. These exercises use breathing, mental concentration, and physical postures to facilitate the flow of energy throughout the body.

Learning Outcomes

By the end of this chapter the student will be able to:

- Differentiate between elements of physical activity and exercise
- Describe benefits of physical exercise
- Describe positive and negative motivating factors for exercise
- Identify strategies to encourage clients to adopt a more active lifestyle
- Discuss strategies to encourage walking activity
- Discuss special physical activity considerations for the elderly client
- Demonstrate tai chi and qigong postures and forms

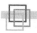

Physical Activity

Movement of energy is essential for a person's well-being. In the physical body, energy flow is associated with the movement of skeletal muscles. In fact, a broad definition of physical activity is "any bodily movement produced by skeletal muscles that results in energy expenditure" (Caspersen et al., 1985, p. 126). Numerous short bouts of moderate physical activity that can be planned into activities of daily living has been called *lifestyle physical activity* (Pender, 2002).

Scientific evidence clearly demonstrates that regular, moderate-intensity physical activity provides substantial health benefits. However, low levels of physical activity continue to be a major public health challenge in almost every population group of developed countries (Dubbert, 2002). Therefore, it is important that integrative health promotion activities include the encouragement and facilitation of physical activity and exercise by children and adults.

Many people erroneously believe that to reap health benefits they must engage in vigorous, continuous exercise, although it is clear that regular moderate physical activity provides substantial health benefits. Pate and colleagues (1995) suggest that 30 minutes or more of moderate-intensity physical activity is needed on most, preferably all, days of the week. Physical activity can be accumulated in relatively short bouts, enough to expend approximately 200 calories per day (e.g., walking briskly at 3 to 4 mph), conditioning exercise or general calisthenics, or home care and general cleaning).

The current emphasis for physical activity is on total daily energy expenditure, which can be achieved in a number of ways. The amount of activity, including the mode, intensity, and duration, is more important than the specific manner in which the activity is performed. Physical activity does not need to be continuous, and Pate and colleagues (1995) propose that most adults do not need to see their physician before starting a moderate-intensity physical activity program.

Even intermittent activity confers substantial benefits. The recommended 30 minutes of activity can be accumulated in short bouts of activity, such as 8 to 10 minutes of walking up the stairs instead of taking the elevator, walking instead of driving short distances, doing calisthenics, or pedaling a stationary cycle while watching television. Gardening, housework, raking leaves, dancing, and playing actively with children can also contribute to the 30-minute-per-day total if performed at an intensity that corresponds to brisk walking. Those who perform lower-intensity activities should do them more often for longer periods of time, or both, and people who prefer more vigorous exercise may choose to walk or participate in more vigorous activities, such as jogging, swimming, or cycling for 30 minutes daily. Sports and recreational activities, such as tennis or golf (without riding a cart), also can be applied to the daily total.

A more active lifestyle for people who lead sedentary lives would benefit the public's health and individual well-being (American College of Sports Medicine, 2000). Persons of all ages can improve their energy circulation and lower their risk for many chronic diseases (Nieman, 1998). Any level of activity above the sedentary state is helpful for weight loss. However, the evidence to date shows that to be beneficial in reducing long-term risk for coronary artery disease, exercise (specifically aerobic exercise) is necessary.

Physical Exercise

Physical exercise has been defined as "a subset of physical activity that is planned, structured, and repetitive and has as a final or intermediate objective towards the improvement or maintenance of physical fitness" (Caspersen et al., 1985, p. 126). Therefore, physical exercise is a specific form of physical activity associated with desired outcomes of fitness, flexibility, and balance.

According to Caspersen, Powell, and Christenson (1985), being physically fit is "the ability to carry out daily tasks with vigor and alertness, without undue fatigue and with ample energy to enjoy leisure-time pursuits and to meet unforeseen emergencies" (pp. 128-129). Physical fitness encompasses cardiorespiratory and muscular endurance, muscular strength, body composition, and flexibility. Strength is the ability of a muscle or muscle group to exert force against resistance (Griffin, 1998). Flexibility is "the capacity of a joint to move freely through a full range of motion without undue stress" (1998, p. 72), while balance involves the ability to maintain equilibrium while standing still or moving (Caspersen et al.,1985).

The capacity for physical performance is determined by the capacity for energy output (aerobic and anaerobic mechanisms), neuromuscular functions (strength, technique, and coordination), and psychosocial factors (motivation, social support) (Allan, 1992). When intense enough to lead to a significant increase in muscle oxygen uptake, exercise is defined as "aerobic." The goal of aerobic exercise is to strengthen the cardiovascular system and increase stamina. In contrast, anaerobic exercise is exercise during which the energy needed is provided without utilization of inspired oxygen. This occurs during short, vigorous bouts of exercise or when the body's oxygen supply capabilities cannot meet the metabolic demands of the exercise.

The heart rate is a simple measure of whether or not exercise is aerobic. "If the pulse reaches or exceeds a level of 60% of the theoretical maximum normal, age-adjusted heart rate (220 minus the person's age), or 0.6 (220 minus age), the exercise is considered aerobic... To assure that exercise intensity remains at a safe level, the pulse rate should remain below 85% of the person's theoretical maximum rate" (Jonas, 1996, p. 177). A formula for calculating a safe rate for aerobic exercise is maximum heart rate – age – resting heart rate × 0.6 and 0.8 resting heart rate.

Treat-Jacobson and Mark (1998) suggest that in order to assess the heart rate, the nurse should:

1. Determine the heart rate one-third to one-half of the way through and immediately after stopping exercise

2. Assess whether the individual can talk comfortably while exercising

3. Rate the sense of effort from 1 to 10 (10 is maximal)

Another approach to calculating desirable exercise intensity is a rating of perceived exertion (RPE), "a subjective measure of exercise intensity that takes into account the client's feelings of exercise fatigue, including musculoskeletal, psychological, and environmental factors" (Griffin, 1998, p. 96). The Borg Scale of Perceived Exertion assigns a numerical value to subjectively perceived exertion between 6 (no exertion at all) and 20 (maximal exertion). RPEs from a graded exercise test can be used independently or in combination with heart rate to prescribe exercise training intensities (Griffin, 1998).

BENEFITS OF EXERCISE

Exercise improves the cardiovascular system; improves the strength, endurance, and flexibility of the muscular system; induces positive changes in the skeletal, digestive, and immune body systems; and lowers serum lipids and blood pressure (Zelasko, 1995). Pender (2002) documents many specific benefits of exercise.

RESEARCH FINDINGS

Physical activity and physical exercise have been found to have a number of beneficial effects for primary, secondary, and tertiary prevention of a number of chronic diseases. Below are a sampling of recent research findings:

- Regular exercise improves psychosocial well-being (Donker, 2000; Sharkey et al., 2000).

- The protective effect of physical exercise is not proportional to frequency or intensity (Donker, 2000).

- "Unequivocal evidence for the favorable effects of physical exercise on cardiovascular morbidity is not yet available, although cardiovascular mortality seems to be reduced" (Sebregts et al., 2000, p. 431).

- In general, physical fitness and activity are related to lower levels of cardiovascular arousal during and following mental stress... helps to buffer the body against the ill effects of mental stress (Nieman, 1998, p. 234), can reduce depression (p. 255), reduce anxiety (p. 257), and improve self-esteem or self-concept (p. 258).

- Even light activity such as walking has been shown to reduce the risk for hypertension in a "dose-related" manner and does so independently of other risk factors (Hayashi et al., 1999). However, "the blood pressure-lowering effect of exercise training depends on a regular schedule of activity" (American College of Sports Medicine, 1993).

- Several studies have found a statistically significant inverse relation between physical activity and the risk of stroke in men and women (Bronner et al., 1995; Hu et al., 2000).

- Despite statistically significant improvements in bone density after exercise, fracture reduction due to exercise remains questionable, but the risk of falls in older persons may be reduced. Exercise must be continued to maintain gains in bone mass (NIH Consensus Panel, 2001; Sharkey et al., 2000), but walking does not prevent bone loss (Nieman, 1998).

- Given that fairly rigorous activity is necessary to maintain bone mass in postmenopausal women, "building greater bone mass in our younger years is probably a more realistic and beneficial method of preventing or delaying the onset of osteoporosis" (Sharkey et al., 2000).

- Carefully controlled exercise in people with osteoarthritis of the knee and hip is associated with increased joint mobility, increased strength, reduced pain, reduced reliance on medication, enhanced proprioception, enhanced activity performance, and reduced disability (Sharkey et al., 2000), although exercise training does not improve the underlying disease process (Nieman, 1998).

■ "In general, exercise programs that facilitate weight loss, trunk strengthening, and the stretching of musculotendinous structures appear to be most helpful in alleviating low back pain" (Patel & Ogle, 2000, p. 1785). It appears that a return to normal, daily activities may be superior to either bed rest or specific back exercises in acute low back pain (Nieman, 1998).

■ There is "convincing support" for the role of regular physical activity in the prevention of noninsulin-dependent diabetes mellitus (NIDDM). For most individuals with NIDDM, regular exercise improves glycemic control. In addition, "regular exercise will reduce the insulin requirements of well-controlled insulin dependent diabetes mellitus [clients] by 30% to 50%" (Nieman, 1998, p. 97), resulting in smaller than usual insulin doses or increased food intake.

■ Moderate exercise provides a short-term boost that appears to reduce the risk of infection over the long-term (Nieman, 1998).

■ Regular exercise reduces the odds of gaining weight with age. But "exercise does not accelerate weight loss significantly when combined with a reducing diet" (Nieman, 1998, p. 234). In addition, "moderate amounts of exercise appear to have little if any effect in countering the 10% to 30% decrease in resting metabolism associated with dieting" (p. 238).

■ "Nearly all studies have shown that death rates for all causes combined are lower in physically active and fit people when compared to those who largely avoid exercise. In practical terms, middle-aged adults who are physically active gain on average about 2 years of life" (Nieman, 1998, p. 295).

Prompting, in the form of weekly brief prompts, is a low-cost strategy for increasing exercise and physical activity among older women (Conn et al., 2003). On the other hand, mass media approaches such as radio and television have not produced physical activity behavior change, despite good recall (Dubbert, 2002).

EXERCISE EPIDEMIOLOGY

Healthy People 2010 sets goals for 30% of adults and adolescents to engage in moderate physical activity, preferably daily, for 30 or more minutes (Pender, 2002). Unfortunately, 41% to 51% of adults are sedentary. "Of those already regularly engaged in either group or solitary exercise, about 50% will discontinue activity at some time in the coming year.... The rate of participation typically drops within the initial 3 to 6 months, then plateaus and continues a gradually decreasing but linear pattern across the next 12 to 24 months. Individuals who are still active after 6 months are likely to remain active a year later" (Dishman et al., 1985, pp. 159, 162). Lack of physical activity starts early in life. By age 10, more than one-third of children have adopted a sedentary lifestyle (Pender, 2002).

Research has shown that exercise participation varies with persons' ethnic, gender, educational, and occupational characteristics. Some examples include (Marcus et al., 1997; Pate et al., 1995):

- African Americans and other ethnic minority populations are less active than white Americans, and this disparity is more pronounced for women.

- People with higher levels of education participate in more leisure-time physical activity than do people with less education. Differences in education and socioeconomic status account for most, if not all, of the differences in leisure-time physical activity associated with race or ethnicity.

- White-collar workers may be more likely to engage in leisure time recreational activities than blue-collar workers. It has been shown that blue-collar workers and smokers are likely dropouts from cardiac rehabilitation exercise programs and corporate exercise programs.

- Negative health status variables (e.g., smokers, being overweight) appear to predict inactivity. Overweight persons are unlikely to continue a fitness program. Knowledge of one's health status may prompt adoption of activity, but it does not appear to facilitate maintenance of activity.

- Men are more likely than women to engage in regular activity, in vigorous exercise, and sports.

- The total amount of time spent in physical activity declines with age.

MOTIVATION

A number of motivational factors that may affect exercise participation and persistence have been identified. However, none of these factors alone appears to be able to predict whether someone will initiate or continue exercise. People drop out of lifestyle activities at a rate of approximately one-half of that typically seen for vigorous exercise (Dishman et al., 1985). It appears that an individual's exercise participation and persistence may be affected by complex and variable interactions among many factors. A number of the most important possible influencing factors include:

Positive Exercise Factors

- Belief in the health benefits of exercise and short-term advantages such as feeling good, improving personal appearance, and increasing self-esteem are strong incentives for physical activity and exercise (Jonas, 1996; Marcus et al., 1997).

- Risk reduction. In contrast, the reduction of risk for future disease or illness is not an incentive. Most regular exercisers do not engage in activity to achieve future risk reduction, and few nonexercisers start for that reason (Jonas, 1996). Many people require a challenge before they realize that a sedentary lifestyle is a threat (Allan, 1992).

- Past participation. Previous participation in exercise or sports activity is related to current participation.

- Social support. The social support of a spouse has been identified as a strong predictor of exercise maintenance for women. Individuals who exercise with their spouses have higher rates of exercise adherence than those who exercise alone (Marcus et al., 1997).

- Self-efficacy. Self-efficacy, the degree of confidence individuals have that they can participate in a healthful behavior across a broad range of specific, salient situations, is an important determinant of physical activity.

- Decisional balance. The balance between pros and cons of exercise has been shown to be an important determinant of participation in physical activity.

- Convenience. Moderate-intensity home-based exercise programs have higher adherence rates and produce fitness and psychological benefits comparable to those produced by higher-intensity group programs, at least among retirees.

- Self-motivation. "Self-motivated persons also appear less sensitive to activity barriers, such as inconvenience or competing lifestyle behaviors" (Dishman et al., 1985, p. 165).

- Perceived exercise enjoyment. Feelings related to well-being and enjoyment seem more important to maintaining activity than concerns about health. Initial involvement may be motivated by knowledge of and belief in the health benefits of physical activity, but continued participation seems to be motivated more by feelings of enjoyment and well-being (Dishman et al., 1985).

- Perception of being in good health.

Motivation for Physical Activity

Methods of motivation for physical activity include (Phillips, Schneider, & Mercer, 2004):

- Education about activity benefits and practice

- Promotion of goal-oriented, gradual activity progression

- Addressing costs and affordability

- Addressing safety

- Adapting activities and equipment for less able-bodied people

- Treating concurrent morbidities

- Facilitating empowerment

- Giving written prescriptions on a prescription pad

- Focusing on accessibility and affordability

- Promoting socialization

- Providing physical and occupational therapy

Negative Exercise Factors

- Environmental barriers. Actual and perceived practical factors such as the safety, availability, and geographic proximity of community facilities, weather, financial considerations, and both work and childcare schedules consistently predict the amount of participation in vigorous activity in men and women.

- Lack of time and energy. Unmarried women report participation in significantly more vigorous activity than married women. Having children is related to perceived lack of

time for exercise. It has been suggested that dropping out may reflect a lack of interest, intention, or commitment, even though the reason given is lack of time (Marcus
et al., 1997).

■ Limited access to training and information about physical activity. Few physicians and
nurses routinely give advice about physical activity, therefore the popular media often
serve, by default, as an important source of information (Marcus et al., 1997).

■ Lack of readiness to exercise. Only about 10% of the population are ready. For example, girls experience a substantial reduction in physical activity during adolescence
(Marcus et al., 1997).

■ Lack of role models. Most women do not have peer role models for appropriate kinds
and levels of physical activity. "Perceived barriers may frequently reflect inadequate
motivation to be active rather than reasons for inactivity. This can be a critical distinction, because no data support the notion that removing stated barriers leads to
increased activity" (Dishman et al., 1985, p. 166).

■ Lack of encouragement by health care providers. "Only a minority of physicians perceive exercise as very important for the average person, and fewer than 50% routinely ask [clients] about their exercise habits... Important barriers to exercise
counseling by physicians include perceived lack of counseling skills, lack of confidence in counseling ability, perceived ineffectiveness of counseling, lack of organizational support, little or no reimbursement for preventive counseling, and limited
availability of materials to aid both the [client] and the physician" (Marcus et al.,
1997, p. 345).

■ Lack of self-regulatory skills. Interventions that teach goal setting, planning, self-
monitoring, self-reward skills, and how to make plans to prevent relapse, can increase
short-term participation among people who intend to exercise (Dishman et al., 1985).

■ Disruption of exercise routine. Unexpected disruption in an activity routine or its setting can interrupt or end even a previously continuous exercise program, but there is
less of an impact by stressful events as the activity habit becomes more established
(Dishman et al., 1985).

RISKS OF EXERCISE

Intrinsic injury may be caused by the nature of the activity or sport (e.g., shin splints in
running) and can be decreased or prevented by the use of proper equipment and correct technique. Extrinsic injury is caused by an external factor (e.g., a cyclist is hit by an automobile)
and overuse injury, which results from trying to go too far, too fast, too frequently, and can be
prevented by choosing a suitable sport and workout schedule, and by maintaining moderation
in distance, intensity, and speed (Jonas, 1996).

Regular exercise presents a definite risk for persons with previous myocardial infarction;
exertion chest pain or pressure, or severe shortness of breath; pulmonary disease, especially
chronic obstructive pulmonary disease; or bone, joint, or other musculoskeletal diseases. In
addition, regular exercise presents a possible risk for persons with hypertension; cigarette
smokers; those with high blood cholesterol; prescription medication users; abusers of drugs or
alcohol; or those with any other chronic illness such as diabetes mellitus.

Given the complexity of positive and negative factors for physical activity and exercise, nursing interventions must be carefully designed and personalized based on individual needs and preferences. The following section will discuss factors to be considered in designing an activity or exercise regimen.

EXERCISE INTERVENTION STRATEGIES

Exercise must be an integral part of personal lifestyle if it is to have optimum effects on health. However, "most interventions have lasted only 3 to 10 weeks" (Dishman et al., 1985, p. 164) despite the fact that it takes adults 20 to 30 weeks of regular physical activity to reach an optimal training level (Allan, 1992).

Despite the obvious multiple health benefits, few professional nurses even try to intervene to promote integration of activity and exercise into a client's lifestyle. Part of the problem may be that relatively few nurses have integrated regular physical exercise into their own lifestyle, even though role modeling an active lifestyle is an important part of effective physical activity counseling by health care providers. Not surprisingly, physically active nurses are more likely to counsel patients regarding physical activity than nurses with sedentary lifestyles.

Another concern is the possible lack of knowledge among health professionals. Many physicians and nurses have not received adequate training about exercise science or behavioral counseling in their educational programs. Due to currently limited curricular content, it is improbable that nurses prepared at the baccalaureate and graduate levels are prepared to deliver health promotion and prevention services, including physical-activity counseling.

The following discussion highlights a number of nursing considerations and strategies that can empower clients to adopt a more active lifestyle.

Goals and Motivation

It is important to consider what goals the person wants to accomplish and why? Realistic goal setting by the client in terms of limits and limitations is essential (e. g., become fit, lose weight, look and feel better, reduce future risk of disease and conditions).

In addition, what is the client's inner motivation? "The only kind of motivation that works in the long run for positive lifestyle and behavior change comes from within... Purely external motivation... almost invariably leads to guilt, anxiety, anger, frustration, and, usually, injury and/or quitting" (Jonas, 1996, p. 181).

Gradual Changes

Changes should be introduced gradually in order to promote permanent change. The previously sedentary person should start with ordinary walking, at a normal pace, for 10 minutes or so, three times a week. After a couple of weeks, the length of each session can be increased, followed by an increase in the frequency of sessions. After several more weeks, the speed with which the exercise is performed can also be increased (Jonas, 1996). The activity should be stopped if untoward symptoms occur. Warm-up exercises should be done for 10 minutes, involve all major body parts, and achieve a heart rate within 20 beats per minute of the target heart rate for the following aerobic exercise (Treat-Jacobson & Mark, 1998). For cool down, 5 to 10 minutes are needed for the body to adjust to a slower pace. Cooling down exercises may include walking slowly, deep breathing, and stretching exercises (Treat-Jacobson & Mark, 1998).

Regularity of Exercise

Regularity is critical to the effectiveness of physical exercise. The focus of the first 2 to 4 weeks of an exercise program should focus on the challenge of making the time. A total of 30 minutes daily of moderate-intensity physical activity should be performed on as many days of the week as possible (Jonas, 1996). A daily routine helps to reinforce participation. Weil (1999, p. 3) suggests "an unthinking routine, such as exercising first thing in the morning before you're really awake and can talk yourself out of it," as a strategy for establishing discipline.

Integrating Activity and Exercise into Daily Life

Activity and/or exercise should be integrated into daily life. Opportunities to get physical are everywhere, and include parking the car in a far corner of the mall parking lot, walking down the hall to speak with a co-worker rather than sending an e-mail message, jumping rope during TV commercials, and cleaning up the house (Weil, 1999). It is important for the client to take control of his or her behavior. The client must have and be aware of options and consider some of the options feasible.

Making Exercise Fun

How can exercise be made to be fun? Exercise actually increases energy. So "if you feel run down, recharge your batteries by moving around" (Weil, 1999, p. 3). Jonas (1996) suggests a number of strategies to make exercise more fun:

- Positive anticipation is very important.
- Set appropriate goals. Avoid doing too much, too soon.
- For distance sports, train by minutes, not miles. Recognize that, in many distance sports in which concentration on technique is not required, time spent is uniquely private, thinking time.
- While exercising, listen to music, the news, or talk shows through a headset.
- Set nonexercise-related goals, like getting an errand or two completed in the course of a workout.
- Periodically reward oneself, with a new piece of clothing, or a long-denied snack treat.
- Exercise outdoors.
- Vary activity from day to day.
- Incorporate activities already enjoyed (e.g., working in the garden, bike-riding with the kids) into an exercise program.

Social Support

A positive therapeutic relationship with the nurse or other health care provider is a strong source of social support. Other sources of social support include a spouse (the spouse's attitude can be more important than that of the participant), other family members, an activity partner, or a friend. Follow-up visits should be scheduled on a regular basis to assess progress and concerns. Manifestations of exercise patterns are identified through the frequency/intensity and strength/harmony of the behaviors (Weil, 1999).

Cognitive-Behavioral Strategies

King (1994) identified a number of cognitive-behavioral strategies that appear useful in promoting at least short-term exercise adherence. These include goal-setting, feedback through progress charts, decision balance sheets, relapse-prevention training, written agreements and contracts, stimulus control strategies, contingency management, face-to-face individual counseling by health care professionals or personal trainers, videotapes, booklets, self-help kits and correspondence courses, telephone-based interventions, and/or recognition of accomplishments through a system of rewards, and provision of qualified, enthusiastic leaders. Health communications that are tailored for the individual have promise as a strategy to promote the adoption and maintenance of physical activity and exercise (Robbins et al., 2001).

Group or class formats have particular advantages and disadvantages that are presented in Box 13-1.

Box 13-1

Advantages and Disadvantages of Using Groups to Promote Exercise

Advantages of group or class formats include:

- Potentially more cost-effective
- On-site supervision
- Visual modeling by the instructor (culturally and demographically similar to the population segment being targeted)
- A set structure with respect to location, exercise format, and time
- Face-to-face encouragement by the instructor
- Potential peer support.
- Social reinforcement, camaraderie, and companionship

Disadvantages of a group format include:

- The inconvenience of getting to class several times a week, along with constraints related to class schedules
- A limited variety of activities, which, in contrast with many people's preferences, typically take place indoors
- Constraints on individualizing the regimen for the individual.
- The expense of fees, equipment, and special attire
- Social costs, such as embarrassment or discouragement, that may develop from the social comparisons that inevitably occur in groups
- Group leader effects. May involve dislike of the leader's style or disruptions in the class or group that inevitably occur with leader absence or turnover

ENVIRONMENTAL AND POLICY APPROACHES TO EXERCISE PROMOTION

Given the documentation of intrapersonal, interpersonal, social/cultural, and physical environmental correlates of physical activity, a multilevel ecologic approach seems to be demanded (Bauman, Sallis, Dzewaltowski, & Owen, 2002).

The health belief model has failed to receive clear support in the literature on adult physical activity correlates (Bauman et al., 2002).

Linkages between individual, environmental, and policy interventions improve the likelihood of impact (Orleans et al., 1999). Many environmental or policy approaches focus on changing aspects of a setting/environment or establishing public policy to promote physical activity or exercise. Some examples are providing security escorts for groups of participants walking in dangerous neighborhoods; installing curtains on the windows in the exercise room to ensure privacy; making free transportation and child care available; adjusting the physical education curriculum in schools to include more class time spent in moderate and vigorous physical activity; addressing physical activity in work sites, places of worship, and to an increasing degree, senior centers and senior residential settings; organizing races and fun runs or walking events to increase community awareness concerning physical activity; providing safe and accessible pedestrian and bicycle lanes available throughout the community; making stairways more open, accessible, and attractive; requiring activity promotion ads on TV and after movies; providing funding for walking or biking trails; subsidizing health club memberships for employees; and providing public transportation that allows residents ready access to community exercise settings (Sallis et al., 1998).

PHYSICAL ACTIVITY FOR WEIGHT REDUCTION

When trying to lose weight, physical activity should be targeted in combination with other behaviors. A combined program of dietary change and regular exercise is more effective at facilitating weight loss than either strategy alone. In addition, successful weight loss may serve as an incentive for maintaining exercise adherence. Regular exercise may also help moderate the weight changes that many smokers fear following smoking cessation and, thus, enhance mood and other psychological outcomes during and after quitting.

WALKING AS PHYSICAL ACTIVITY

"Walking requires no special equipment, facilities, or new skills. It is also safe and relatively easy to maintain. Intensity, duration, and frequency are easily regulated and adjusted" (Treat-Jacobson & Mark, 1998, p. 28). Zelasko (1995) and Jonas (1996) suggest an emphasis on consistency first, then duration, intensity, and frequency. Workouts should be measured in minutes not miles, with a goal of maintaining a lifetime of increased physical activity. Strategies to encourage walking activity are presented below:

- Wear well-fitting lace-type shoes that provide good support and shock absorption. "Proper fit means that the shoe should be shaped like one's foot; it should touch one's foot in as many places as possible, except over the toes; it should be flexible under the ball of the foot; and it should have a firm heel counter to keep the heel down in the shoe" (Jonas, 1996, p. 188).

- Wear thick socks that will absorb perspiration and protect the feet.

- Wear comfortable, loose-fitting clothing appropriate to the temperature and weather.

- Walk at a rate designed to bring the heart rate to target levels; 3 to 3.5 mph may be a good training pace for the average person.

- Walk in an easy, balanced position, head upright, looking ahead rather than directly at the ground, arms swinging easily with each stride, using a slight push-off step with the rear foot and leaning forward just slightly with each step. Take long, easy steps from the hip, landing on the heel and rolling over the foot in a smooth motion. Avoid reaching for too long a step.

- Walk continuously, frequent stops and starts interfere with the aerobic effect.

- Walk in an interesting area at a suitable time of day. Try to set aside the same time each day for the walk. Walk with others, if desired.

- When walking up or down steep hills, lean forward slightly and shorten the stride a bit to maintain a balanced pace.

- Start slowly, but gradually increase distance and time until desired maximums are achieved. Keeping a log of accomplishments enhances motivation.

- Cool down with a flexibility program, a slower paced walk for another block or two, or some gently conditioning exercises.

SPECIAL CONSIDERATIONS FOR THE ELDERLY CLIENT

Physical activity is one of the most significant health interventions in the lives of older individuals (O'Brien & Vertinsky, 1991). Benefits within weeks include short-term enhancement of physical, social, and emotional well-being. Intervention studies generally provide support for positive cardiovascular changes with exercise, although results are inconsistent (Houde & Melillo, 2002). There are also numerous long-term contributions to prolonged good health, including:

- Resistance to illness

- Optimization of self-care and functional independence

- Reduced mortality risk

- Reduced bone loss in postmenopausal women

- Overall increased quality of life with extended longevity

- Stress reduction

- Better sleep

- Muscle relaxation and improvement in joint mobility

- Positive mood states

- Improved self-image and self-concept

■ Short-term improvements in memory, intelligence, and cognitive speed

■ Higher levels of self-efficacy, internal locus of control, and sense of life control

However, many older individuals are afraid to exercise. Nigg and colleagues (1999), in a study using the transtheoretical model (TTM), found that most older individuals were in pre-contemplation for exercise (See Chapter 8, *Promoting Individual Behavior Change*, for discussion of the transtheoretical model). Among older women, factors such as fear of "wearing out" the body, concern about the likelihood of serious injury, and the threat of sudden death caused by physical exertion contribute to an avoidance of exercise. Many older people do not believe that they can improve their health through exercise and question their ability to participate in exercise. However, research indicates that by strengthening self-efficacy and outcome expectations, exercise participation by older individuals can be increased (Resnick et al., 2000).

A wellness program for the elderly should include activities designed to improve strength, increase (shoulder, trunk, and hip) flexibility, promote endurance, improve balance and coordination, be enjoyable, and fit into the person's lifestyle (May, 1990). May (1990) suggests guidelines for an overall fitness program for well older individuals that are listed in Box 13-2.

Box 13-2

Guidelines for a Fitness Program for Healthy Older Individuals

A fitness program for healthy older individuals should be:

■ Safe, in that the potential for injury is minimized

■ Designed to improve muscle strength, flexibility, endurance, coordination, balance, and functional capabilities

■ At an intensity level to provide a training effect

■ Designed to include a variety of slow and fast activities including a warm-up and cool-down period

■ Structured to allow participants to lower the level of participation, if desired

■ Designed to give participants an understanding of the purpose of the exercise and what sensations may be elicited

■ Performed regularly, at least three to five times per week

■ Performed for at least 30 minutes and preferably 1 hour each time

■ Designed to fit within the lifestyle and interests of the client to encourage consistency of participation over time.

It is unclear which physical activity interventions are most effective among older adults. Van der Bij and colleagues (2002) evaluated 38 randomized controlled trials. All three of the types of interventions identified, home-based, group-based, and educational resulted in small and short-lived changes in physical activity, but participation declined the longer the duration of the intervention. It was not evident that behavioral reinforcement strategies were beneficial. The authors concluded that comparative studies evaluating the effectiveness of diverse interventions are needed.

Resnick (1999) suggests that exercise programs for older individuals can be designed using a seven-step approach. The steps are presented in Box 13-3.

Box 13-3

A Seven-Step Approach to Exercise Programs for Older Individuals

- Step 1: Education
- Step 2: Exercise prescreening
- Step 3: Setting goals or making a contract
- Step 4: Exposure to exercise
- Step 5: Exposure to role models
- Step 6: Verbal encouragement
- Step 7: Verbal reinforcement and rewards

Physical activity and/or exercise to prevent disease is consistent with the disease worldview. In contrast, moving energy through energy exercise is consistent with the person worldview.

Energy Exercise

According to Ballentine (1999), "some forms of exercise are really exercising the energy body rather than the physical body" (p. 357). These include the Chinese movement forms of tai chi and qigong.

TAI CHI (CHOREOGRAPHY OF BODY AND MIND)

Tai chi, (pronounced "tie chee", and also known as tai chi chuan) can be translated as "the ultimate" or "supreme ultimate" which means improving and progressing toward the unlimited (Shaller, 1998). "Tai chi integrates the connections between mind, body, and spirit in a quest for the highest form of harmony in life through the combination of exercise and meditation" (Bottomley, 1997, pp. 134, 136). While meditation aims to increase yang and reduce and diminish yin, the goal of exercise is to reduce Yang and to increase and enhance yin. Theory proposes that the combined practice of meditation, breathing, and exercise balances these opposing, yet complementary, forces of equal strength energies, promoting health. See Chapter 3, *The Meaning of Health Care: Health Belief Systems*, for an additional discussion of yin/yang.

There are five main schools of tai chi, each named after the style's founding family: Chen, Yang, Sun, Wu (Jian Qian), and Wu (He Qin). The relaxed, evenly paced, and graceful Yang style is the most popular style being practiced today. There are 24, 48, 88, and 108 forms, and Li and colleagues have recently proposed an easy eight-form sequence that is suitable for elderly adults (Li, Fisher, Harmer, & Shirai, 2003).

Tai chi involves a series of fluid, continuous, graceful, dance-like postures, and the performance of movements known as "forms," performed in a slow, rhythmical, and well-controlled manner. These body movements are integrated by mind concentration, balance shifting of body weight, muscle relaxation, and breathing control. Tai chi is a convenient exercise that can be practiced in any place, at any time, and without any equipment (Chen & Snyder, 1999). The emphasis on softness, continuity, and relaxation allows the chi to move freely along meridians.

Examples of tai chi exercises are depicted in Figure 13-1.

Tai chi is regarded as a method of "moving meditation." While outwardly at rest, and with inner peacefulness and quiet, the meditator uses abdominal or "inner" breathing and mental concentration to facilitate the flow of energy throughout the body. Inhalation "stores" energy while exhalation "releases" energy (Bottomley, 1997).

Principles of Tai Chi Movement

Principles of tai chi movement include (Shaller, 1998):

1. Wear loose-fitting clothes and soft shoes or bare feet.

2. The movements are best learned from an instructor in a group setting. Once the movements are learned, the form can be performed alone or in a group.

3. Begin and maintain complete relaxation with natural breathing.

4. Stand with the sacrum pressed slightly forward and with the head and torso erect as if suspended from above by wire.

5. Shoulders are relaxed with slight drooping; fingers are spread apart and slightly cupped.

6. Concentration is on the soles of the feet or the *t'an t'ien* (area slightly below the umbilicus).

7. Knees are slightly bent with the weight being shifted from right to left and forward and back.

8. Movements are slow and fluid, performed meditatively. The emphasis is on softness, continuity, and relaxation. Postures and movements should be performed with the feeling of "swimming through very heavy air."

9. Circulation of chi can be noted by the amount of tingling felt in the fingers and hands.

10. Practice should be approximately 25 to 30 minutes daily.

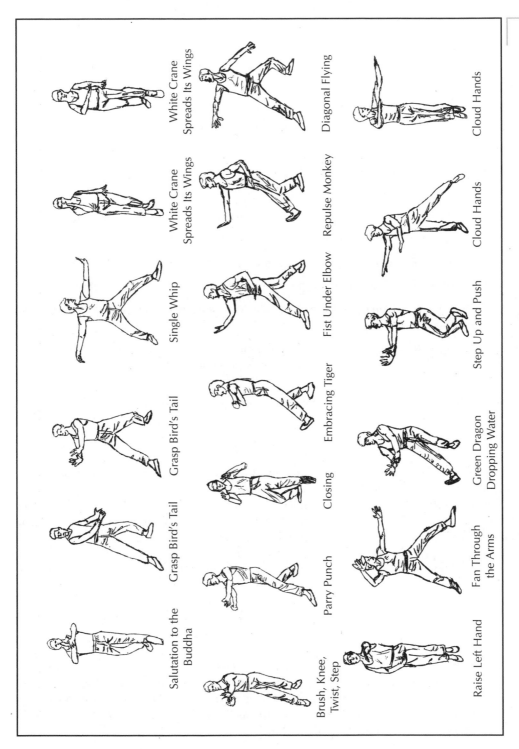

White Crane
Spreads Its Wings

White Crane
Spreads Its Wings

Single Whip

Grasp Bird's Tail

Grasp Bird's Tail

Salutation to the
Buddha

Diagonal Flying

Repulse Monkey

Fist Under Elbow

Embracing Tiger

Closing

Parry Punch

Brush, Knee,
Twist, Step

Cloud Hands

Cloud Hands

Step Up and Push

Green Dragon
Dropping Water

Fan Through
the Arms

Raise Left Hand

Figure 13-1. Double stance tai chi exercises (reprinted with permission from Bottomley, J. M. (1997). Tai chi: Choreography of the mind. In Davis, C. M. (Ed.), *Complementary therapies in rehabilitation*. Thorofare, NJ: SLACK Incorporated).

Uses for Tai Chi Movement

Potential uses for tai chi (Bottomley, 1997; Olsen, 1990) include:

- Strengthening and toning the muscles of the lower body, which enhances trunk control, strengthens the lower back, and expands the base of support.

- Improving balance. Balance, muscular strength, and aerobic power are three components of physical fitness that are important for the preservation of function.

- Improving flexibility and posture.

- Improving cardiorespiratory fitness.

- Improving blood and lymph circulation.

- Improving rotation of the trunk and coordination of isolated extremity motions.

- Helping to facilitate awareness of movement and position.

- Warding off illness and fatigue through increased energy flow.

- Cultivating poise and a tranquil spirit.

- Aiding waste elimination through gentle leg-raising movements that massage and strengthen the intestines.

- Calming both body and mind, and relieving stress and anxiety. The stress-reducing effect of tai chi is comparable to the physiological changes produced by moderate exercise (Bottomley, 1997).

- Opening joints, especially the knees, alleviating inflammatory diseases such as arthritis and rheumatism.

- Increasing longevity, good health, vigor, mental alertness, and creativity (Bottomley, 1997).

Research studies on tai chi support improved balance, postural stability, decreased falls, enhanced cardiovascular and ventilatory functions, and reduced pain in people of all ages (Chen & Snyder, 1999), as well as foster social support, independence, and autonomy in the elderly (Jancewicz, 2001). Tai chi chuan is beneficial to cardiorespiratory function, strength, balance, flexibility, microcirculation, and psychological profile. It can be prescribed as an alternative exercise program for selected patients with cardiovascular, orthopedic, or neurological diseases, and can reduce the risk of falls in elderly individuals (Lan, Lai, & Chen, 2002).

Below are abstracts of two tai chi research studies:

1. An 8-week tai chi pilot study was conducted with a sample of 19 patients diagnosed with multiple sclerosis to explore psychosocial and physical benefits. Walking speed increased by 21% and hamstring flexibility increased by 28%. Patients experienced improvements in vitality, social functioning, mental health, and ability to carry out physical and emotional roles. The authors concluded that "tai chi and other health promotion programs offer help toward achieving the goals of increasing access to services, maximizing independence, and improving quality of life for people with chronic disabling conditions" (Husted et al., 1999).

2. A 6-month pilot study was conducted with a sample of 94 healthy, physically inactive older adults to determine whether a tai chi exercise program can improve self-reported physical functioning limitations. The sample was divided into 49 experimental participants and a control group of 45. The experimental group attended two 60-minute sessions each week for 6 months. Overall, the tai chi participants reported improvement in daily activities such as walking and lifting and in moderate-vigorous activities such as running. Compared to the tai chi group, the control group did not show any statistically significant improvement on any of the measures. It was concluded that the 6-month tai chi exercise program was effective for improving functional status in healthy, physically inactive older adults (Li et al., 2001).

A programmed tai chi chuan exercise intervention is beneficial for retarding bone loss in weight-bearing bones in early postmenopausal women (Chan et al., 2004). In a study with 34 relatively sedentary, normotensive middle-aged women, dynamic balance was significantly improved following a three times per week, 12-week tai chi exercise program, and there were significant decreases in both mean systolic and diastolic blood pressure (Thornton, Sykes, & Tang, 2004).

Qigong (Chi Gung)

Another method of energy exercise is qigong (also known as chi gung). Qigong is one of three aspects, along with herbs and acupuncture, of traditional Chinese medicine (Ai et al., 2001). "The term qigong is the phonetic juxtaposition of two Chinese characters: *qi*, meaning 'flow of air' in a literal sense, or 'vital energy' in a symbolic sense; and *gong* meaning perseverant practice" (Ai et al., 2001, p. 83). In comparison with tai chi, which focuses primarily on identifying the chi within the body, qigong specializes in mentally generating, balancing or harmonizing, and utilizing this energy (Carnie, 1997).

Qigong is an ancient Chinese exercise that combines movement, meditation, and breath regulation to stimulate and balance the flow of qi, or vital life energy, along the acupuncture meridians. Qigong practice can range from simple calisthenics-type movements with breath coordination to complex exercises where brain wave frequency, heart rate, and other organ functions are altered intentionally. When practiced regularly, qigong is believed to improve blood circulation, enhance immune function, cultivate inner strength, calm the mind, and promote relaxation, awareness, and healing (Burton Goldberg Group, 1995). Qigong is a method that can be used to cure and prevent diseases, to promote health, and to avoid premature aging while prolonging life.

The several branches of qigong (Carnie, 1997; Burton Goldberg Group, 1995) include:

- *Mental Qigong.* Where the primary emphasis is on teaching control of the mind so that the brain is active and alert. Personal self-healing and health maintenance practice is called internal qigong, which can be performed with little or no movement (quiescent). When internal qigong includes movement, it is called dynamic qigong.

- *Medical Qigong.* Used for healing oneself and, at advanced levels, healing others. The practitioner learns how to move chi throughout the body in order for it to flow properly (internal qigong). The primary idea here is that physical movement is essential for the movement of chi. When a qigong master or practitioner projects or emits his or her own qi to serve or heal another, it is considered external qigong.

- *Martial Qigong.* Concentrates on learning how to fight and how to defend oneself. This training covers ways to increase one's muscular strength and endurance by using internal energy.

- *Spiritual Chi Gung.* One tries to learn how to control one's emotions and spirit by cultivating will, patience, and endurance in order to learn to live longer as well as to reach spiritual enlightenment (Carnie, 1997).

Qigong enhances a number of physiological mechanisms (Burton Goldberg Group, 1995), including:

- Initiating the "relaxation response" that decreases the sympathetic function of the autonomic nervous system (triggered by any form of mental focus that frees the mind from its many distractions). This decreases heart rate and blood pressure, dilates the blood capillaries, and optimizes the delivery of oxygen to the tissues.

- Altering the neurochemistry profile moderating pain, depression, and addictive cravings, as well as optimizing immune capability.

- Enhancing the efficiency of the immune system through increased rate and flow of the lymphatic fluid.

- Improving resistance to disease and infection by accelerating the elimination of toxic metabolites (metabolic byproducts) from the interstitial spaces in the tissues, organs, and glands through the lymphatic system.

- Increasing the efficiency of cell metabolism and tissue regeneration through increased circulation of oxygen and nutrient rich blood to the brain, organs, and tissues.

- Coordinating the right and left brain hemisphere dominance promoting deeper sleep, reduced anxiety, and mental clarity.

- Inducing alpha and, in some cases, theta brain waves, which reduce heart rate and blood pressure, facilitating relaxation, mental focus, and even paranormal skills; this optimizes the body's self regulative mechanisms by decreasing the activity of the sympathetic nervous system.

- Moderating the function of the hypothalamus, pituitary, and pineal glands, as well as the cerebrospinal fluid system of the brain and spinal cord, which mediates pain and mood and enhances immune function.

Qigong exercises are done in short movement groups that are repeated many times, in contrast to the flow of positions in tai chi. Repetitions of coordinated physical motions with mental concentration and directive efforts move the qi in the body. The mind moves the chi and the chi moves the blood and oxygen (Berman & Larson, 1994).

Chi supply can be increased in several ways. The first way is the simplest and involves contracting muscles in a series of exercises called wai dan. The next method, called *nei dan*, is the most advanced and involves using your mind. The third method requires a trained acupuncturist, and the final method consists of various forms of massage (Carnie, 1997).

Wai dan involves using a variety of physical postures in order to create a surplus of chi in the arms and legs. Once the chi builds up to a high enough level, it will clear through most any tension or blockage. In still wai dan (zhan zhuang), a particular position is held while the muscles are relaxed. In a typical position, a person might stand with feet shoulder width apart and knees slightly bent while also having the arms extended straight out at the sides at shoulder height, palms facing forward and elbows slightly bent. After standing in this position for up to 20 minutes, the arms will feel quite fatigued. When the arms are lowered, the energy that has built up in the shoulders will flow down into the arms and eventually circulate through the body. According to Chinese medical statistics, about 80% of clients who practice these positions are healed of their medical problems (Carnie, 1997).

Moving wai dan involves repeatedly tensing and relaxing various muscle groups while moving from one position to another. There should be as little tension in the muscles as possible so the chi has the greatest chance of moving through the various meridians. In one exercise resembling a bird flapping its wings as it flies, the person stands in a comfortable position with feet about shoulder width apart and arms hanging loosely at the sides. The arms are slowly raised until they are level with the shoulders while concentrating the mind on the feeling as each muscle moves. Palms should be facing down. Once the arms have reached shoulder height, they should be lowered back down to the sides as slowly as possible. The exercise should be repeated until the arms and shoulders feel like they are starting to warm up (Carnie, 1997).

Nei dan, on the other hand, builds chi by using mental effort. It is generally considered more complex and challenging to learn than wai dan, but is more effective once it is learned. Nei dan works by building up abdominal chi through a series of breathing exercises. Once the chi has built up in this area, the mind controls and circulates the chi throughout the body (Carnie, 1997).

It is best to study qigong with a qualified teacher to avoid side effects (Sancier, 1996), but almost anyone can learn and practice the exercises. Following are some suggestions for qigong practice (Burton Goldberg Group, 1995):

- Take it easy, don't strive for any particular result, and don't rush. Excess effort and trying too hard go against the natural benefits of qigong.

- Although qigong may seem simplistic, a dedication to these practices can mobilize one's inherent healing forces.

- Qigong can be performed standing, walking, sitting, or lying down. Qigong exercises can even be performed by those confined to bed or a wheelchair.

- Results come over time, so don't overdo it or expect too much too soon.

- If performed correctly, qigong is safe to practice as often as desired.

- Feel free to make up an individualized routine and to change the practices to suit personal needs, likes, and limitations.

- Always approach each practice with an intention to relax. The mind should be directed toward quiet indifference.

■ Regulate the breath so that both the inhalation and exhalation are slow and deep, but not urgent or exaggerated.

There are few research studies of qigong in the English language literature. However, two abstracts of qigong studies are presented below:

1. Twenty-six adult patients (aged 18 to 65 years) with complex regional pain syndrome type I (a disease involving malfunction of the sympathetic nervous system following minor tissue or nerve injury) were randomly assigned to experimental and control groups. Each patient assigned to the experimental group received six sessions (40 minutes, twice a week) of qigong training with two recognized Asian qigong masters. After 3 weeks of formal instruction, participants were told to continue their qigong exercises on a daily basis at home for an additional 7 weeks. Each patient assigned to the control group received 6 sessions of simulated qigong training. In the experimental group, 82% reported less pain by the end of the first training session compared with 45% of control patients. By the last training session, 91% of qigong patients reported analgesia compared with 36% of control patients. Anxiety was reduced in both groups over time, but the reduction was significantly greater in the experimental group. The authors concluded that qigong training resulted in transient pain reduction and long-term anxiety reduction (Wu et al., 1999).

2. To explore the effectiveness of qigong therapy on detoxification of heroin addicts (N = 34) compared to medication treatment (lofexidine-HCl) (N = 26) and treatment only of severe withdrawal symptoms (N = 26), male heroin addicts in the People's Republic of China (aged 18 to 52) were randomly assigned to one of the three groups. The qigong group practiced pan gu qigong and received qi (chi) adjustments daily from a qigong master. The medication group was on a 10-day gradual reduction method. The control group received only basic care and medications to treat severe withdrawal symptoms. Reduction of withdrawal symptoms occurred more rapidly in the qigong group than in the other groups. From day 1, the qigong group had significantly lower mean symptom scores (p < .01) and lower anxiety scores (p < .01). It was concluded that qigong may be an effective alternative for heroin detoxification without side effects (Li et al., 2002).

Integrative Health Promotion

ASSESSMENT

The process of using activity and exercise in integrative health promotion should begin with client assessment. Four important areas for an initial assessment of the client include 1) the purpose for proposing an activity or exercise modality; 2) energy ebb and flow; 3) client readiness for activity or exercise; and 4) client priorities.

Determining the purpose for proposing an activity/exercise intervention is an important initial consideration. The purpose for the intervention is basic to determining the most appropriate modality. For example, if the purpose is risk reduction for cardiac problems in an obese client, the appropriate modality might be an aerobic exercise regimen, whereas primary prevention of falls in the elderly suggests a tai chi exercise intervention.

An initial assessment of energy ebb and flow will determine if energy augmentation is needed, or if energy is blocked in any area. Touch for health can be used to assess local energy blockages, and qigong is very effective in smoothing energy flow. See Table 4-10 for appropriate energetic patterning modalities to clear, convey, conserve, course, convert, and/or connect energy. Additionally, an initial assessment of energy ebb and flow provides a baseline for evaluating outcomes of any intervention.

Client readiness for adoption of activity/exercise is another important area to assess. As discussed in Chapter 8, *Promoting Individual Behavior Change*, the TTM suggests that there are five stages of behavior change: precontemplation, contemplation, preparation, action, and maintenance. Given the proposal that stage-specific factors to promote adoption can be mobilized through intervention methods, the stage of readiness provides a guide for appropriate intervention approaches. For example, during the contemplation stage of behavior change, consciousness raising through increased information or confrontation might be appropriate strategies. In contrast, stimulus control, emphasizing activities that precede activity and exercise can be helpful during the action and maintenance stages of change. Rodgers and colleagues (2001), in a cross-sectional study, found the same pattern of change among the TTM variables across stages of exercise behavior in three populations (high school students, university undergraduate students, and employed adults), supporting the claim that "the pattern of change among TTM variables across the stages is the same regardless of the population examined" (Rodgers et al., 2001, p. 40).

Client priorities are another important area for assessment. Does the client consider the adoption of an activity or exercise program to be important? If not, the nurse might consider using a precontemplation strategy to encourage reconsideration. But, if the client does not value activity or exercise behavior, external pressure by the nurse is useless. If the client is internally motivated, what are the reasons that the client values adoption of an activity or exercise program? An understanding of the client's motivation is essential to selection of appropriate strategies and effective support.

DEVELOPMENT OF A PLAN

The process of using activity and exercise in integrative health promotion should continue with development of a plan. Four important areas for development of a plan with the client include 1) mutuality with the client; 2) individualizing the plan for each client; 3) targeting interventions toward the stage of readiness of the client; and 4) choosing an appropriate modality.

As discussed in Chapter 10, *The Essence of the Healing Helping Relationship*, presence, respect, listening, and reciprocy are some of the key elements of a healing relationship. Reciprocy involves a mutual exchange and shared control, status, and power in the nurse-client relationship. The role of the nurse is to share information and facilitate desired lifestyle behavior change rather than to prescribe or attempt to control client behavior.

Behavior change strategies need to be individualized for each client. Because of the complex mix of purpose, motivation, perceived self-efficacy, and strengths or constraints, each intervention must be careful crafted for the specific individual. Based on basic assessment data, the nurse can not only select the most appropriate intervention, but can combine the modality with a plan for support and follow-up.

The need to target interventions toward the stage of readiness was discussed above. In many cases there are alternative interventions that may be equally effective in achieving the desired outcome. The selection of a specific intervention modality depends on a number of the factors discussed above. One modality or a combination of several modalities may initially be planned. However, on the basis of continued monitoring and evaluation, this plan may be modified and other modalities substituted.

IMPLEMENTATION OF THE PLAN

The process of using activity and exercise in integrative health promotion should continue with implementation of the plan. Three important areas for implementation of the plan with the client include 1) consistency; 2) meaningful involvement; and 3) building in maintenance.

Earlier in this chapter it was suggested that 30 minutes or more of moderate-intensity physical activity is desirable on most, and preferably all, days of the week. Consistency in the performance of activity or exercise is needed to achieve desired outcomes. A regular routine is also helpful for maintaining the behavior, even when other priorities intrude. Meaningful involvement of the client in the activity/exercise is essential to its consistent performance.

Given that almost half of adults are sedentary and that participation in exercise programs often drops within the initial 3 to 6 months, it is essential that attention be paid to maintenance of an exercise program once it has been started. This requires knowledge by the nurse and client of the conditions that promote relapse and stabilizing change through the development of non self-defeating responses. Counterconditioning is one strategy that can address negative emotional associations that may arise. For example, if exercise becomes boring, some strategies that the nurse can suggest include encouraging a varied routine, walking outside (whenever weather permits), and at least occasional exercise with a partner.

EVALUATION

Finally, the process of using activity and exercise in integrative health promotion should continue with evaluation of the plan. Two important areas for evaluation of the plan with the client include 1) assessing progress and 2) modifying as needed.

Evaluation should address two assessment factors. Regular observations should determine if there been change toward desired outcomes when progress is compared with baseline data. Reassessment of purpose, priorities, and motivation are also needed. If necessary, the plan may need to be modified. Relapse and recycling through the stages of change occur frequently with activity or exercise behaviors. During relapse, the client will probably regress to an earlier stage. This will necessitate a reconsideration of appropriate strategies, and possibly a change in intervention modalities. In other words, nursing assessment, planning, intervention, and evaluation to promote activity/exercise adoption are components of a continuous process.

Movement of energy is essential for well-being. Physical activity and exercise move the energy body as well as the physical body and provide significant health benefits and reduced health risks. Yet, lack of physical activity starts early in life, and at least half of all adults, including nurses, do not exercise. Also of concern is the sharp drop in participation in exercise programs within the initial 3 to 6 months. This chapter has emphasized the need for development and testing of theory-based interventions to promote physical activity initiation and maintenance at individual, environmental, and policy levels. Professional nurses need to role model and actively promote regular and sustained activity or exercise by clients.

Chapter Key Points

- Movement of energy is essential for a person's well-being.

- Exercise is a specific form of physical activity associated with desired outcomes of fitness, flexibility, and balance.

- Regular moderate physical activity provides substantial health benefits.

- Nursing strategies to empower clients to adopt a more active lifestyle include consideration of the clients' goals and motivation, introducing changes gradually, promoting regularity of activity, integrating the activity into daily life, making exercise fun, and having the client take control of his or her behavior.

- Walking is an ideal physical activity that requires no special equipment, facilities, or new skills.

- The Chinese movement forms of tai chi and qigong exercise the energy body and promote harmony through the combination of exercise and meditation.

References

Ai, A. L., Peterson, C., Gillespie, B., Bolling, S. F., Jessup, M. G., Behling, A., & Pierce, F. (2001). Designing clinical trials on energy healing: Ancient art encounters medical science. *Alternative Therapies in Health and Medicine, 7*, 83-90.

Allan, J. D. (1992). Exercise program. In G. M. Bulechek, & J. C. McCloskey (Eds.), *Nursing interventions: Essential nursing treatments* (2nd ed., pp. 406-424). Philadelphia: W. B. Saunders.

American College of Sports Medicine. (1993). Physical activity, physical fitness and hypertension. *Medicine and Science in Sports and Exercise, 25*, i-x.

American College of Sports Medicine. (2000). *Guidelines for exercise testing and prescription* (6th ed.). Philadelphia: Lippincott, Williams & Wilkins.

Ballentine, R. (1999). *Radical healing.* New York: Harmony.

Bauman, A. E., Sallis, J. F., Dzewaltowski, D. A., & Owen, N. (2002). Toward a better understanding of the influences on physical activity. *American Journal of Preventive Medicine, 23*, 5-14.

Berman, B. M., & Larson, D. B. (Eds). (1994). *Alternative medicine: Expanding medical horizons.* Washington, DC: U.S. Government Printing Office.

Bottomley, J. M. (1997). Tai chi. Choreography of body & mind. In C. M. Davis, (Ed.), *Complementary therapies in rehabilitation* (pp. 133-156). Thorofare, NJ: SLACK Incorporated.

Bronner, L. L., Kanter, D. S., & Manson, J. E. (1995). Primary prevention of stroke. *New England Journal of Medicine, 333*, 1392-1400.

Burton Goldberg Group. (1995). *Alternative medicine: The definitive guide*. Fife, WA: Future Medicine.

Carnie, L. V. (1997). *Chi gung. Chinese healing, energy, and natural magick*. St. Paul, MN: Llewellyn.

Caspersen, C. J., Powell, K. E., & Christenson, G. M. (1985). Physical activity, exercise, and physical fitness: Definitions and distinctions for health-related research. *Public Health Reports, 100*, 126-131.

Chan, K., Qin, M., Woo, J., Au, S., Chay, W., Lee, K., & Lee, S. (2004). A randomized, prospective study of the effects of tai chi chan exercise on bone mineral density in postmenopausal women. *Archives of Physical Medical Rehabilitation, 85*, 717-722.

Chen, K., & Snyder, M. (1999). A research-based use of tai chi/movement therapy as a nursing intervention. *Journal of Holistic Nursing, 17*, 267-279.

Clark, C. C. (1996). *Wellness practitioner*. New York: Springer.

Conn, V. S., Burks, K. J., Minor, M. A., & Mehr, D. R. (2003). Randomized trial of 2 interventions to increase older women's exercise. *American Journal of Health Behavior, 27*, 380-388.

Dishman, R. K., Sallis, J. F., & Orenstein, D. R. (1985). The determinants of physical activity and exercise. *Public Health Reports, 100*, 158-171.

Donker, F. J. (2000). Cardiac rehabilitation: A review of current developments. *Clinical Psychological Review, 20*, 923-43.

Dubbert, P. M. (2002). Physical activity and exercise: Recent advances and current challenges. *Journal of Consulting and Clinical Psychology, 70*, 526-536.

Griffin, J. C. (1998). *Client-centered exercise prescription*. Champaign, IL: Human Kinetics.

Hayashi, T., Tsumura, K., Suematsu, C., Okada, K., Fujii, S., & Endo, G. (1999). Walking to work and the risk for hypertension in men: The Osaka health survey. *Annals of Internal Medicine, 131*, 21-26.

Houde, S. C., & Melillo, K. D. (2002). Cardiovascular health and physical activity in older adults: An integrative review of research methodology and results. *Journal of Advanced Nursing, 38*, 219-234.

Hu, F. B., Stampfer, W. J., Colditz, G. A., Ascherio, A., Rexrode, K. M., Willett, W. C., & Manson, J. E. (2000). Physical activity and risk of stroke in women. *Journal of the American Medical Association, 283*, 2961-2967.

Husted, C., Pham, L., Hekking, A., & Niederman, R. (1999). Improving quality of life for people with chronic conditions: The example of tai chi and multiple sclerosis. *Alternative Therapies in Health and Medicine, 5*(5), 70-74.

Jancewicz, A. (2001). Tai chi chuan's role in maintaining independence in ageing people with chronic disease. *Journal of Bodywork and Movement Therapies, 5*, 70-77.

Jonas, S. (1996). Exercise. In S. H. Woolf, S. Jonas, & R. S. Lawrence. (Eds.), *Health promotion and disease prevention in clinical practice* (pp. 176-192). Baltimore: Williams & Wilkins.

King, A. C. (1994). Clinical and community interventions to promote and support physical activity participation. In R. K. Dishman (Ed.), *Advances in exercise adherence* (pp. 183-235). Champaign ,IL: Human Kinetics.

Lan, C., Lai, J., & Chen, S. (2000). Tai chi chuan. An ancient wisdom on exercise and health promotion. *Sports Medicine, 32*, 217-224.

Li, F., Harmer, P., McAuley, E., Duncan, T. E., Duncan, S. C., Chaumeton, N., & Fisher, K. J. (2001). An evaluation of the effects of tai chi exercise on physical function among older persons: A randomized controlled trial. *Annals of Behavioral Medicine, 23*, 139-46

Li, F., Fisher, J., Harmer, P., & Shirai, M. (2003). A simpler eight-form easy tai chi for elderly adults. *Journal of Aging and Physical Activity, 11*, 206-218.

Li, M., Chen, K., & Mo, Z. (2002). Use of qigong therapy in the detoxification of heroin addicts. *Altern Ther Health Med, 8*, 50-59.

Marcus, B. H., Bock, B. C., & Pinto, B. M. (1997). Initiation and maintenance of exercise behavior. In D. S. Gochman (Ed.), *Handbook of health behavior research*, (Vol. 2, pp. 335-352). New York: Plenum Press.

May, B. J. (1990). Principles of exercise for the elderly. In J. V. Basmajian, & S. L. Wolf (Eds.), *Therapeutic exercise* (5th ed., pp. 279-298). Baltimore: Williams & Wilkins.

Nieman, D. C. (1998). *The exercise-health connection.* Champaign, IL: Human Kinetics.

Nigg, C. R., Burbank, P. M., Padula, C., Dufresne, R., Rossi, J. S., Velicer, W. F., et al. (1999). Stages of change across ten health risk behaviors for older adults. *Gerontologist, 4*, 473-82.

NIH Consensus Development Panel on Osteoporosis Prevention, Diagnosis, and Therapy. (2001). Osteoporosis prevention, diagnosis, and therapy. *Journal of the American Medical Association, 285*, 785-795.

O'Brien, S. J., & Vertinsky, P. A. (1991). Unfit survivors: Exercise as a resource for aging women. *Gerontologist, 31*, 347-357.

Olsen , K. G. (1990). *The encyclopedia of alternative health care.* New York: Pocket Books.

Orleans, C. T., Gruman, J., Ulmer, C., Emont, S. L., & Hollendonner, J. K. (1999). Rating our progress in population health promotion: Report card on six behaviors. *American Journal of Health Promotion, 14*, 75-82.

Pate, R.R., Pratt, M., Blair, S. N., Haskell, W. L., Macera C. A., & Bouchard, C. (1995). Physical activity and public health: A recommendation from the Centers for Disease Control and Prevention and the American College of Sports Medicine. *Journal of the American Medical Association, 273*, 402-407.

Patel, A.T., & Ogle, A. A. (2000). Diagnosis and management of acute low back pain. *American Family Physician, 61*, 1779-1786, 1789-90.

Pender, N. J., Murdaugh, C. L., & Parsons, M. A. (2002). *Health promotion in nursing practice* (4th ed.). Upper Saddle River, NJ: Prentice Hall.

Phillips, E. M., Schneider, J. C., & Mercer, G. R. (2004). Motivating elders to initiate and maintain exercise. *Archives of Physical Medicine Rehabilitation, 85* (Supp. 3), S52-57.

Resnick, B. (1999, March). Exercise for the older adult: The seven step approach to wellness. *Advance for Nurses*, 20-21.

Resnick, B., Palmer, M. H., Jenkins, L. S., & Spellbring, A. M. (2000). Path analysis of efficacy expectations and exercise behavior in older adults. *Journal of Advvanced Nursing, 31*, 1309-15.

Robbins, L. B., Pender, N. J., Conn, V. S., Frenn, M. D., Neuberger, G. B., Nies, M. A., et al. (2001). Physical activity research in nursing. *Journal of Nursing Scholarship, 33*, 315-321.

Rodgers, W. M., Courneya, K. S., & Bayduza, A. L. (2001). Examination of the transtheoretical model and exercise in 3 populations. *American Journal of Health Behavior, 25*, 33-41.

Sallis, J. F., Bauman, A., & Pratt, M. (1998). Environmental and policy interventions to promote physical activity. *Am J Prev Med, 15*, 379-397.

Sancier, K. M. (1996). Medical applications of qigong. *Alterntive Therapies in Health and Medicine, 2*, 40-46.

Sebregts, E. H. W. J., Falger, P. R. J., & Bar, F. W. H. M. (2000). Risk factor modification though nonpharmacological interventions in patients with coronary heart disease. *Journal of Psychosomatic Research, 48*, 425-441.

Shaller, K. (1998). Tai chi/movement therapy. In M. Snyder & R. Linduist. (Eds.), *Complementary/alternative therapies in nursing* (pp. 37-47). New York: Springer.

Sharkey, N. A., Williams, N. I., and Guerin, J. B. (2000). The role of exercise in the prevention and treatment of osteoporosis and osteoarthritis. *Nursing Clinics of North America, 35*, 209-221.

Thornton, E. W., Sykes, K. S.,& Tang, W. K. (2004). Health benefits of tai chi exercise: Improved balance and blood pressure in middle-aged women. *Health Promotion International, 19*, 33-38.

Treat-Jacobson, D., & Mark, D. L. (1998). Exercise. In M. Snyder & R. Lindquist (Eds.), *Complementary/alternative therapies in nursing* (pp. 23-35). New York: Springer.

Van der Bij, A. K., Laurant, M. G. H., & Wensing, M. (2002). Effectiveness of physical activity interventions for older adults: A review. *American Journal of Prevntitive Medicine, 22*, 120-133.

Weil, A. (1999, April). Exercise: The best health tonic. *Self-Healing*, 2-3.

Wu, W., Bandilla, E., Ciccone, D. S., Yang, J., Cheng, S. S., Carner, N., et al. (1999). Effects of qigong on late-stage complex regional pain syndrome. *Alternative Therapies in Health and Medicine, 5*(1), 45-54.

Zelasko, C. J. (1995). Exercise for weight loss: What are the facts? *Journal of the American Dietetic Association, 95*, 1414-1417.

Additional Information

ASSOCIATIONS AND CREDENTIALING

Tai Chi

There is no national agency for licensing or credentialing in the United States. Tai chi associations are as varied as the styles and systems.

Internet Links

www.chebucto.ns.ca/Philosophy/Taichi/other

www.nih.gov/nia/new/press/taichi

http://frank.mtsu.edu/~jpurcell/Taichi/tc-links.htm

Qigong

National Qigong Association USA
PO Box 20218
Boulder, CO 80308
Tel: (888) 218-7788
www.nqa.org

Currently there is no official credentialing or licensing of qigong instructors in the United States or guidelines for what is required to be called a Master of Qigong therapist. The

National Qigong Association is working to establish a recommended minimum curriculum, hours of training, and ethical guidelines for both general qigong and medical qigong therapy.

The Qigong Institute
561 Berkeley Avenue
Menlo Park, CA 94025
www.qigonginstitute.org

RELEASING BLOCKED ENERGY
Touch and Bodywork Techniques

Abstract

Touch, used with sensitivity, allows the clinician to locate areas of muscle tension, reduce pain, soothe injured muscles, stimulate blood and lymphatic circulation, and promote deep relaxation. Bodywork techniques, with touch as their fundamental medium, discussed in this chapter include massage therapies, acupressure, and various postural/movement reeducation therapies. Additional information about organizational resources and certification for each of the therapies is located at the end of the chapter.

Learning Outcomes

By the end of the chapter the student should be able to:

- Identify the therapeutic effects of massage

- Differentiate between types of soft tissue manipulation used in massage strokes

- Compare and contrast types of massage from European and Chinese traditions

- Describe techniques for reflexology, shiatsu, Touch for Health, jin shin do, and self-acupressure

- Differentiate between techniques for the Alexander method, the Feldenkrais method, Trager integration, and the structural integration (Rolfing) method of postural movement or re-education

Touch is tactile communication from one person to another for the primary purposes of the transmission and receipt of signals of recognition, acceptance, protection, and caring concern. Used as a verb, touch means to make contact with. To be touched by something also has the meaning of being emotionally affected. Physical touch is reciprocal, such that whom or what a person touches also touches the person (Mackey, 2001; Routasalo, 1999).

Sensitive touch can convey a sense of caring, which is an essential element in a therapeutic relationship. Touch also has a comforting and calming effect. Touch used with sensitivity allows the clinician to receive useful information about the body, such as locating areas of muscle tension and other soft tissue problems. Bodywork helps to reduce pain, soothe injured muscles, stimulate blood and lymphatic circulation, and promote deep relaxation (Berman & Larson, 1994). Bodywork techniques (with touch as their fundamental medium) discussed in this chapter include massage therapy, acupressure, and postural or movement re-education therapies.

Massage Therapy

Massage, a word that comes from both the Greek *masso*, to knead, and the Arabic *mass*, to press gently (Olsen, 1990), is a systematic, therapeutic stroking and kneading of the skin and muscle. Through the systematic and scientific manipulation of the soft tissues of the body, soft-tissue massage blends mechanical proficiency and artistic sensibility to aid the ability of the body to heal itself. Specifically, the purposes of massage include promotion of relaxation, reduction of stress, improving skin and muscle tone, stimulating venous and lymphatic circulation, and producing therapeutic effects on the respiratory and nervous systems, and the subtle interactions between all body systems (Huebscher, 1998).

MASSAGE METHODS

Traditional European methods are the dominant approaches to massage practiced in the United States. Massage is supported by the physiology-based theory that muscle tension, whether from normal activity or from awkward movement or stress, contributes to muscle fatigue and pain by compressing nerve fibers in the muscle. Prolonged muscle contraction interferes with the elimination of chemical wastes in the muscles and surrounding tissues, and can cause frequent nerve and muscle pain (Berman & Larson, 1994). Massaging soft tissue and muscles speeds up the metabolic re-absorption or release of the fluid toxins. Massage may be indicated for personal growth, balance, and emotional release as well as for release of muscle tension.

Based on traditional Western concepts of anatomy and physiology, the basic categories of soft tissue manipulation used in massage (Clark, 1996; D'Epiro, 1997; Olsen, 1990) include effleurage, petrissage, kneading, tapotement, touch, vibration, brushing, range of motion, and nerve compression:

- *Effleurage.* Consists of light stroking, firm and gentle movements. Slow, rhythmic, gliding strokes are often used to begin and end a session. Gradual compression on the skin encourages relaxation by reducing muscle tone, firm pressure speeds blood and lymph flow to reduce swelling, and rapid strokes enhance muscle tone. Centripetal effleurage moves toward the heart, stimulating circulation, and rotary or spiral effleurage stimulates the smaller blood vessels in the skin.

- *Petrissage.* Consists of firm friction stroking, both deep and superficial. Confined to fleshy areas, this technique is more powerful than kneading. Folds of skin, subcutaneous tissue, and muscle are compressed, lifted, and rolled against underlying tissue in a circular manner to lengthen contracted or adherent fibrous tissue, soothe muscle spasm, and propel motion of body fluids, which relieves swelling.

- *Kneading.* Consists of a rhythmic lifting and squeezing of flesh. It involves slow, circular squeezing of soft tissue against underlying bone to improve swelling and inflammation. A more energetic motion is intended to reduce muscle spasm and elongate tissues.

- *Tapotement.* Consists of percussive motions such as lightly hitting the skin with cupped hands (clapping), the ulnar edge of the hand (hacking), loosely flexed fingers (tapping), or closed fists over muscles and the fleshy parts of the body to induce cutaneous reflexes and vasodilation. It results in increased muscle tone and distribution of accumulated interstitial fluid, so swelling is diminished. The movement is done parallel to the muscle fibers to prevent trauma or spasm. This stroke is especially effective on tight muscles in the shoulders or neck.

- *Vibration.* Consists of rapid shaking and pulsating, done by hand or with a machine. A fine, tremulous movement, sometimes only fluttering above a body part, can be used for its soothing effect. When more crude and vigorous than tapotement, both hands are shaken while pressed against the skin to condense swollen tissue and diminish edema.

- *Touch.* Consists of simple placing or molding of the hand over a part of the body. If desired by the recipient, the physical contact of holding the hand or touching the shoulder while interacting can be very effective in reducing the muscle tension associated with anxiety and encouraging relaxation.

- *Brushing.* Consists of light fingertip contact done slowly and rhythmically to spread general sensations over the body. This is often done as a finishing stroke, but pressure should be strong enough to avoid a tickling sensation.

- *Range of motion.* Consists of passive exercising by rotating, flexing, and extending body and limbs to mobilize joints and boost secretion of synovial fluids.

- *Nerve compression.* Consists of exerting firm pressure to relieve knots or pain at nerve points.

In addition to the European methods described above, traditional Chinese massage can be used to treat and relieve many medical conditions through both "tonification" (energizing) and "sedation" techniques. Traditional Chinese massage is based on the principle that chi must flow harmoniously through the meridians for proper functioning of the muscles and organ systems. Symptoms occur when chi is blocked, stagnant, or excessive. Massage can remove energy blocks or excesses and restore harmony. Berman and Larson (1994) list some of the major massage methods:

- *Ma.* Rubbing with palm or fingertips.
- *Pai.* Tapping with palm or fingertips.

- *Tao.* Strong pinching with thumb and fingertip.

- *An.* Rapid and rhythmical pressing with thumb, palm, or back of the clenched hand.

- *Nie.* Twisting, with both thumbs and tips of the index fingers grasping and twisting the area being treated.

- *Ning.* Pinching and lifting in a stationary position.

- *Na.* Moving, while performing ning.

- *Tui.* Pushing, often with slight vibratory effect.

TYPES OF MASSAGE

Berman and Larson (1994) describe a number of massage traditions that are based on traditional European methods, including:

- *Swedish massage.* Involves use of long gliding strokes, kneading, and friction techniques on the more superficial muscles, generally in the direction of blood flow toward the heart, sometimes combined with active and passive movements of the joints. This type of massage is used to promote general relaxation, improve circulation and range of motion, and relieve muscle tension.

- *Deep tissue massage.* Involves use of slow strokes, direct pressure, or friction directed across the grain of the muscles with the fingers, thumbs, or elbows. It is applied with greater pressure and to deeper layers of muscle than Swedish massage. It is used to release chronic patterns of muscular tension.

- *Neuromuscular massage.* A form of deep massage that is applied specifically to individual muscles. It is used to increase blood flow, release trigger points (intense knots of muscle tension that refer pain to other parts of the body), and release pressure on nerves caused by soft tissues. It is often used to reduce pain.

- *Manual lymph drainage.* A form of deep tissue massage that uses firm rhythmic strokes to direct lymphatic fluid from the tissues into the lymphatic ducts and back to the heart. It is primarily used for conditions of the extremities related to poor lymph flow such as edema, inflammation, and neuropathies.

PRINCIPLES FOR MASSAGE PRACTICE

Before starting therapeutic massage, observation and palpation, using a firm but light touch, should be used to assess areas of tenseness or immobility, tenderness, changes in temperature, or edema. This information will help to determine areas and methods for massage emphasis. Mackey (2001) stresses that in addition to being aware of the client, the environment, and precautions, the nurse needs to be self-aware, centered, confident, relaxed, and self-prepared. The nurse should take care of her hands, wrists, and fingers by stretching and strengthening the muscles regularly. Permission to touch should always be obtained.

Care should be taken to ensure client privacy and a comfortable room temperature during the procedure. The nurse should be careful to use correct body mechanics to avoid personal fatigue and strain. The hands should be warm, and fingernails should be short and trimmed.

Use of a lubricating oil or lotion will prevent a feeling of burning due to skin friction. The techniques of massage can be combined with other methods, such as aromatherapy and music therapy, to induce relaxation and relieve muscle tension. Basic massage techniques to promote circulation and relaxation can be practiced by all nurses. However, advanced techniques for other therapeutic effects or for a full body massage require additional continuing education and training (see sources at the end of the chapter).

Massage has been found to be therapeutic for hospitalized cancer patients, according to a recent massage study detailed in Box 14-1.

Box 14-1

Massage Study Abstract

In a quasi-experimental design without random assignment to groups, 41 primarily male cancer patients hospitalized for chemotherapy or radiation therapy received either three 15- to 30-minute treatments with light Swedish effleurage and petrissage massage within 1 week (the experimental treatment), or 20 minutes of "deliberate focused communication" (the control treatment) with the same nurse. Compared with scores on admission, at the end of 1 week, "mean scores for pain, sleep quality, symptom distress, and anxiety improved from baseline for the subjects who received therapeutic massage; only anxiety improved from baseline for participants in the comparison group." However, lack of random assignment to groups and a sample comprised primarily of Caucasian men prevents generalizability of these findings. The authors stress the need for randomized clinical trials to determine the efficacy of therapeutic massage in decreasing symptoms in hospitalized patients.

Source: Adapted from Smith, M. C., Kemp, J., Hemphill, L., & Vojir, C. P. (2002). Outcomes of therapeutic massage for hospitalized cancer patients. *Journal of Nursing Scholarship, 34,* 257-262.

Lloyd (1995, p. 30) describes a procedure for neck massage based on effleurage and kneading methods. Lloyd stresses that the experience of administering and receiving massage increases confidence and understanding of what feels good. The procedure for neck massage is described in Box 14-2.

It is believed that massage has many therapeutic effects, including (Berman & Larson, 1994; Moyer et al., 2004; Smith et al., 2003):

- A sedative effect on the nervous system and promotion of voluntary muscle relaxation
- Promoting recovery from fatigue produced by excessive exercise
- Help in breaking up scar tissue and lessening fibrosis and adhesions that develop as a result of injury and immobilization
- Relief from certain types of pain

Box 14-2

A Procedure for Neck Massage

- Stand behind seated client.
- Lightly place your hands on the client's shoulders.
- Using a kneading motion, begin to pick up flesh between your thumb and fingers.
- Keep strokes smooth and rhythmic.
- Move outward from the base of the neck along the shoulder.
- Ask the client for feedback on any sore spots and the degree of pressure he or she likes.
- Using the same kneading motion, work from the base of the neck up the base of the skull.
- Using a circular motion, work your fingertips out along the base of the skull to the ears.
- Ask the client to drop her or his head forward. Support the forehead with your hand. Using your thumb and index finger, use a circular and pinching motion on either side of cervical spine.
- With your index and middle finger on either side of the spine, rub up and down.
- For headache, use a circular motion on the temple region and stroking across the forehead.
- To finish, very gently stroke from top of the head, down the neck, and along the shoulders several times.

- Treatment of chronic inflammatory conditions by increasing lymphatic circulation
- Reduction of swelling from fractures
- Increased blood flow through the muscles, affecting circulation through the capillaries, veins, and arteries
- Loosened mucus and promote drainage of sinus fluids from the lungs by using percussive and vibratory techniques
- Increased peristaltic action in the intestines to promote fecal elimination
- Altered psychological and neurological complications associated with chemotherapy during bone marrow transplant (Smith, Reeder, Daniel, Baramee, & Hagman, 2003)

Single applications of massage therapy can reduce state anxiety, blood pressure, and heart rate, but not negative mood, immediate assessment of pain, and cortisol level. Reductions of trait anxiety and depression are the largest effects, with a course of treatment providing benefits similar in magnitude to those of psychotherapy (Moyer, Rounds, & Hannum, 2004).

In contrast to the many therapeutic effects of massage, there are few contraindications. Hill (1995) suggests that the contraindications to massage are primarily skin lesions, blood clots or bruises, fractures, severe arthritic pain, and fever. General precautions also should be exercised in cases of severe pain or an acute condition with unknown cause, enlarged varicose veins, burns, infections, new surgery, and pregnancy (Mackey, 2001).

When presenting symptoms are considered to be secondary manifestations of dysfunction elsewhere in the body, a form of touch known as acupressure may be an appropriate alternative.

Acupressure

Acupressure massage is defined as the application of finger pressure to any of 657 specific sites or points along the body's 14 energy meridians for the purpose of relieving tension and re-establishing the flow of energy along the meridian lines. A meridian is one of a series of channels running longitudinally on the body. These pathways are conduits for the body's circulating energy, or chi. Each pathway is associated with particular organs and psychological/physical functions. The various acupressure points (acupoints) are located on their respective meridians. These areas are particularly sensitive to bioelectrical impulses in the body (Kahn & Saulo, 1994).

In disease and pain, there is disruption in this energy pattern and organization caused by an accumulation, blockage, or loss of energy. The essential energy is contingent on adequate blood flow. Accupressure massage enhances circulation of both blood and lymph, which increases the dispersion of nutrients and aids in the disposal of metabolic wastes.

The clinician uses finger pressure on acupoints to balance the energy "body," thus bringing about optimal function. The purpose is to stimulate the body's own recuperative powers. "In most people, when all pathways are open and energy flow is unhindered, the body's energy can be balanced. Balance brings good health, vitality, and a sense of well-being" (Olsen, 1990, p. 48). There are specific acupressure points to relieve common ailments such as asthma, arthritis, constipation, insomnia, nosebleeds, sciatica, bedwetting, dizziness, fatigue, sore throat, and impotence (Olsen, 1990). Acupressure also can be used to support other treatments or to give temporary relief for both chronic and functional problems such as back pain, hypoglycemia, migraines, and menstrual cramps. Hand or mechanical (e.g., Acuband) pressure on P6, the Neiguan point on the pericardial meridian, has been used effectively to treat nausea and vomiting and prevent motion sickness (Stern et al., 2001). Additionally, in a blind, randomized trial, 24 healthy adult males received either pressure on acupoints, stroking along the meridians, or a control stimulation. The acupoint group had significantly lower diastolic and mean arterial pressures when compared with the two other groups, supporting the assertion that pressure on acupoints can significantly influence the cardiovascular system (Felhendler & Lisander, 1999).

Acupressure is effective as a health maintenance method with regular, periodic sessions (once a week or once a month, for example) to reduce stress, increase circulation, and "tune up" energy. Accupressure is also used for general preventive health care, warding off upper respiratory infections, improving muscle tone, and increasing energy levels (Kahn & Saulo, 1994).

All acupressure therapies use finger pressure on specific meridian points (acupoints), to stimulate or to sedate them (Berman & Larson, 1994). In the following section, myotherapy, reflexology, shiatsu, Touch for Health, and jin shin do will be presented as examples of specific acupressure methods. Guidelines for self-acupressure will also be discussed.

TRIGGER POINT/MYOTHERAPY

Trigger point technique is similar to shiatsu or acupressure. Trigger points are tender, congested spots on muscle tissue or fascia that may radiate pain to other areas. Practitioners of this modality apply pressure to specific points on the body to relieve tension.

REFLEXOLOGY

This accupressure method is often called zone therapy. The body, according to reflexology theory, is divided into 10 zones running longitudinally from the head to the feet, with five zones on each side, each corresponding to one of the five toes. In addition to the longitudinal zones, there are transverse zones that enable clinicians to draw up a grid for the identification of reflex points. There are also "cross-reflexes," in which a relationship exists between different points on each side of the body (Booth, 1994). Specific "zones" on the feet are related to specific organs. Thus, every part of the body, including organs and glands, can be affected by stimulating the appropriate reflex areas on the hands or the feet. When the energy flow through these zones is impeded, disease can result.

Reflexology stimulates deep relaxation, improves the blood supply, and promotes the unblocking of nerve impulses to normalize and balance the entire body. Reflexology provides tactile stimuli that are carried by large, type-A, beta-sensory fibers that can depress the transmission of pain signals. This produces local, lateral inhibition via the dorsal horn of the spinal cord (Stephenson & Dalton, 2003). Stimulating blocked or congested reflexes through massage of the appropriate area on the foot can release the stagnation and congestion related to a particular structure and allow energy to flow to it. Any congestion shown by tenderness in the extremities should correspond to a disorder in the body (Lynn, 1996). The emphasis is on targeting the breakup of lactic acid and calcium crystals accumulated around the 7,200 nerve endings in each foot (Berman & Larson, 1994). Blood circulation and the nervous system are stimulated, and this promotes self-healing and restores homeostasis within the body.

Clark (1996) and Mackey (2001) describe a number of strategies to improve reflexology technique:

1. Prior to attempting reflexology, strength and sensitivity of the fingers need to be developed—particularly the thumb. Practice in sensing a thread under the page of a book is a good exercise. When that can be sensed, try two pages, then three, and so on. Different materials such as dental floss, rubber bands, and seeds of different sizes can also be used. To estimate the pressure needed, practice pressing a bathroom scale to 20 to 25 pounds of pressure.

2. As with other body therapies, it is not wise to practice reflexology when feeling depleted or ill oneself, because it is possible to drain energy from the client.

3. Use information gathered from the client's history, palpatory assessment, and intuition to determine areas for reflexology. Reflex points on the left hand or foot have zones corresponding to the organs and glands on the left side of the body and the same for the right side.

4. Pressure in reflexology should evoke a "good hurt" or pressure that is comfortably tolerated. Start with a light pressure with the fingers and thumb, and move to deeper pressure when the appropriate area is located. Once the appropriate amount of pressure is found, hold it until a rhythmic pulsation is felt or until the client experiences a release of stress and tension. Observe for a change to a deeper breathing pattern, change to a better skin tone, relaxation in facial expression, and/or the client's words. For very painful spots, return to them again and again rather than trying to relieve the pain all at once; too much work all at once may bruise the capillaries.

Reflexology is not intended as diagnostic or as a treatment for a specific illness (Kunz & Kunz, 1995). In a blind study in which two reflexologists examined the feet of each of 18 adults and rated the probability that each of six conditions was present, inter-rater reliability scores were very low. It was concluded that the results did not support relexology techniques as a valid method of diagnosis (White et al., 2000). The main benefit of reflexology is the release of stress and tension. Other reported benefits include relief of pain, release of kidney stones, and recovery from the effects of stroke, sinusitis, sciatica, and menstrual disorders (Berman & Larson, 1994). Regular use has a general toning effect, which enhances other treatments and one's vitality and feelings of well-being. However, reflexology can produce side effects, which are referred to as healing crises (Lynn, 1996). Contraindications to reflexology include circulatory disorders of the lower limb, pregnancy, renal calculi, gallstones, and pacemakers (Booth, 1994). Box 14-3 presents a reflexology study abstract.

Box 14-3

Reflexology Study

Two hundred and twenty patients with migraine and/or tension headache were treated for a maximum of 6 months by 78 reflexologists systematically drawn from the membership lists of five alternative therapist associations in Denmark. Data collection methods included headache diaries, questionnaires, and qualitative interviews. Medication was continued as needed. At the 3-month follow-up, 81% of patients reported that they were helped by the treatments or were cured of their headache problems. Nineteen percent of those who had formerly taken drugs to control their headaches were able to stop medication support following participation in the study. The investigators indicated that additional studies are needed.

Source: Adapted from Launso, L., Brendstrup, E., & Arnberg, S. (1999). An exploratory study of reflexological treatment for headache. *Alternative Therapies in Health and Medicine, 5*(3), 57-65.

SHIATSU

Meridians were discussed earlier in this chapter. The technique of using finger pressure on specific points is also used in a form of massage known as shiatsu. Shiatsu relies largely on sequenced applications of pressure applied from one end of each meridian to the other. Shiatsu is "literally, finger (shi) pressure (atsu); a rhythmic series of finger pressures over the entire body along energetic meridians, or pathways, that also includes stretching and tapping methods. Points are held only 3 to 5 seconds" (Olsen, 1990).

The client reclines, usually lying on the back and then the abdomen, for approximately equal periods as the clinician uses thumb pressure to stimulate the point through a combination of direct pressure and transference of chi to the point from the clinician's thumb. "An extremely soothing intervention is to place one hand on the lower abdomen (hara) of the patient and the other on the 'third eye' area on the center of the forehead" (Hare, 1988, p. 72). "Barefoot shiatsu" can use foot pressure to stimulate the meridian points.

Sessions, which can be stimulating as well as relaxing, typically treat the meridians of the entire body in an attempt to induce relaxation, harmony, and balance (Berman & Larson, 1994; Olsen, 1990). In a study in which 66 individuals with lower back pain received four shiatsu treatments, pain and anxiety were significantly decreased over time (2 days after treatment) (Brady et al., 2001).

TOUCH FOR HEALTH (APPLIED KINESIOLOGY)

Using the acupuncture meridian system in addition to acupressure touch and massage, Touch for Health (TFH), or applied kinesiology, focuses on the relationship of muscle strength to energy flow. In this approach, each muscle corresponds to a related organ or bodily process. The theory is that if a particular muscle is strong, this indicates that the energy flow, neurological impulses, circulation, and lymphatic drainage to the muscle and corresponding organ are also strong. TFH is not testing the mechanical strength of the muscle, but rather the energy in the meridian associated with that muscle and the ability of the body to replenish energy (Clark, 1996). Energy flow is assessed through testing one muscle on each meridian pathway, identifying imbalances that are then corrected through acupressure massage techniques. Muscles that previously tested weak are found to be strong once the energy balance is restored (Gottesman, 1992).

Six different types of balancing techniques within THF (Gottesman, 1992, pp. 315-316) are:

1. Massaging the skin over the spinous process (the center portion of the vertebrae) at the level indicated by muscle testing, moving the skin over the bone in a headward to footward fashion for 10 to 20 seconds.

2. Gentle massage of the neurolymphatic points to stimulate the reflexes.

3. Stroking meridian pathways, over clothing if desired, which also has the effect of rebalancing the energy flow. Coming within 2 inches of the meridian is all that is necessary.

4. Sustained stationary touch to the neurovascular points.

5. Sustained stationary touch to the acupressure holding points.

6. Massaging the origin and insertion points of the muscle toward one another in a quick jiggling motion using hard, heavy pressure.

In the process of TFH, one muscle is manually tested on each side of the body to see if it locks, indicating energy is flowing, or is weak or "gives way," indicating an energy blockage. Then, the balancing techniques are performed one at a time, followed by a repeat of the muscle test to determine whether a correction has been made. If the muscle does not lock solidly and hold effortlessly in place, the next technique is performed and the muscle test is repeated. This procedure is repeated until 14 muscles have been tested and balanced on each side of the body. Once the tester has massaged, stroked, or touched the appropriate points for any weak muscles, the result is an immediate strengthening of the muscle, which can be seen and felt as the muscle locks solidly in place and holds effortlessly when tested. This indicates that the proper energy flow to the muscle has been restored. This also stimulates the organ sharing the same meridian (Gottesman, 1992).

TFH techniques can be used for self-care to improve health and obtain optimal-level wellness. Putting a hand across one's forehead, which covers the neurovascular points, enhances emotional stress release. This has a very relaxing effect and facilitates objectivity and problem solving. Additionally, stroking of the meridians can be incorporated into the bath or shower by washing with the proper flow of the meridians, down the inside of the arms, up the outside of the arms, up the inside of the legs, and down the outside. Stroking meridians can also be used as a pain relief technique by using the meridian closest to the painful area (Gottesman, 1992, pp. 317-318).

Theory predicts that when energy is out of balance over a period of time, physical illness is manifested. TFH is a method for identifying and correcting imbalances in the energy system before they become illness. TFH can be thought of as a "manual biofeedback technique that assists individuals to develop their intuitive ability through sensing and feeling their body signals" (Gottesman, 1992, pp. 311, 313). Muscle testing also can be used to bring unconscious material into consciousness, and to enhance flexibility, balance, coordination, range and ease of motion, and body symmetry. Through the testing and balancing procedure, changes occur posturally and structurally as habitual patterns of muscle tension are broken down. Other benefits claimed for TFH, as yet not supported by a body of evidence, are increased energy, increased resistance to illness, accelerated healing when sick or injured, improved ability to tolerate stress, decreased pain and tension, and alleviation of mood swings (Gottesman, 1992).

JIN SHIN DO

In comparison with TFH, which tests for areas of energy weakness, jin shin do (JSD), another form of acupressure, most often focuses on the parts of the body with an excess of energy, with the goal of releasing undesired blocked energy and restoring balance to body, mind, and spirit (Mik & Treppmann, 1997).

The English translation of jin shin do is "way of the compassionate spirit." Developed in the 1970s by Iona Marsaa Teeguardenn, an American psychotherapist, it is a synthesis of Western psychology, Taoist philosophy, and traditional Chinese medicine (Mik & Treppmann, 1997).

Jin shin do consists of a pattern of gentle, prolonged point-holding of key acupressure points on selected meridians and channels. The so-called local point of a blockage is held with one finger for 1 to 5 minutes, while the other hand successively touches two or three energetically connected distal points on other parts of the body to release the tension in the local point. Time devoted to therapy should be limited to one hour per week (Olsen, 1990).

JSD treatments are done in a meditative state to balance energy and body systems. The process of JSD starts with a thorough history of physical and/or emotional problems in order to detect patterns of disharmony. For the manual examination, the client preferably lies supine and the therapist starts from the neck and shoulders. Since each person has an individual distribution of tension and "armorings" (repressed, locked-in emotions), similar symptoms are not necessarily caused by the same tension patterns in different people (Mik & Treppmann, 1997).

Mik and Treppmann (1997) place special emphasis on self-care of the JSD practitioner. They point out that many professionals tend to "burn out" because they pour their energy into trying to cure or fix their patients, take too much responsibility for the outcome, and often feel as if they don't get anything back. However, "as JSD therapists, first of all, we are required to take good care of ourselves.... It is important for the therapist to be in a comfortable place, as his/her energy highly affects the state of the recipient and the outcome of a treatment.... It is the therapist's compassion and empathy that is required.... We don't have to fix anything for anyone. Our role is more that of an amplifying catalyst. We don't channel energy from outside of us, we simply support redistribution of what there is. The recipient and his/her energy do the job" (pp. 260, 264). This approach requires being nonjudgmental and present to each experience as it happens.

Applications of JSD are specific to the symptoms being addressed. Treatments are believed to be especially effective in improving disorders of function. Symptoms of low back pain often are accompanied by breathing or digestion problems. All three of these difficulties are affected by JSD energy release. As a gentle relaxation technique, JSD also can be used to relieve stress. With a series of treatments, the "armorings" can be released and experienced (Mik & Treppmann, 1997). However, JSD is contraindicated for patients in radiation therapy. Additionally, combining JSD with other energy therapies at the same time might alter the outcome of both. It is safer not to mix energy approaches but apply different approaches after a sufficient treatment-free interval.

SELF-MASSAGE

Any of the preceding methods can be used for accupressure self-massage.

In the preceding section, a number of approaches were discussed that use accupressure touch and/or massage to move body energy. In this section, four therapies that use postural or movement re-education as the mechanism to alter the flow of energy through the body, including Alexander technique, Feldenkrais method, Trager integration, and Rolfing, will be discussed.

Postural/Movement Re-education Therapies

Postural or movement re-education techniques use as their approach the re-education of the body through movement and physical touch. Patients are taught how to retrain their bodies to come into alignment to release and change postural faults, to improve coordination and balance, and to relieve structural and functional stress. A major principle underlying the

Alexander technique, Feldenkrais method, and Trager integration, is that awareness has to be experienced rather than taught verbally. The awareness may then lead to more effective use of one's whole self (Berman & Larson, 1994).

ALEXANDER TECHNIQUE

The Alexander technique uses lessons to re-educate the body and mind to overcome poor habits of posture and movement and to reduce physical and mental tension. A Shakespearean actor developed this technique after he realized that bad posture was responsible for his own chronic voice loss. F. M. Alexander felt that understanding is necessary to break habits, and that understanding occurs with repetition of small, simple movements. Consequently, simple, efficient movements designed to improve balance, posture, and coordination and to provide pain relief are taught in this technique.

The Alexander method is a body dynamics approach, especially in respect to the head, neck, and shoulders. It is assumed that the body reacts to gravity and the stresses of modern life with learned stress responses of poor posture and inhibited movements. The key to the lessons is learning a new repertoire of posture and movement. The clinician calls attention to certain ways of holding, which interfere with an innate ease of movement. Clients then use awareness of body position, action, and movement to distinguish between poor and fluid movements, allowing use of the body with less tension and more awareness and efficiency (Berman & Larson, 1994; Olsen, 1990). A study evaluating the Alexander technique is abstracted in Box 14-4.

Box 14-4

Alexander Technique Study

To test the effect of the Alexander technique on the management of disability and feelings of depression in patients with Parkinson's disease, seven volunteers received a median of 12 lessons in the Alexander technique. Post-lessons, the subjects were significantly ($p<0.05$) less depressed. They had a significantly more positive body concept and had significantly less difficulty performing daily activities. It was concluded that further, controlled research is desirable.

Source: Stailbrass, C. (1997). An evaluation of the Alexander technique for the management of disability in Parkinson's disease—A preliminary study. *Clinical Rehabilitation, 11*, 8-12.

The challenge of the Alexander technique is the need for continued practice. Results for this healing modality very much rest on the motivation and discipline of the client. Lessons are only introductions, reminders, and feedback on progress and improvement in use of the technique (Olsen, 1990).

FELDENKRAIS METHOD

Moshe Feldenkrais was a physicist, a mechanical engineer, and a black-belt judo practitioner. He developed his method when he was told that a worsening chronic knee injury might cause him to be wheelchair bound in the future. Through the use of his method he was able to successfully rehabilitate his knee.

The Feldenkrais method "uses movement as a model and means to facilitate creating a new sense of one's self as a physical being" (Olsen, 1990, p. 138). The keys to the Feldenkrais method are awareness, touch, and discussion to assist clients to create freer, more efficient movement. Awareness involves an attentiveness to both internal experience and external environment, developed through experience of the skeleton and its muscles, and their orientation and movement in space. There is no attempt to structurally alter the body.

The Feldenkrais approach begins by inviting the individual to choose to participate, while trust in the clinician is purposefully fostered. The clinician takes on the roles of teacher, facilitator, and guide to assist the individual using verbal, visual, and kinesthetic information. Rather than first evaluating the client and then treating with massage and strengthening or range of motion exercises, the client is "invited to learn" using the discovery model. "The [client] is asked to explore a new focus of movement by attending to altered kinesthetic cues during a desired action. Evaluation is not performed separately from the learning process. The therapist constantly observes and adapts stimuli in order for the patient to maximally explore and adapt during a particular session; to experience, at best, a sense of success or, at least, the novelty of discovery" (Jackson-Wyatt, 1997, pp. 189, 191).

The notion of "self-image" is central to the Feldenkrais method. It is believed that if the negative habitual patterns of movement are interrupted, the body will learn to function with greater ease, fluidity, and motion. This would, in turn, improve one's self-image and simultaneously increase awareness and health (Berman & Larson, 1994). The starting point for self-observation is to help the client discover his or her current habitual responses in a particular situation. Intervention cues are initially small, gentle, and paced so that the learner perceives that "this feels doable and worth doing again" (Jackson-Wyatt, 1997).

Feldenkrais takes two forms. In individual hands-on sessions of "functional integration," the clinician's touch is used to improve the client's breathing and body alignment. In a series of classes of slow, nonaerobic motions ("awareness through movement"), clients "relearn" the proper ways their bodies should move.

Functional integration, which uses positioning, contact, pressure, and movement, combined with verbal and visual stimuli, is used as a strategy when the individual is not able, for whatever reason, to actively initiate the exploration (Jackson-Wyatt, 1997). In this method, words and gentle, noninvasive touch are used to guide a client to an awareness of existing and alternative movement patterns. The use of touch is for communication, not correction, and no special techniques of pressing or stroking are used (Berman & Larson, 1994).

Awareness through movement, which uses primarily verbal and visual stimuli, "is the approach of choice as long as the learner is prepared to initiate the movement experiment that will create new awareness and a variety of responses that are different from the habitual actions" (Jackson-Wyatt, 1997, pp. 195-196). This verbally directed form of the Feldenkrais method consists of gentle exploratory movement sequences organized around a specific human function (such as reaching, bending, or walking) with the intention of increasing awareness of multiple possibilities of action. Thinking, sensory perception, and imagery are also involved in examining each function (Berman & Larson, 1994). The method is frequently used to help reduce stress and tension, to alleviate chronic pain, and to help athletes and others improve their balance and coordination (Kahn & Saulo, 1994).

Feldenkrais attempts to give the brain, and therefore the body, new messages, new images, and patterns for movement. The task is to help clients free themselves from old patterns of distorted position and movement and learn to transmit new patterns and ways of moving to their bodies. The goal is to regain the potential to move with grace and freedom. Clients take responsibility for themselves, but cleverness, not force, stretches and releases muscles and reorganizes how to move body parts (Olsen, 1990). Thus, the method "imparts a sense of exploration, experimentation, and innovation that allows each person to find his or her optimal style of movement" (Berman & Larson, 1994, p. 101).

As with most touch and bodywork methods, only limited clinical studies have been conducted to document outcomes of the Feldenkrais method (Berman & Larson, 1994). However, an abstract of one randomized, controlled study is presented in Box 14-6.

TRAGER PSYCHOPHYSICAL INTEGRATION

The intention of Tragering is to allow the client to give up unconscious muscular control and relax deeply in order to increase flexibility and joint range of motion (Berman & Larson, 1994). Clinicians use light, gentle, nonintrusive hand and mind movements to break up and release deep-seated physical and mental patterns that restrict range of motion of the muscles. "Trager targets the unconscious mind, the central nervous system, rather than the local tissue. It goes directly to the source of the disturbance" (Stone, 1997, p. 201).

Key is the ability of clinicians to perform their work in a relaxed, meditative state, or "hook-up," which is intended to enhance sensory, kinesthetic, and other pleasurable experiences for the client (Olsen, 1990). The emphasis for the clinician is on mindfulness while moving. Mindfulness is the high level of conscious awareness and focus that the clinician assumes while working. This almost meditative state of alertness, sensitivity, and nonjudgment allows a clear open connection between the clinician and the client (Stone, 1997).

This method of movement reeducation is distinguished by compressions, elongations, light bounces, rhythmic rocking, and shaking movements to the client's head, torso, and appendages, which loosen joints, ease movement, and release chronic patterns of tension. These actions cause clients to begin to experience freedom of movement of their body parts. The clinician feels how the client is holding his or her body. "The Trager practitioner uses his or her hands with the aim of influencing deep-seated psychophysiological patterns in the client's mind and interrupting the projection of those patterns into body tissues" (Berman & Larson, 1994, p. 132).

A session consists of gentle passive movements of the client while lying on a treatment table. The Trager approach is "based in feeling, not in doing... The fluffing, jiggling, lengthening, and shimmering of muscle tissue is communicated to the patient's mind" (Stone, 1997, p. 200). The emphasis of this subtle approach is on comfort, gentleness, effortlessness, playfulness, and gentle, painless movements. Balance, gait, and strengthening may also be addressed. Each session, viewed not only as a treatment but also a lesson, is modified and adapted to fit the needs of the individual.

After each session, homework is assigned in Mentastics, a series of mentally directed, active, effortless, physical movements developed to maintain and enhance a sense of lightness, freedom, and flexibility. Mentastics is the active, self-guided version of the passive, individualized Trager session. Exercises are chosen to support progress made at each particular session (Olsen, 1990). The lesson is in how to feel movement in a manner that is correct for that body, thus increasing body awareness. Employing the weight of the body, a person is instructed to initiate a movement and then "let go." This release and allowing the weight of the body part to carry the motion to completion with mindfulness helps separate Mentastics movements from exercise (Stone, 1997).

The goals of Trager work are general functional improvement, creating a feeling of pleasure in being able to move body parts more freely, decreased muscular tension, improved body alignment, renewed and greater ease of movement, the experience of total relaxation and peace, and a sense of functional integration (Stone, 1997). Despite lack of research-based evidence of its effectiveness, Trager work has been indicated for those who want to learn to relax, improve posture, prevent pain, reduce tension, or move with greater ease. Box 14-5 describes a pilot study using the Trager approach.

Box 14-5

A Feldenkrais Method Study

To investigate whether physiotherapy or Feldenkrais interventions resulted in a reduction in neck and shoulder complaints, 97 female industrial workers were randomized to 1) a physiotherapy group treated for 50 minutes twice a week in groups of five to eight subjects and a program of home exercises according to the ergonomic program of the physical therapists of the occupational health service; 2) a Feldenkrais group with 50 minute per week interventions done individually four times, in a group of seven to eight subjects 12 times, and eight exercises for home practice on audio cassette; and 3) a control group that received no intervention but were promised participation in group exercise after termination of the study. The two interventions lasted 16 weeks during paid working time. An average of 1.5 months after the interventions, the Feldenkrais group showed significant decreases in complaints from neck and shoulders and in disability during leisure time. The other two groups showed no change (physiotherapy) or worsening of complaints (control). The authors concluded that more randomized and controlled studies with a longer follow up period are needed.

Source: Lundblad, I., Elert, J., & Gerdle, B. (1999). Randomized controlled trial of physiotherapy and Feldenkrais interventions in female workers with neck-shoulder complaints. *Journal of Occupational Rehabilitation, 9,* 179-194.

STRUCTURAL INTEGRATION (ROLFING)

In a study with 33 volunteers with a self-reported history of at least one headache per week for at least 6 months, analysis of variance demonstrated significant improvement in health-related quality of life for the medication and Trager group, and the medication and attention control group (compared with the medication-only control group), and reduction in medication usage for the Trager group. Participants randomized to Trager demonstrated a significant decrease in the frequency of headaches, and a 44% decrease in medication usage (Foster et al., 2004).

Structural integration, or Rolfing, consists of a series of 10 basic bodywork sessions of deep connective tissue manipulation involving stretching the fascia sheaths (sheets of connective tissue) by applying sliding pressure to the affected area with fingers, thumbs, and occasionally elbows. Bones support the body, and muscles connect the bones; the enwrapping fascias that support and hold not only the normal relationship of bone and muscle but also whatever postural misalignment the body might adopt. For example, when the body attempts to distribute the stress of an injury, the result is likely to be shortened and thickened fascias, which may in turn lead to symptoms somewhere other than the site of the original trauma (Berman & Larson, 1994). Manipulation of the fascias frequently elicits a strong emotional response, such as crying from clients.

The aim is to increase muscular length and overall balance for optimal posture. By aligning and structurally and functionally integrating the body's major anatomic segments (head, neck, shoulders, torso, pelvis, and legs) in balance with gravity, it is believed that the body will be able to use energy more efficiently (Olsen, 1990). Major offshoots of structural integration include Aston patterning, developed by Judith Aston, and Hellerwork, developed by Joseph Heller.

Rolfers recommend 10 sessions to obtain the maximum benefit from Rolfing. The sessions last approximately 1 hour and can be spaced anywhere from once a week to once a month. There is also a five session advanced series and a Rolfing movement series. Progressive tissue unfolding and restructuring keeps the client in balance between each session. Psychotherapy or a Rolfing movement session between manipulation sessions might also help the client process and integrate changes. After the initial 10 sessions, some people return for periodic tune-up work or a mini series of two or three sessions (Bernau-Eigen, 1998).

There are varied benefits of Rolfing. "Changes have the potential to affect the total well being of the person" (Bernau-Eigen, 1998, p. 240). General benefits include:

- Reduced chronic stress

- Increased flexibility

- Better circulation (older people comment on this effect)

- Pain relief

- A sense of expansion and feeling taller and lighter

- Greater self-acceptance

- Positive postural changes

- More energy

- A sense of support

The emphasis in this chapter has been on the use of touch to locate areas of muscle tension, reduce pain, soothe injured muscles, stimulate blood and lymphatic circulation, and promote deep relaxation. Noninvasive therapeutic modalities discussed include massage therapies, acupressure approaches such as reflexology, shiatsu, and TFH, and various postural/movement reeducation therapies. An extensive training program leading to certification is necessary for competent practice of many of these modalities (see additional information at the end of the chapter).

Chapter Key Points

- Sensitive touch can convey a sense of caring, which is an essential element in the therapeutic relationship.

- Bodywork in all its forms helps to reduce pain, soothe injured muscles, stimulate blood and lymphatic circulation, and promote deep relaxation.

- Types of massage include Swedish, deep tissue, neuromuscular, and manual lymph drainage from European traditions, and traditional Chinese methods.

- Types of acupressure include trigger point/myotherapy, reflexology, shiatsu, TFH, jin shin do, and self-acupressure.

- Forms of postural movement/reeducation include the Alexander technique, Feldenkrais method, Trager integration, and structural integration (Rolfing).

References

Berman, B. M., & Larson, D. B. (Eds). (1994). *Alternative medicine: Expanding medical horizons*. Washington, DC: U.S. Government Printing Office.

Bernau-Eigen, M. (1998). Rolfing: A somatic approach to the integration of human structures. *Nurse Practitioner Forum, 9*, 235-242.

Booth, B. (1994). Reflexology. *Nursing Times, 90*, 38-40.

Brady, L. H., Henry, K., Luth, J. F., & Casper-Bruett, K. K. (2001). The effects of shiatsu on lower back pain. *Journal of Holistic Nursing, 19*, 57-70.

Clark, C. C. (1996). *Wellness practitioner: Concepts, research and strategies* (2nd ed.). New York: Springer.

D'Epiro, N. W. (Ed.). (1997, October). Herbal medicine: What works, what's safe. *Patient Care*, 49-77.

Felhendler, D., & Lisander, B. (1999). Effects of non-invasive stimulation of acupoints on the cardiovascular system. *Complementary Therapies in Medicine, 7*, 231-234.

Foster, K.A., Liskin, J., Cen, S., Abbott, A., Armisen, V., Globe, D., et al. (2004). The Trager approach in the treatment of Chronic headache: A pilot study. *Alternative Therapies in Health and Medicine, 10*, 40-46.

Gottesman, C. (1992). Energy balancing through Touch for Health. *Journal of Holistic Nursing, 10*, 306-323.

Iare, M. L. (1988). Shiatsu acupressure in nursing practice. *Advances in Nursing Science, 2*, 68-74.

Hill, C. F. (1995). Massage in intensive care nursing: A literature review. *Complementary Therapies in Medicine, 3,* 100-104.

Huebscher, R. (1998). An overview of massage: Part I. *Nurse Practitioner Forum, 9,* 197-199.

Jackson-Wyatt, O. (1997). Feldenkrais method and rehabilitation: A paradigm shift incorporating a perception of learning. In C. M. Davis (Ed.), *Complementary therapies in rehabilitation* (pp. 189-196). Thorofare, NJ: SLACK Incorporated.

Kahn, S., & Saulo, M. (1994). *Healing. A nurse's guide to self-care and renewal.* Albany, NY: Delmar.

Kunz, K., & Kunz, B. (1995). Understanding the science and art of reflexology. *Alternative and Complementary Therapies, 1,* 183-186.

Lloyd, K. (1995, January). The power to heal colleagues and clients with a two-minute massage. *Lamp,* 30.

Lundblad, I., Elert, J., & Gerdle, B. (1999). Randomized controlled trial of physiotherapy and Feldenkrais interventions in female workers with neck-shoulder complaints. *Journal of Occupational Rehabilitation, 9,* 179-194.

Lynn, J. (1996). Using complementary therapies. Reflexology. *Professional Nurse, 11,* 321-22.

Mackey, B. T. (2001). Massage therapy and reflexology awareness. *Nursing Clinics of North America, 39,* 159-169.

Mik, G. H., & Treppmann, U. (1997). Jin shin do. In C. M. Davis (Ed.), *Complementary therapies in rehabilitation* (pp. 257-265). Thorofare, NJ: SLACK Incorporated.

Moyer, C. A., Rounds, J., & Hannum, J. W., (2004). A meta-analysis of massage therapy research. *Psychological Bulletin, 130,* 3-18.

Olsen, K. G. (1990). *The encyclopedia of alternative health care.* New York: Pocket Books.

Routasalo, P. (1999). Physical touch in nursing studies: A literature review. *Journal of Advanced Nursing, 30,* 843-850.

Smith, M. C., Kemp, J., Hemphill, L., & Vojir, C. P. (2002). Outcomes of therapeutic massage for hospitalized cancer patients. *Journal of Nursing Scholarship, 34,* 257-262.

Smith, M. C., Reeder, F., Daniel, L., Baramee, J., & Hagman, J. (2003). Outcomes of touch therapies during bone marrow transplant. *Alternative Therapies in Health and Medicine, 9,* 40-49.

Stailbrass, C. (1997). An evaluation of the Alexander technique for the management of disability in Parkinson's disease—A preliminary study. *Clinical Rehabilitation, 11,* 8-12.

Stephenson, N. L. N., & Dalton, J. A. (2003). Using reflexology for pain management. *Journal of Holistic Nursing, 21,* 179-191.

Stern, R. M., Jokerst, M. D., Muth, E. R., & Hollis, C. (2001). Acupressure relieves the symptoms of motion sickness and reduces abnormal gastric activity. *Alternative Therapies in Health and Medicine, 7,* 91-94.

Stone, A. R. (1997). The Trager approach. In C. M. Davis (Ed.), *Complementary therapies in rehabilitation* (pp. 199-212). Thorofare, NJ: SLACK Incorporated.

White, A. R., Williamson, J., Hart, A., & Ernst, E. (2000). A blinded investigation into the accuracy of reflexology charts. *Complementary Therapies in Medicine, 8,* 166-172.

Additional Information

ASSOCIATIONS AND CREDENTIALING

Massage

American Massage Therapy Association
820 Davis Street Suite 100
Evanston, IL 60201
Tel: (847) 864-0123
www.amtamassage.org

National Association of Nurse Massage Therapists
Tel: (800) 262-4017
www.nanmt.org

Massage therapists are currently licensed by 29 states, the District of Columbia, and a number of localities. Most states require 500 or more classroom hours of training from a recognized training program and passing an examination. The National Certification Board for Therapeutic Massage and Bodywork (NCBTMB) developed an exam that most states have adopted for their licensing examination. Those certified can use the title NCBTMB. The Commission on Massage Therapy Accreditation, and the Accrediting Commission of Career Schools and Colleges of Technology and the Accrediting Council for Continuing Education and Training also accredit massage training programs.

Trager Approach

The Trager Institute
21 Locust Avenue
Mill Valley, CA 94941
Tel: (415) 388-2688
www.trager.com

Trager practitioners are not regulated by any state. However, some states may require practitioners to obtain a massage license. Trager practitioners are certified by the Trager Institute, which monitors training and continued competency. To become a practitioner, an individual must experience the work from a certified practitioner before entering the training track. After a week-long initial training the student must complete and log at least 30 practice sessions, receive at least 10 sessions, and attend additional tutorials to be eligible for the intermediate training. Achieving practitioner status typically takes 1 to 2 years.

Rolfing

Rolf Institute of Structural Integration
205 Canyon Blvd.
Boulder, CO 80302
Tel: (800) 530-8875
www.rolf.org

The Rolf Institute is the sole certifying body for Rolfers.

Feldenkrais Method

Feldenkrais Guild of North America
524 Ellsworth St. SW
PO Box 489
Albany, OR 97321
Tel: (541) 926-0981
www.feldenkrais.com

The training required to be a certified Feldenkrais practitioner requires 160 days of training spread over a period of over 3 years. The educational director of training programs grants initial certification after students have passed a supervised clinic.

Certification must be maintained through continuing education requirements on a bi-annual basis.

Alexander Technique

The American Society for the Alexander Technique (ASAT)
3010 Hennepin Avenue South, Suite 10
Minneapolis, MN 55408
Tel: (800) 473-0620
www.alexandertech.com

Alexander Technique International (ATI)
USA Regional Office
1692 Massachusetts Avenue
Cambridge, MA 02138
Tel: (617) 497-2342

Both of these organizations certify teachers of the Alexander technique. In the United States, there are 18 ASAT-approved teacher training courses and five training courses affiliated with ATI. To become a certified ASAT teacher, an individual must complete 1,600 hours of training over a minimum of 3 years at an ASAT-approved teacher training course.

Applied Kinesiology

The International College of Applied Kinesiology (ICAK)
6405 Metcalf Avenue, Suite 503
Shawnee Mission, KS 66202
Tel: (913) 384-5336
www.icakusa.com

There is no specific degree for Applied Kinesiology; rather, it is practiced by those already possessing a doctorate degree (such as DC, DO, MD, and others) and a license to diagnose. The ICAK provides various levels of certification for physicians.

Reflexology

International Institute of Reflexology
PO Box 12642
St. Petersburg, FL 33733
Tel: (727) 343-4811
www.reflexology-usa.net

No formal credentialing exists for reflexology. Certification is provided by certain educational institutions specializing in this training, which can range from 100 to 1,000 hours of instruction.

Acupressure

American Oriental Bodywork Therapy Association (AOBTA)
Laurel Oak Corporate Center
1010 Haddonfield Berlin Road, Suite 408
Voorhees, NJ 08043
Tel: (856) 782-1616
www.AOBTA.org

The hands-on nature of acupressure has put acupressure under the auspices of massage therapy. The National Committee on Certification for Acupressure and traditional Eastern medicine recently created national examination and credentialing standards for oriental bodywork and acupressure. Among the many requirements are a minimum of 500 hours of training including at least 100 hours of anatomy. Although the industry standard is 500 hours of training, each state has different requirements for licensure.

REDUCING ENERGY DEPLETION
Relaxation and Stress Reduction

Abstract

The goals of stress management are to help people deal with short-lived stressful events and to defuse the effects of chronic stress. The parasympathetic nervous system helps to compensate for periods of high arousal and stress. All of the techniques described in this chapter, including different forms of meditation, breathing, yoga, biofeedback, and guided imagery, are designed to induce a positive parasympathetic state and reduce stress responses through relaxation. Additional information about organizational resources and certification for each of the therapies is located at the end of the chapter.

Learning Outcomes

By the end of the chapter the student will be able to:

- Describe symptoms of stress
- Differentiate between concentrative and mindfulness meditation
- Discuss how to elicit the relaxation response
- Differentiate between a body scan to practice mindfulness meditation and progressive muscle relaxation
- Describe the "essential breath" technique
- Discuss the use of yoga as a preparation for meditation
- Describe different types of biofeedback instrumentation

The Stress Response

At the beginning of the 19th century, the Harvard physiologist Walter B. Cannon first described the "fight-or-flight response," the internal adaptive response of the body to a change perceived as a threat. In this response, the body secretes catecholamines—stress hormones—that prepare a person under threat to fight or run. Epinephrine (adrenaline), which is produced by the adrenal glands, is the best known of these hormones.

The fight-or-flight response was essential to survival in a time when human beings faced physical threats, such as wild animals, that caused acute stress and could be dealt with effectively by either fighting or running away. By contrast, today's stresses, such as weather, noise, crowding, time pressures, performance standards, threats to security and self-esteem, lack of exercise, poor nutrition, and perception of an experience as stressful, are not resolvable through fight-or-flight. It is one's reaction to stressful experiences that can create a stress response.

There are two forms of stress: *short-term* (acute) and *long-term* (chronic). Acute stress, caused by stressors such as a near miss on the highway or the reaction to a sudden loud noise, is associated with a cascade of physiological changes that prepare the body for fight or flight. During acute stress, heart rate, blood pressure, and muscle tension all rise sharply; the stomach and intestines become less active; and the blood level of glucose rises for quick energy. The physiological responses are associated with psychological responses, such as racing thoughts, anxiety, and even panic.

Under conditions of chronic, long-term stress, the typical and normal responses that occur during short-term stress are abnormally extended and can contribute to the development of chronic disease. With chronic stress, the immune system tends to be suppressed or become less active, the blood cholesterol level rises, and calcium is lost from the bones. When protracted, the normal short-term increases in blood pressure can become hypertension, increased muscle tension can lead to headaches or aggravate pain, unusual changes in the activity of the intestinal tract can lead to diarrhea or spasms, and increases in heart rate can raise the risk of an arrhythmia. In addition, depressed immunity may make an individual susceptible to colds and the flu or possibly to more serious diseases. Indeed, more than 80% of all illnesses have stress-related etiologies (Bottomley, 1997).

Pelletier (1993) describes a number of symptoms associated with chronic, long-term stress:

- Cognitive symptoms such as anxious thoughts, poor concentration, and difficulty with memory.

- Emotional symptoms such as feelings of tension, irritability, restlessness, and depression.

- Behavioral symptoms such as sleep problems, crying, and changes in drinking, eating, or smoking behaviors.

- Physiological symptoms such as grinding teeth, sweating, nausea, constipation, tiredness, and weight loss or gain.

- Social symptoms such as withdrawal and change in the quality of relationships.

Stress responses are regulated by the autonomic nervous system, a part of the nervous system not usually under voluntary control. The sympathetic branch of the autonomic nervous

system regulates the kind of arousal described above. The parasympathe
nomic nervous system, on the other hand, induces relaxation and he
periods of high arousal. The goals of stress management are to help pe
term stressful events and to defuse the effects of chronic stress. All of the
in this chapter are designed to induce a positive parasympathetic st;
responses through relaxation.

Relaxation

Relaxation begins with an inward focus and a mental retreat from one's surroundings. When thoughts are stilled, muscular relaxation and stress reduction follow. Given that the relaxation response can be elicited by any one of a number of Eastern and Western practices (Horowitz, 1999), there is a great deal of room for individual choice from among the possible techniques. In fact, there is no evidence of a clear benefit of one relaxation technique over another. It is possible that client preference is the most important consideration in the effectiveness of any intervention (Snyder & Chlan, 1999).

There are a number of possible uses of relaxation therapy, including to:

- Decrease anxiety
- Promote sleep
- Reduce or prevent the physiological and psychological effects of stress
- Serve as a coping device or skill
- Reduce the perception of pain and enhance the effectiveness of pain relief measures
- Alleviate muscle tension
- Increase suggestibility
- Combat fatigue
- Increase perceived energy
- Warm or cool parts of the body
- Slow the heartbeat
- Decrease blood pressure (Zahourek, 1988)

However, despite the numerous indications, there are several precautions for relaxation that should be considered. These include making an illness worse by indiscriminate symptom removal or masking other illnesses; providing superficial relief, particularly with psychiatric difficulties, or promoting withdrawal, intensifying anxiety or panic; causing a counterproductive physiological response, a hypotensive state, or an unwanted drug reaction; or intensifying pain because of the focus on the body (Zahourek, 1988).

Olsen (1990, p. 262) clearly describes the possible consequences of profound relaxation:

"Done to an extreme, one can get too relaxed, one's mind too plastic. Profound relaxation over a prolonged period heightens suggestibility.... Stimulated too often or too fast, the new emotional awareness may be too intense. The individual becomes one raw nerve, suffering the impact of things and people inordinately in everyday life.... Some people may become addicted to the seeming euphoria or relaxation and withdraw from active life—physically and/or emotionally. Meditation or another form of relaxation becomes a shield, a way not to deal with real life."

In moderation, any one of the approaches to meditation can be a useful approach to induce relaxation. The next section will describe the relaxation response, autogenic training, and transcendental meditation as examples of the concentrative type of meditation, and progressive muscle relaxation as an example of the mindfulness type of meditation.

MEDITATION

The word *meditate* comes from the Sanskrit word, *medha*, meaning wisdom. Meditation simply means getting in touch with our inner wisdom (Gimbel, 1998).

According to Kuhn (1999, p. 199), meditation is defined in several ways: "a systematic and continued focusing of the attention on a single target perception—a sound or mantra—or continually holding a specific attention set; or a technique that allows a person to investigate the process of his or her consciousness and experiences to discover the more basic underlying qualities of existence; or simply any activity that keeps the attention pleasantly anchored in the present moment."

As a person continues to meditate, the general trend is toward greater calm, positive emotions and perceptual and introspective sensitivity. Exactly how meditation produces its many effects remains unclear. However, possible physiological processes include lowered arousal and increased hemispheric synchronization. Possible psychological mechanisms include relaxation, desensitization, development of self-control skills, insight and self-understanding (Walsh, 1996). However, Walsh (1996, p. 119) expresses concern that "more attention has been given to heart rate than . . . transpersonal goals such as enhanced concentration, ethics, love, compassion, generosity, wisdom, and service."

Many meditative and religious disciplines have moral, psychological, social, and spiritual requests for those who join their tradition. In Buddhism this includes the Noble Eightfold or Middle Path, as follows (Lowenstein, 2002):

- Right Understanding and Perception

- Right Thought and Aspiration

- Right Speech

- Right Action and Conduct

- Right Means of Livelihood

- Right Effort and Endeavor

- Right Mindfulness-Concentration

- Right Concentration-Contemplation

Wright (2001) identifies and rebuts several misconceptions about meditation that create obstacles to its practice. For example, one misconception is that meditation is somehow a sin because it is connected to Eastern mysticism. In fact, meditation "can be found in all religions" (2001, p. 96). Its universal nature transcends all religions and all cultures. Another misconception is that the mantra is of utmost importance and must be especially selected for the individual by a holy man. Wright (2001, p. 96) states that "in reality the choices for mantras are endless, and their importance is minimal." Yet another misconception experienced by adults is that meditation must be done perfectly. Actually, "there is no way to get it wrong. Meditation is the only state I know in which one's intent is to have no intention" (2001, p. 97). Finally, "is the idea that if one does not see God or is not levitating then he or she is doing it wrong" (2001, p. 97).

There are two basic approaches to meditation: concentrative and mindfulness meditation.

Concentrative (Reflective) Meditation

Concentrative meditation involves focus, or "awareness without thought" (Fugh-Berman, 1997, p. 167). Focus is attained in one of the following ways:

1. *Mental meditation.* Concentration on a word or phrase, commonly called a mantra.

2. *Physical repetition.* Concentration on breathing or the sound of one's feet hitting the ground in jogging.

3. *Problem contemplation.* Attempts to solve a problem with paradoxical components. Zen terms this the "koan."

4. *Visual concentration.* Akin to imagery, with the focus on an image.

Two specific concentrative meditation techniques that are widely used are the relaxation response and Transcendental Meditation (Maharishi Vedic Education Development Corporation)

The Relaxation Response

The relaxation response, which is based on mental meditation to achieve focus, consists of muscle relaxation, relaxed breathing, and repetition of the focus word/phrase. One set of instructions (Benson, 1993, p. 240) used to elicit the relaxation response is described below:

- Step 1. Pick a focus word or short phrase that's firmly rooted in your personal belief system. For example, a nonreligious individual might choose a neutral word like one, or peace or love, while a religious Christian person desiring to use a prayer could pick the opening words of Psalm 23, "The Lord is my shepherd," and a religious Jewish person could choose Shalom.

- Step 2. Sit quietly in a comfortable position.

- Step 3. Close your eyes.

- Step 4. Relax your muscles.

- Step 5. Breathe slowly and naturally, repeating your focus word or phrase silently as you exhale.

- Step 6. Throughout, assume a passive attitude. Don't worry about how well you're doing. When other thoughts come to mind, simply say to yourself, "Oh, well," and gently return to the repetition.

- Step 7. Continue for 10 to 20 minutes. You may open your eyes to check the time, but do not use an alarm. When you finish, sit quietly for a minute or so, at first with your eyes closed but later with your eyes open. Then do not stand for 1 or 2 minutes.

- Step 8. Practice the technique once or twice a day.

Benson and colleagues have found that the relaxation response also can be elicited by physical repetition during exercise. They found that adding the relaxation response to running decreased the metabolic rate and stimulated a mild euphoria (jogger's high) within the first mile or two. The following are steps to elicit the relaxation response during walking or jogging (Benson, 1993, pp. 254-255):

- Step 1. Get into sufficiently good condition so that you can jog or walk without becoming excessively short of breath.

- Step 2. Do your usual warm-up exercises before you jog or walk.

- Step 3. As you exercise, keep your eyes fully open, but attend to your breathing. After you fall into a regular pattern of breathing, focus in particular on its in-and-out rhythm. As you breathe in, say to yourself, silently, "in," when you exhale, say "out." In effect, the words in and out become your mental devices or focus words, in the same way that you would use your personal focus words or phrases with other relaxation response methods. If this in/out rhythm is uncomfortable for you (you might feel that your breathing is too fast or too slow), you may focus on something else. For example, you can become aware of your feet hitting the ground, silently repeating, "One, two, one, two" or "left, right, left, right." Alternatively, focusing on a faith-oriented word or phrase during exercise may be helpful and perhaps make exercise more satisfying.

- Step 4. Remember to maintain a passive attitude, simply disregarding disruptive thoughts. When they occur, think to yourself, "Oh, well," and return to your repetitive focus word or phrase.

- Step 5. After you complete your exercise, return to your normal after-exercise routine.

The relaxation response comprises an assortment of physiological changes, including a decrease below resting levels in oxygen consumption, heart rate, breathing rate, and muscle tension, plus a decrease in blood pressure in some people, and a shift from normal waking brain wave patterns to a pattern in which slower brain waves predominate (Benson, 1993). The relaxation response was developed to help people recognize that "stressors have multiple meanings, not all necessarily negative, and that one can work, through increased awareness, to get away from the victim role and from self-destructive cognitive and behavior patterns" (Horowitz, 1999, p. 15).

The relaxation response can be very useful in enhancing health, to the extent that any disorder is caused or made worse by stress. However, Canter (2003, p. 1049) asserts that a review of the literature indicates "current evidence for the therapeutic effectiveness of any type of meditation is weak."

"The nonjudgmental mindset required of the relaxation response attained via meditation facilitates the realization that one's identity entails more than pain. Mastery attained through the voluntary self-regulation of meditation (focused breathing, body scans, etc.) may help partly by increasing confidence in one's ability to have some control over symptoms or at least developing attitudes that render symptoms more bearable" (Horowitz, 1999, p. 14).

Benson (1993, p. 248) states that "at The New England Deaconness Hospital we have taught the relaxation response to people with muscle tension pains (which can include some headaches), infertility, insomnia, psychological problems, cardiac arrhythmia, premenstrual syndrome, and several common symptoms related to cancer and AIDS (anticipatory nausea and vomiting of chemotherapy). For these conditions, there is good evidence that the relaxation response can undo some or all of the damage caused by stress and have a significant clinical impact."

Outcomes of the relaxation response include:

- Slowed rate of breathing
- Slowed heart rate
- Relaxed muscles (muscle ache may be gone)
- Slight welling of tears in the eyes
- Sensation of warmth in hands and feet
- Feeling peaceful and calm but also more alert and less fatigued

The relaxation response can be elicited through a variety of techniques that share an emphasis on a repetitive mental focus and a passive attitude. Another such concentrative meditation technique is autogenic training.

Autogenic Training

Autogenic means self-generated. Developed in Germany by physician J. H. Schultz, autogenic training is a kind of self-hypnosis, a highly systematized series of attention-focusing exercises designed to generate deep relaxation and enhance one's recuperative and self-healing powers. (Olsen, 1990).

In autogenic training, there is a focus on "feelings of heaviness and cultivating a sense of warmth in the limbs, combined with a passive focus on breathing… [the] attitude toward the exercises should be one of passive concentration—not intense or compulsive, but rather of a 'let it happen' nature" (Benson, 1993, p. 242). Simple phrases are used to cue the body to elicit the relaxation response. The phrases should theoretically elicit specific physiological responses; for example the phrase, "My arms are heavy and warm," is meant to increase blood flow to the arms. Benson suggests that the client be instructed to get comfortable and have someone slowly read the instructions in Box 15-1, or make a tape recording to use until the process has been memorized.

Box 15-1

Autogenic Training to Elicit the Relaxation Response

"Close your eyes and focus on the sensations of breathing. Imagine your breath rolling in and out like ocean waves. Think quietly to yourself, 'My breath is calm and effortless...calm and effortless....' Repeat the phrase to yourself as you imagine waves of relaxation flowing through your body—through your chest and shoulders, into your arms and back, and into your hips and legs. Feel a sense of tranquility moving through your entire body. Continue for several minutes....

"Now focus on your arms and hands. Think to yourself, 'My arms are heavy and warm. Warmth is flowing gently through my arms into my wrists, hands, and fingers. My arms and hands are heavy and warm.' Stay with these thoughts and the feelings in your arms and hands for several minutes....

"Now bring your focus to your legs for a few minutes. Imagine warmth and heaviness flowing from your arms down into your legs. Think to yourself: 'My legs are becoming heavy and warm. Warmth is flowing through my feet...down into my toes. My legs and feet are heavy and warm.'

"Now scan your body for any points of tension, and if you find some, let them go limp, your muscles relaxed. Notice how heavy, warm, and limp your body has become. Think to yourself: 'All my muscles are letting go. I'm getting more and more relaxed.'

"Finally, take a deep breath, feeling the air fill your lungs and down into your abdomen. As you breathe out, think, 'I am calm.... I am calm....' Do this for a few moments, feeling the peacefulness throughout your body.

"Then, as your practice session ends, count to three, taking a deep breath, and exhaling with each number. Open your eyes and get up slowly. Stretch before going back to everyday activities" (Benson, 1993, p. 244).

Source: Benson, H. (1993) The relaxation response. In D. Goleman & J. Gurin (Eds.), *Mind-body medicine: How to use your mind for better health*. Yonkers, NY: Consumer Reports. Used with permission of the author.

There are six basic meditative exercises that can be used to increase resistance to stressors, reduce or eliminate sleep disorders, and modify pain reactions (Clark, 1996). It may take up to 10 months to master the six exercises. The exercises focus on:

■ Relaxing the neuromuscular system

■ Relaxing the vascular system

■ Regulating and adjusting the heart rate

■ The breathing mechanism

- Creating warmth in the abdomen
- Cooling the forehead

After mastery of the first set of exercises has been achieved, several advanced exercises can be studied (Olsen, 1990). These include:

- *Autogenic meditation.* A series of structured meditations designed to help reach more deeply into the unconscious mind.
- *Autogenic modification.* Directed toward a specific organ or body part to promote functional changes in order to overcome chronic conditions.
- *Autogenic neutralization.* Uncovers particularly introspective psychophysical blockages using stream-of-consciousness verbalization to trigger more powerful or intense releases.

In addition to the relaxation response, with or without autogenic training, another concentrative meditation technique that is widely used is Transcendental Meditation.

Transcendental Meditation

There are two basic components to Transcendental Meditation (TM). First, the silent repetition of a sound, called a mantra, to minimize distracting thoughts, and second, the passive disregard of thoughts that do intrude, followed by a return to the repetition (Benson, 1993). TM is simple. To prevent distracting thoughts a client is given a mantra (a word or sound) to repeat silently over and over again while sitting in a comfortable position. The mantra is selected not for its meaning but strictly for its sound. Clients are instructed to be passive and, if thoughts other than the mantra come to mind, to notice them and return to the mantra. A TM client is asked to practice for 20 minutes in the morning and again in the evening (Berman & Larson, 1994). Transcendental Meditation is "not a philosophy and does not require specific beliefs or changes in behavior or lifestyle" (Kreitzer, 1998, p. 127).

Mindfulness Meditation

In comparison with concentrative meditation, mindfulness meditation is a type of receptive meditation. With receptive meditation, instead of focusing on one sound or image, one clears the mind of all thoughts, "cultivating silence" (Gimbel, 1998).

Mindfulness meditation was developed at the Stress Reduction Clinic at the University of Massachusetts Medical Center in Worcester by Kabat-Zinn and colleagues. Based on the Buddhist practice of vipassana meditation, the goal of this meditative practice is to increase insight by becoming a detached observer of the stream of changing thoughts, feelings, drives, and visions until their nature and origin is recognized. The process includes eliciting the relaxation response, centering on breath, and then focusing attention freely from one perception to the next. In this form of meditation, no thought or sensation is considered an intrusion (Kreitzer, 1998).

Insight or mindfulness meditation means to see clearly (Pettinati, 2001). Much more than a technique, it is a practice and a discipline that affects the individual's way of being in the world, increasing self-awareness, patience, relaxation, and an ability to live more in the present moment (Zahourek, 1988). An expectant, nonstriving attitude of loving acceptance (passive volition) is desired (Kolkmeier, 1995). Without becoming emotionally involved, the individual remains present and aware of unpleasant and painful sensations when these are present, as opposed to ignoring or escaping from them (McDowell, 1995).

According to McDowall (1995), the critical aspects of the practice of mindfulness include:

1. Nonjudging (impartial) witness to your experience

2. Patience (some things must unfold in their own time)

3. Beginners mind (free of expectations from past experience)

4. Trust (in yourself and your feelings)

5. Nonstriving (no goal other than to be yourself)

6. Acceptance (a willingness to see things the way they are)

7. Letting go (refers both to pleasant and unpleasant experiences/thoughts)

Progressive Muscle Relaxation

The meditation approaches discussed thus far focus primarily on mental relaxation strategies, with secondary effects on body tension. In contrast, the technique of progressive muscle relaxation (PMR) can induce the relaxation response directly through its effect on muscle tension.

Developed by Jacobson, an American physiologist, PMR is defined as "the progressive tensing and relaxing of successive muscle groups" (Snyder, 1998, p. 1). Eventually, by discriminating between the feelings experienced when a muscle group is relaxed and when it is tensed, an individual can sense muscle tension without having to progress through the tensing and relaxing of specific muscle groups. To facilitate the PMR experience, the client should be encouraged to:

- Lie down on his or her back, with arms along the sides of the body, in a quiet room. "This technique can be done in any large chair that supports your head and neck, but is best done lying on your back on a firm but soft surface, such as a thick carpet or workout mat (a bed is too soft—you're more likely to glide off to sleep)" (Benson, 1993, p. 246).

- Make sure there will be no interruptions.

- Loosen any clothing that's uncomfortably tight, and take off shoes, and glasses or contact lenses

- Quiet music and reduced lighting may be helpful.

- Use the bathroom before sessions. Sessions, particularly initial ones, may last 45 to 60 minutes.

- Assume a passive attitude. "You are taught to recognize even the slightest muscle contractions so that you can release them and achieve a deep degree of muscular relaxation" (Benson, 1993, p. 242).

- The tightening and relaxing of the muscle groups should last about 5 to 7 seconds for each group. Check for relaxation before moving to the next muscle group.

- Either have someone read the instructions at a slow, easygoing pace, or make a tape for yourself.

- Practice sessions of at least 15 minutes once or twice each day should become part of your routine.

Benson (1993, pp. 246-7) describes a basic script for progressive muscle relaxation as presented in Box 15-2.

Box 15-2

A Basic Script for Progressive Muscle Relaxation

"First, tense the muscles throughout your body, from head to toe. Tighten your feet and legs, tense your arms and hands, clench your jaw, and contract your stomach. Hold the tension while you sense the feelings of strain and tightness. Study the tension and notice the difference between how the muscle feels when it is tensed and when it is relaxed. Then take a deep breath, hold it, and exhale long and slowly as you relax all your muscles, letting go of the tension. Notice the sense of relief as you relax.

"Now you're going to tense and relax individual groups of muscles, keeping the rest of your body as relaxed as you can. You'll hold the tension for a few seconds in each part of your body while you get a clear sense of what the tension feels like; then breath deeply, hold the breath for a moment, and let go of the tension as you exhale.

"Start by making your hands into tight fists. Feel the tension through your hands and arms. Relax and let go of the tension. Now press your arms down against the surface they're resting on. Feel the tension. Hold it . . . and let go. Let your arms and hands go limp.

"Shrug your shoulders tight, up toward your head, feeling the tension through your neck and shoulders. Hold . . . then release, letting go. Drop your shoulders down, free of tension.

"Now wrinkle your forehead, sensing the tightness. Hold . . . release, letting your forehead be smooth and relaxed. Shut your eyes as tight as you can. Hold . . . and let go. Now open your mouth as wide as you can. Hold it . . . and gently relax, letting your lips touch softly. Then clench your jaw, teeth tight together. Hold . . . and relax. Let the muscles of your face be soft and relaxed, at ease.

"Take a few moments to sense the relaxation throughout your arms and shoulders, up through your face. Now take a deep breath, filling your lungs down through your abdomen. Hold your breath while you feel the tension through your chest. Then exhale and let your chest relax, your breath natural and easy. Suck in your stomach, holding the muscles tight . . . and relax. Arch your back . . . hold . . . and ease your back down gently, letting it relax. Feel the relaxation spreading through your whole upper body.

"Now tense your hips and buttocks, pressing your legs and heels against the surface beneath you . . . hold . . . and relax. Curl your toes down, so they point away from your knees . . . hold . . . and let go of the tension, relaxing your legs and feet. Then bend your toes back up toward your knees . . . hold . . . and relax.

continued

Box 15-2 CONTINUED

"Now feel your whole body at rest, letting go of more tension with each breath...your face relaxed and soft...your arms and shoulders easy...stomach, chest, and back soft and relaxed...your legs and feet resting at ease...your whole body soft and relaxed.

"Take time to enjoy this state of relaxation for several minutes, feeling the deep calm and peace. When you're ready to get up, move slowly, first sitting, and then gradually standing up."

Source: Benson, H. (1993) The relaxation response. In D. Goleman & J. Gurin (Eds.), *Mind-body medicine: How to use your mind for better health.* Yonkers, NY: Consumer Reports. Used with permission of the author.

Although the procedure is very gentle, Snyder (1998) describes several cautions for PMR:

- May affect the pharmacokinetics of medications so that a lower dose is needed
- May produce a hypotensive state
- The client may have heightened awareness of pain in muscles

In an exploratory study, relaxation exercises (including progressive muscle relaxation, breathing exercises, guided imagery, and listening to soft music) lasting approximately 20 minutes were conducted with a group of 39 patients on a hospital general psychiatric unit. There was a significant reduction in anxiety. The author recommends future research with a larger, randomly selected sample and a control group (Weber, 1996).

Nineteen participants undergoing organ transplant experienced improvement from baseline symptom scores for depression and anxiety after a mindfulness meditation intervention. Global and health-related quality of life scores, however, were not improved (Gross, Kreitzer, Russas, Treesak, Frazier, & Hertz, 2004).

As discussed above, meditation techniques to promote relaxation can be very powerful. Another technique to promote relaxation is conscious, proper breathing.

Breathing

Achterberg and colleagues (1994) indicate that being conscious of one's breathing is a powerful way to achieve relaxation. In addition, "proper breathing improves circulation, normalizes muscle tone, and enhances clear thinking. These effects often result in a more positive mood" (Wang & Snyder, 1998, p. 16). Nineteen participants undergoing organ transplant experienced improvement from baseline symptom scores for depression and anxiety after a mindfulness meditation intervention. Global and heath-related quality of life scores however, were not improved (Gross, Kreitzer, Russas, Treesak, Frazier, and Hertz, 2004).

Or 5 consecutive weeks.

Jahnke (1997, pp. 86-98) describes a breathing technique that he calls the "essential breath." This technique uses abdominal breathing. Practice usually is needed before really satisfying and full breaths are experienced. Elements of the "essential breath" technique are presented in Box 15-3.

Box 15-3

Elements of the Essential Breath Technique

1. Essential breath:
   - Adjust posture so that the lungs, chest, and abdomen can expand freely (standing or sitting erect; lying down).
   - Breathe in through the nose, filling the lower portion of the lungs first (abdomen expands).
   - Allow the upper lobes of the lungs to fill (ribs and chest cavity expands to reach fullness) providing an enormous sense of satisfaction.
   - Rest for an instant.
   - Exhale slowly through the nose—rushing of warmth or flowing feeling throughout body.
   - Try 10 as you fall asleep and 10 before you rise.
   - Repeat.

2. Remembering breath
   - Done every time you can remember to do it.
   - Focus on a purposeful, positive thought.

3. Sigh of relief
   - Audible sigh expressing restfulness and trust (visualize peace and safety) or loud groan freeing accumulated frustration, anxiety, and other tensions (visualize traffic jams, the boss, too much work) on exhalation
   - Do several times.

4. Gathering breath
   - Sit down with the hands in the lap or stand with hands dangling at the sides.
   - Begin to inhale and move the hands outward and upward as if you are scooping something useful, even precious, from the air around you.
   - When the hands are slightly above and in front of you, inhalation should be complete.
   - Bring hands, side by side, palms facing you, toward your head.
   - Move the hands slowly down in front of your face, in front of your chest, in front of your abdomen while exhaling.
   - When the hands reach the navel area, linger for a moment.
   - Repeat.

Proper breathing is a powerful relaxation technique, even when used alone. Breathing (pranayama) also is an essential part of other relaxation techniques such as yoga.

YOGA

Hindu texts define yoga as a means of deliverance from suffering, pain, and sorrow "by mastering that which disturbs one's peace and harmony on the path to perfect union with God or the universal spirit" (Olsen, 1990, p. 312). The meaning of the word yoga is "union," the integration of physical, mental, and spiritual energies that enhance health and well-being (Berman & Larson, 1994).

"Classical yoga is organized into eight 'limbs' [paths] that provide a complete system of physical, mental, and spiritual health. The eight limbs of yoga are systematically arranged to outline specific lifestyle, hygiene, and detoxification regimens, as well as physical and psychological practices that can lead to a more integrated personal development. Ultimately, yoga helps prepare one for heightened vitality and spiritual awareness" (Berman & Larson, 1994, p. 469). The paths include *ethical* (yamas and hiyamas), *physical* (pranayamas and asanas), *mental* (dharma), *supramental* (dyyama), and *god-consciousness* (samadhi). Some of the most common yoga practices or branches are:

- *Bhakti.* For those seeking the pathway to God through devotion and love.

- *Jnana.* The yoga of knowledge has as its goal to attain prajna, or transcendental wisdom through meditation and thought; this is the yoga of the intellect.

- *Karma.* A yoga of service in action, emphasizing doing for others as a remembrance of God, and surrendering the rewards to God.

- *Raja.* Its object is to realize directly the absolute self by stilling the mind through concentrated meditative effort (via asanas and pranayama breathing exercises) so the light of the internal spirit can shine through.

- *Mantra* or *Nada.* Focuses on vibrations and radiations of life energy using sound.

- *Kundalini.* Awakens the primal force through contemplation and/or tantra, a sexual way to raise kundalini.

- *Hatha.* Seeks integration of different aspects of self to attain a relaxed health and harmony of mind and body. Identified with the sun (ha) and moon (tha), it is sometimes called the gentle yoga. Breathing routines and asanas focus on mastery over the body and the chakras, or energy centers, in the body (Olsen, 1990, pp. 315-316).

For the most part, the West has adopted three aspects of entirely different yoga practices: the breathing techniques of pranayoga, meditation, and the postures (or asanas) of hatha yoga.

Pranayama, or yogic breathing, is an ancient practice of deep breathing techniques. Prana in Sanskrit means universal energy. Prana is brought into the body through the breath. Pranayama literally means regulation or control of prana, or life force through various deep breathing techniques. The connection of the breath and the mind is a basic principle of yoga.

Gimbel (1998, p. 251) describes a pranayama for balancing and stress reduction as follows: "Take in a few cleansing breaths, inhaling through the nose and exhaling through the mouth. Move into the three-part breath, breathing into your diaphragm, the middle lungs, and the upper lungs. Combine this breath with the yogic sound, which is created by dragging the air across the back of the throat, with a 'saaa' sound on the inhalation and 'haa' sound on the exhalation. Take several complete breaths, inviting the exhalation to be a real letting go, letting go of any physical or mental tension, and each inhalation bringing you deeper into the present moment. Invite your mind to become totally absorbed in the breath. Invite any extraneous thoughts that may come into your awareness to float by without attachment as if they were flowing downstream in a bubbling brook."

To begin pranayama:

■ Take a billows breath, blowing out through the mouth, totally emptying the lungs to start from a place of freshness.

■ Inhale through the nose, using your yogic sound to a count of four.

■ Hold the breath without holding tension in the body to a count of eight.

■ Exhale through the nose using your yogic sound, to a count of eight.

■ Repeat the cycle, continuing your pranayama for at least 7 minutes.

Pranayama is often performed as a preparation for meditation. The final stage of yoga is samadhi, or spiritual realization, the culmination of a long, disciplined and dedicated practice. In samadhi, one is said to enter a fourth state of consciousness, separate from and beyond the ordinary states of waking, dream, and sleep (Berman & Larson, 1994).

Among the approaches to yoga are hatha (self-transformation primarily through physical disciplines), raja (primarily mental discipline), jnana (emphasis on discriminative knowledge by which the real is distinguished from the unreal or illusionary), karma (self-transcending action in the world in the form of selfless service), bhakti (love and devotion focusing on the higher reality conceived as a divine personality), and tantra (nondualist approach that seeks to utilize all human experience and convert it into a trigger for self-transcendence; there is a particular acknowledgment of the hidden transformative potential of sexuality) (Criswell & Patel, 2003).

For many people, asana (which means ease in Sanskrit), the yogic postures known as Hatha yoga, are the element most commonly associated with yoga. Asana "includes a variety of physical postures and exercises that create immediate changes in the body.... Meditative asanas (corpse, child's posture, posterior stretch) bring the spine and head into perfect alignment, promoting proper blood flow throughout the body and bringing the mind into a state of relaxation and stillness that facilitates increased concentration during meditation. At the same time, these asanas keep the glands, lungs, and heart properly energized. Therapeutic asanas (cobra, locust, spinal twist, and shoulder stand) are geared toward improving health and physical well-being, and have been commonly prescribed for clients with back, neck, and joint pain.... Although yoga postures may involve very little movement, the mind is involved in the performance of every asana, to provide discipline, awareness, and a relaxed openness. The discipline and awareness help maintain the posture, and the relaxation and openness help stimulate the circulation of prana (life energy).... According to the Yoga

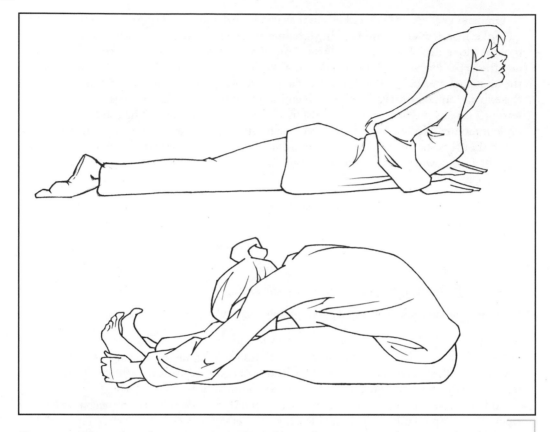

Figure 15-1. Examples of yoga exercises: The cobra and posterior stretch (reprinted with permission from Burton Goldberg Group. (1995). *Alternative medicine: The definitive guide.* Fife, WA: Future Medicine).

Sutras, a properly executed asana creates a balance between movement and stillness—exertion and surrender—the precise state of a healthy body" (Berman & Larson, 1994). Figure 15-1 shows the correct posture for the posterior stretch and the cobra positions.

However, the yoga poses, if done incorrectly, for too long, or too strenuously, can cause physical damage, particularly to the back. Aerobic yoga requires all the cautions of doing aerobics, including a complete cardiovascular and structural evaluation to determine whether, how hard, and how long to exercise; stretching before and after the workout; and including warm-up, cool-down, and relaxation periods in the routine (Olsen, 1990).

A typical yoga session as practiced in the United States lasts 20 minutes to an hour. Some people practice daily at home, while others practice one to three times a week in a class. A session usually begins with gentle postures to relax tension in the muscles and joints, then moves to more difficult postures. Every movement should be made gently and slowly, and clients are urged not to stretch beyond what is comfortable for them. Rather, practice should be "easeful." Emphasis is placed on breathing slowly from deep in the abdomen. Specific pranayama breathing exercises also are an important part of the practice. Guided (or self-guided) relaxation, meditation, and sometimes visualization follow the asanas. The session frequently ends with chanting, such as a repeating Om shanti ("Let there be peace"), to bring the body and mind into a deeper state of relaxation (Berman & Larson, 1994).

Kuhn (1999) describes several contraindications of yoga:

- *Sciatica.* Do not do forward bends or intense stretching.

- *Menstruation.* Do not do inverted poses.

- *Hypertension.* Do not do breath retentions or inverted poses.

- *Glaucoma* or *ear congestion.* Do not do breath retentions or inverted poses.

- *Pregnancy.* Do not do breath retentions, inverted poses, or breath suspensions.

Box 15-4 presents a yoga study abstract.

Box 15-4

Yoga Study

Twenty-eight volunteers with mild depression were randomly assigned to either a yoga course or a wait-list control group. The yoga group attended a 1-hour Iyenger yoga class each week. The yoga group demonstrated significant decreases in self-reported symptoms of depression and trait anxiety. Changes were also observed in acute mood, with subjects reporting decreased levels of negative mood and fatigue following yoga classes. Finally, there was a trend for higher morning cortisol levels in the yoga group.

Source: Adapted from Woolery, Meyers, Sternlieb, & Zeltzer, 2004.

Yoga can be self-taught through books or tapes, or by a yoga teacher. There is no national certification.

BIOFEEDBACK

Biofeedback, meaning "life-feedback," refers to any technique that uses noninvasive, simple, electronic devices to give a person immediate and continuing signals of changes in a body function of which the person is usually not conscious. The instruments measure, amplify, and display involuntary physiological processes in order to provide information, but nothing is done to people. The machine and the training itself do not stimulate the brain or change muscle activity. "Using the machine is like stepping on the bathroom scale or looking in a mirror. It tells you how you are doing" (Olsen, 1990, p. 112).

Biofeedback works by way of operant conditioning. It is believed that a new association between a stimulus and a response is developed. The response is instrumental in producing a reward or removing a negative stimulus. Reinforcement then shapes subsequent behavior and function.

There are several different types of biofeedback instrumentation, including:

- Electromyographic (EMG) biofeedback. A modality for measuring and displaying muscle activity, used primarily where any modification of muscular behavior is indicated.

- Skin resistance/conductivity monitors such as galvanic skin response (GSR). GSR registers general levels of autonomic arousal. Activity increases during "tension" and reduces during relaxation.

- Skin temperature monitors. Register skin temperature changes related to vasodilation/vasoconstriction, an indication of the stress response in some people.

- Electroencephalographic (EEG) monitors. Register brain wave activity, enabling trainees to generate wave forms such as alpha waves, associated with a relaxed state.

- Heart and pulse rate or rhythm monitors.

In addition to instrumentation for feedback purposes, treatment techniques often include guided imagery training or progressive muscle relaxation, which are forms of autogenic relaxation techniques. Deep breathing techniques have been shown to effectively regulate mental states and are often employed in combination with biofeedback techniques to enhance a state of relaxation. Among the best tools to assist a client in decreasing muscle tension are deep breathing techniques focusing in on the abdominal region, music, relaxation tapes, and progressive relaxation exercises (Bottomley, 1997).

Clinical training sessions generally last 15 to 40 minutes, several times per week, for a few weeks to a few months (Bray, 1998). The technique, which includes several stages, is presented in Box 15-5.

Box 15-5

Biofeedback Training Technique

1. Contact:
   - The explanation of biofeedback should clarify that it involves the learning of a skill, is not an instant answer, and will take time and practice. The key factors for success are high motivation and compliance.
   - A baseline of assessment data should be established.

continued

Box 15-5 continued

2. Initial sessions:

- Involve familiarization with the instrument. An autonomic body response is measured using instrumentation. The signals are interpreted, and the client is guided through the techniques that are designed to achieve the desired response. When ready, a stressor should be added so that the client can learn how to return the pattern to normal.

3. Follow-up sessions:

- Emphasize practice. Keep practice simple, meaningful and interesting. The client should learn to recognize the desired pattern during the practice sessions.
- Help to motivate.

4. Completion of training:

- Can the client self-regulate without the instrumentation and integrate the process into everyday life?"

Source: Bray, D. (1998). Biofeedback. *Complementary Therapies in Nursing and Midwifery, 4,* 23. Used with the permission from Harcourt Publishers.

The benefits or strengths of biofeedback include:

- Teaching a person how to change and control his or her body's vital functions.
- Allowing people to take responsibility for controlling their own health. "The method enables people to take an active part in their own recovery. It fosters self-reliance, independence, and responsibility for improvement in health" (Bray, 1998, p. 24).
- Strengthening the immune system by relaxing the stress response.

However, there are several cautions to biofeedback, including (Steefel, 1995):

- Severe psychopathology (acute psychosis, major affective disorder, history of disassociation experience, and borderline personality disorders).
- Need for clinician coordination when the client is taking insulin, thyroid replacement or seizure medications, or anti-hypertensives.
- Unexpected sensations, images, experiences, emotional feelings, and thoughts sometimes occur during biofeedback training.

GUIDED IMAGERY

Guided imagery is defined as "the process of purposeful use of mental images by working with another person… to achieve a desired therapeutic goal" (Bazzo & Moeller, 1999, p. 319).

Guided imagery involves the "deliberate formation of a mental representation while in a deeply relaxed state" (Giedt, 1997, p. 115). The client is led with specific words, symbols, and ideas to elicit a mental image. Additionally, devices such as commercial audiotapes of verbal suggestions, music or sounds of nature, pictures of objects or places, aromas from scented oils or candles, or another person giving suggestions in a soft, pleasant voice to assist in relaxation and image formation may be used to facilitate relaxation.

There are different forms of imagery. In active imagery there is a conscious and deliberate effort to construct concrete and symbolic images. These may be general healing images such as events, persons, or things; light, warmth, or heat; or a wise entity or inner guide. This approach may be most helpful when used to address symptoms. In contrast, in receptive imagery, images are allowed to "bubble up" into the conscious mind without conscious creation. This approach may be helpful to understand the emotional meanings of symptoms. Additionally, there are different imagery processes. In process imagery the imagery moves "step by step toward the goal one wishes to achieve... Mechanics or action must follow a pattern consonant with physical reality" (Achtenberg et al., 1994, p. 41). In contrast, in end state imagery, the client imagines the final, healed state. However, at present, research has not advanced sufficiently to determine absolutely what kind of imagery works best with which kind of client, symptom, or with which diagnostic category (Zahourek, 1988).

Achtenberg and colleagues (1994, p. 50) describe a general format for an imagery session as follows:

1. Identify the problem, disease, or goal of imagery.

2. Begin with several minutes of relaxing, meditating, or attention on breath.

3. Develop images of the problem or disease, inner healing resources, external (or treatment) healing resources.

4. End with images of the desired state of well-being.

"Images are thoughts that draw on the senses; they may involve one, several, or all of the following senses: sound, taste, movement (kinesthesis), vision, touch, and inner sensation, or the 'felt sense'" (Achterberg et al., 1994, p. 38). It is important to remember that mental imagery is not just the creation of a picture but is integrated thoroughly with the individual's entire physiological pattern. "The imagination may be the hypothetical bridge between conscious processing of information and physiologic change" (Hoekstra, 1994, p. 9).

A number of examples of therapeutic images can be found in the literature. To induce relaxation, some examples include "a beach at dawn, hearing the waves, feeling the warm sand beneath the body, smelling the salty sea breeze, seeing the colors of the horizon change from purple to red to golden as the sun emerges from the water" (Gimbel, 1998, p. 245), a lush green meadow, blue sky, puffy clouds, fresh and crisp mountain air, singing birds, grass that feels like a pillow, and a babbling brook. For healing, images might include good monsters eating bad ones, or an immune system actively attacking and destroying cancer cells; while for ego building an internal rose developing from a tightly closed bud to a beautiful glorious flower might be an effective image.

Characteristics that lend imagery great value for healing are (Burton Goldberg Group, 1995):

- Imagery directly affects physiology. Individuals can use imagery to control sympathetic nervous system stress responses.

- Through the mental processes of association and synthesis, imagery provides insight and perspective into health. Individuals can use imagery to understand and control their patterns of thinking.

- Relaxation makes the mind more receptive to new information.

- Imagery has an intimate relationship with emotions, which are often at the root of many common health conditions.

- Imagery can help to find meaning in events and situations.

As a result of these characteristics, the purposes or applications of imagery may include any of the following (Achtenberg et al., 1994; Zahourek, 1988):

- To tune in or become sensitive to (or "diagnose") what is going on inside the body.

- To send new or healing messages to the body which may promote healing, without raising unrealistic expectations for disease "cure."

- To complement or enhance other therapies.

- To alter physiological responses, such as blood flow.

- To change behaviors or attitudes.

- As mental preparation for treatment procedures.

- Promote relaxation.

- To reduce fear, anxiety, and pain.

- For habit control.

- For problem solving or goal development, ego building (strong, capable, and motivated), or to explore inner processes (improve problem-solving, develop insight).

- For behavior rehearsal (phobias).

- To facilitate peaceful dying (death imagery).

In contrast to some other modalities, there have been a number of studies of guided imagery. There is extensive evidence that there is a relationship between imagery of bodily change and actual bodily change, although studies are still needed to document whether imagery has an ultimate impact on health or on the course of disease. Thirty-three adults with symptomatic asthma received individual imagery instruction (week 1) and follow-up (weeks 4, 9, and 15). Participants were given 7 imagery exercises to select from and practiced 3 times a day for a total of 15 minutes. Eight of 17 (47%) participants in the imagery group reduced or discontinued their medications. Three of 16 (19%) in the control group reduced their medications as well. It was concluded that the efficacy of imagery needs further exploration (Epstein et al., 2004). In one review of 46 studies published between 1966 and 1998, it was concluded that "there is preliminary evidence for the effectiveness of guided imagery in the management of stress, anxiety, and depression, and for the reduction of blood pressure, pain, and the side effects of chemotherapy.... [However], there is a need for systematic, well-designed studies" (Eller, 1999, p. 57). Clinical reports suggest that the technique may help treat a wide range of conditions including:

- Chronic pain
- Allergies
- High blood pressure
- Irregular heartbeats
- Autoimmune diseases
- Cold and flu symptoms
- Stress-related gastrointestinal, reproductive, and urinary complaints.
- "Speed healing after an injury" (Rossman, 1993, pp. 297-298).
- Stimulating immune function by increasing numbers of natural killer cells.

Box 15-6 presents a guided imagery study abstract.

Box 15-6

Guided Imagery Study

In this pilot study, guided imagery instructional tapes were listened to in the morning and in the evening every day perioperatively for coronary artery bypass graft surgery and for 7 days postoperatively by 50 subjects in the intervention group. 50 subjects in the control group listened to music-only tapes at the same times. Findings demonstrated clinically relevant improvement with reduced pain, fatigue, anxiety, narcotic use, length of stay (LOS), and increased patient satisfaction in the intervention group.

Source: Adapted from Deisch, P., Soukup, M., Adams, P., & Wild, M. C. (2000). Guided imagery: Replication study using coronary artery bypass graft patients. *Nursing Clinics of North America, 35*(2), 417-425.

A specific type of guided imagery is interactive guided imagery, in which "the guide facilitates the process for the client, and the client describes and shares images rather than having the guide present images to work with" (Shames, 1996, p. 72).

Interactive Guided Imagery

The term *interactive guided imagery* was coined by the Academy for Guided Imagery in Mill Valley, CA. "The individual creates his or her own experience and images while the facilitator, or guide, assists the individual in dialoguing with the images to gain insight into a particular health problem or emotional issue" (Gimbel, 1998, p. 245). It is assumed that an effective imagery intervention is one that is specific to the client's personality, to their preferences for relaxation and specific settings, and to the desired outcomes. Imagery is learned more rapidly with guidance and is perfected with practice. Independent of the method of intervention, the nurse should assist with the interpretation or processing of the images and emotional responses. In addition, practicing imagery oneself is extremely helpful in guiding others (Post-White, 1998).

An example of interactive guided imagery is the inner advisor technique. An inner advisor is a representation of the inner knowledge and innate wisdom we all possess, but to which we may not have conscious access. In a relaxed state, the individual invites an image of a wise, caring figure to come into their mind. The image can be anything, plant, animal, or rock, as long as it "feels" supportive, caring, and wise. The facilitator, or guide, then assists the individual in dialoguing with the image about a particular health concern or other issue. This technique can be extremely useful in helping individuals to gain a better understanding of their issues and to bring about resolution (Gimbel, 1998).

The modern use of therapeutic imagery usually entails a 20- to 25-minute session that begins with a relaxation exercise to help focus attention and "center" the mind. During a typical session of imagery, the client focuses on a predetermined image designed to help to control a particular symptom (active imagery) or the client allows his or her mind to provide images that give insight into a particular problem (receptive imagery). It is helpful to use as many senses as possible during guided imagery sessions (Rossman, 1993). Dossey (1997) stresses that the sessions need to be pleasant, and that the guide should not interpret for the client. The person in actual control of the imagery is the client (Sodergren, 1985). However, Sodergren (1985, p. 122) cautions that "the nurse with little knowledge of psychotherapy should use caution in helping patients interpret symbolic material."

Post-White (1998) presents a technique for general guided interactive imagery. The first step is to help the client to achieve a relaxed state by:

- Finding a comfortable sitting or reclining position, but not lying down.

- Uncrossing the extremities.

- Closing the eyes or focusing on one spot or object in the room.

- Focusing on breathing with abdominal muscles; with each breath saying to themselves "in" and "out."

- Feeling the body becoming heavy and warm from the top of the head to the tips of the fingers and toes.

- If thoughts roam, bringing the mind back to thinking of one's breathing and relaxed body.

Specific suggestions for the imagery session (Post-White, 1998, p. 109) include:

1. In your mind, go to a place you enjoy and feel good.

2. What do you see, hear, taste, smell, and feel?

3. Take a few deep breaths and enjoy being there.

4. Now imagine yourself the way you want to be (describe the desired goal specifically).

5. Imagine what steps you will need to take to be the way you want to be.

6. Practice these steps now—in this place where you feel good.

7. What is the first thing you are doing to help you be the way you want to be?

8. What will you do next?

9. When you reach your goal of the way you want to be, feel yourself, touch yourself, embrace yourself, listen to the sounds surrounding you"

After the actual imagery experience, Post-White (1998) suggests that the nurse summarize the process and reinforce practice. Examples of language might be:

1. Remember that you can return to this place, this feeling, this way of being...anytime you want.

2. You can feel this way again by focusing on your breathing, relaxing, and imagining yourself in your special place.

3. Come back to this place and envision yourself the way you want to be every day.

Finally, the client should be helped to return to the present. Examples of language might be:

1. When you are ready you may return to the room we are in.

2. You will feel relaxed and refreshed and be ready to resume your activities.

3. You may open your eyes and tell me about your experience when you are ready

In Table 15-1, Dossey and colleagues (1995, pp. 619-622) suggest a number of words and phrases to empower interactive guided imagery.

Table 15-1

Words to Empower Guided Imagery

WORDS	DEFINITION
Metaphors	Implied comparisons (relaxation as a "warm waterfall").
Truisms	Statements that the intellectual mind accepts as accurate or as true ("as you take your next breath, oxygen is flowing into your lungs and into every cell in your body").

continued

Table
15-1

Words to Empower Guided Imagery (continued)

Embedded commands	Short phrases that stand out in a sentence because of changes in quality of voice, pitch, and tone ("you can relax more deeply...if you want to").
Linkage	Diversion of intellectual thoughts by connecting certain statements, behaviors, and actions with thoughts ("once more...relax more deeply...and really sink into the surface of the chair...feeling yourself being supported by this surface").
Therapeutic double-bind	Relaxation through involvement in the intellectual process of making different choices ("as you are stretched out in the chair...you might be able to relax more deeply by changing the position of your arms...or your head...or your feet").
Synesthesia	Cross-sensing, combination of several senses simultaneously ("can you hear the color of the wind").
Reframing	Ability to contact the part of a behavior/s that may be preventing or prohibiting healthier behaviors or thoughts ("I dread the pain" to "I am opening and softening around the discomfort and it is floating away").
Mirroring	Repetition of the client's words or descriptions rather than using your own.

Source: Dossey, B. M., Keegan, L., Guzzetta, C. E., & Kolkmeier, L. G. (Eds.). (1995). *Holistic nursing: Handbook for practice* (2nd ed.). Sudbury, MA: Jones and Bartlett.

The emphasis in this chapter has been on noninvasive modalities, including different forms of meditation, breathing, yoga, biofeedback, and guided imagery, that are designed to reduce chronic stress responses through relaxation. Biofeedback and yoga should be supervised by an experienced health professional who has been certified for practice. In contrast, meditation, breathing, and guided imagery practices require no special training or certification. These techniques also can be easily taught to clients for their own self-care to promote health and well-being.

Chapter Key Points

- The internal adaptive response of the body to a change perceived as a threat is known as stress. It is one's reaction to stressful experiences that can create a stress response.

- The parasympathetic nervous system induces relaxation and helps to compensate for periods of high arousal.

- The goals of stress management are to help persons deal with short-lived stressful events and to defuse the effects of chronic stress.

- All of the techniques described in this chapter are designed to induce a positive parasympathetic state and reduce stress responses through relaxation.

References

Achterberg, J., Dossey, B., & Kolkmeier, L. (1994). *Rituals of healing: Using imagery for health and wellness.* New York: Bantam.

Bazzo, D. J., & Moeller, R. A. (1999). Imagine this! Infinite uses of guided imagery in women's health. *Journal of Holistic Nursing, 17,* 317-330.

Benson, H. (1993). The relaxation response. In D. Goleman & J. Gurin, (Eds.), *Mind body medicine. How to use your mind for better health* (pp. 233-257). Yonkers, NY: Consumer Reports Books.

Berman, B. M., & Larson, D. B. (Eds.). (1994). *Alternative medicine: Expanding medical horizons.* Washington, DC: U.S. Government Printing Office.

Bottomley, J. M. (1997). Biofeedback: Connecting the body and mind. In C. M. Davis (Ed.), *Complementary therapies in rehabilitation* (pp. 101-123). Thorofare, NJ: SLACK Incorporated.

Bray, D. (1998). Biofeedback. *Complementary Therapies in Nursing & Midwifery, 4,* 22-24.

Burton Goldberg Group. (1995). *Alternative medicine: The definitive guide.* Fife, WA: Future Medicine.

Canter, P. H. (2003). The therapeutic effects of meditation. *British Medical Journal, 326,* 1049-1050.

Clark, C. C. (1996). *Wellness practitioner.* New York: Springer.

Criswell, E., & Parel, K. C. (2003). The yoga path: Awakening from the dream. In S. G. Mijaras. *Modern psychology and ancient wisdom: Psychological healing practices from the world's religious traditions* (pp. 201-225). New York: Haworth.

Deisch, P., Soukup, M., Adams, P., & Wild, M. C. (2000). Guided imagery: Replication study using coronary artery bypass graft patients. *Nursing Clinicsof North America, 35*(2), 417-425.

Dossey, B. M. (1997). Imagery. In B. M. Dossey (Ed.), *Core curriculum for holistic nursing.* Gaithersburg, MD: Aspen.

Dossey, B. M., Keegan, L., Guzzetta, C. E., & Kolkmeier, L. G. (Eds.). (1995). *Holistic nursing: Handbook for practice* (2nd ed.). Gaithersburg, MD: Aspen.

Eller, L. S. (1999). Guided imagery interventions for symptom management. In J. J. Fitzpatrick (Ed.), *Annual review of nursing research.* New York: Springer.

Epstein, G. N., Italper, J. P., Barrett, E. A. M., Birdsall, C., McGee, M., Baron, K. P., & Lowenstein, S. (2004). A pilot study of mind-body changes in adults with asthma who practice mental imagery. *Alternative Therapies in Health and Medicine, 10,* 66-71.

Fugh-Berman, A. (1997). *Alternative medicine—What works: A comprehensive, easy-to-read, review of the scientific literature, pro and con.* Baltimore, MD: Williams & Wilkins.

Garfinkel, M. S., Singhal, A., Katz, W. A., Allan, D. A., Reshetar, R., & Schumacher, H. R. (1998). Yoga-based intervention for carpal tunnel syndrome. *Journal of the American Medical Association, 280,* 1601-1603.

Giedt, J. F. (1997). Guided imagery. A psychoneuroimmunological intervention in holistic nursing practice. *Journal of Holistic Nursing, 15,* 112-127.

Gimbel, M. A. (1998). Yoga, meditation, and imagery: Clinical applications. *Nurse Practitioner Forum, 9,* 243-255.

Gross, C. R., Kreitzer, M. J., Russas, V., Treesak, C., Frazier, P. A., & Hertz, M.I. (2004). Mindfulness meditation to reduce symptoms after organ transplant: A pilot study. *Alternative Therapies in Health and Medicine, 10,* 58-66.

Hoekstra, L. S. (1994). Exploring the scientific bases of holistic nursing. *Nursing Connections, 7,* 5-14.

Horowitz, S. (1999). Aromatherapy: Modern applications of essential oils. *Alternative and Complementary Therapies, 5,* 199-203.

Jahnke, R. (1997). *The healer within: The four essential self-care methods for creating optimal health.* San Francisco: Harper Collins.

Kolkmeier, L. G. (1995). Relaxation: Opening the door to change. In B. M. Dossey, L. Keegan, C. E. Guzzetta, & L. G. Kolkmeier (Eds.), *Holistic nursing: Handbook for practice* (2nd ed.). Gaithersburg, MD: Aspen.

Kreitzer, M. J. (1998). Meditation. In M. Snyder (Ed.), *Independent nursing interventions* (pp. 123-137). New York: John Wiley & Sons.

Kuhn, M. A. (1999). *Complementary therapies for health care providers.* Philadelphia: Lippincott Williams & Wilkins.

Lowenstein, K. G. (2002). Meditation and self-regulatory techniques. In S. Shannon (Ed.), *The Handbook of complementary and alternative therapies in mental health* (pp. 159-178). San Deigo: Academic Press.

McDowell, B. (1995). Body-mind medicine: From the relaxation response to mindfulness. *Alternative and Complementary Therapies, 1*(2), 80-87.

Olsen, K. G. (1990). *The encyclopedia of alternative health care.* New York: Pocket Books.

Pelletier, K. R. (1993). Between mind and body: Stress, emotions, and health. In D. Goleman & J. Gurin (Eds.), *Mind body medicine. How to use your mind for better health* (pp. 19-38). Yonkers, NY: Consumer Reports Books.

Pettinati, P. M. (2001). Meditation, yoga, and guided imagery. *Nursing Clinics of North America, 16,* 47-56.

Post-White, J. (1998). Imagery. In M. Snyder, & R. Lindquist (Eds.), *Complementary/alternative therapies in nursing* (pp. 103-122). New York: Springer.

Rossman, M. (1993). Imagery: Learning to use the mind's eye. In D. Goleman, & J. Gurin (Eds.), *Mind/body medicine. How to use your mind for better health* (pp. 291-300). Yonkers, NY: Consumers Union.

Shames, K. H. (1996). *Creative imagery in nursing*. Albany, NY: Delmar.

Snyder, M. (1998). Progressive muscle relaxation. In M. Snyder & R. Lindquist (Eds.), *Complementary/alternative therapies in nursing* (pp. 1-13). New York: Springer.

Snyder, M., & Chlan, L. (1999). Music therapy. In J. J. Fitzpatrick (Ed.), *Annual review of nursing research*. New York: Springer.

Sodergren, K. M. (1985). Guided imagery. In M. Snyder (Eds.), *Independent nursing interventions* (pp. 103-124). New York: John Wiley & Sons.

Steefel, L. (1995). Establishing a biofeedback program in your clinical practice. *Alternative and Complementary Therapies, 1*, 103-108.

Walsh, R. (1996). Meditation promotes well-being. In S. Barbour & K. L. Swisher (Eds.), *Health and fitness: Opposing viewpoints* (pp. 114-119). San Diego, CA: Greenhaven.

Wang, J. J., & Snyder, M. (1998). Breathing. In M. Snyder & R. Lindquist (Eds.), *Complementary/alternative therapies in nursing* (pp. 15-21). New York: Springer.

Weber, S. (1996). The effects of relaxation exercises on anxiety levels in psychiatric inpatients. *Journal of Holistic Nursing, 14*, 196-205.

Woolery, A., Myers W., Sternlieb, B., & Zelter, L. (2004). A yoga intervention for young adults with elevated symptoms of depression. *Alternative Therapies in Health and Medicine, 10*, 60-63.

Wright, L. D. (2001). Meditation: Myths and misconceptions. *Alternative Therapies in Health and Medicine, 7*, 96-97.

Zahourek, R. P. (Ed.). (1988). *Relaxation and imagery: Communication and intervention*. Philadelphia: W. B. Saunders.

Additional Information

ASSOCIATIONS AND CREDENTIALING

Meditation

Center for Mindfulness in Medicine, Healthcare, and Society
University of Massachusetts Medical Center
Worchester, MA 01655
Tel: (508) 856-5849
www.mbst.com

Offers training and workshops for health professionals interested in teaching mindfulness-based stress reduction. There is no formal credentialing.

The Transcendental Meditation Program
Tel: (800) LEARN TM
www.tm.org
Formally recognizes TM instructors.

Biofeedback

Association for Applied Psychophysiology and Biofeedback
10200 West 33th Avenue #304
Wheat Ridge, CO 80033
Tel: (303) 422-8894

Biofeedback Certification Institute of America (BCIA)
Tel: (303) 420-2902

Many private biofeedback schools train and certify clinicians, but BCIA is the only certifying agency. Certification includes a rigorous examination and supervised training. They do
not monitor practitioners.

Guided Imagery

The Academy for Guided Imagery
PO Box 2070
Mill Valley, CA 94942
Tel: (800) 726-2070
www.interactiveimagery.com

Certification program is based on 150 hours of academy-approved training, including
direct observation and a written examination.

Relaxation

No formal credentialing of relaxation therapies is currently available.
For information:
American Holistic Nursing Association
PO Box 2130
Flagstaff, AZ 86003
Tel: (800) 278-AHNA
www.ahna.org

National Institute for the Clinical Application of Behavioral Medicine
Tel: (800) 743-2226
www.nicabm.org

Yoga

The American Yoga Association
513 S. Orange Avenue
Sarasota, FL 34236
Tel: (800) 226-5859

Himalayan Institute Teachers Association
RR1, Box 400
Honesdale, PA 18431
Tel: (717) 253-5551 ext 1305
www.himalayainstitute.org

Presently, each style of yoga or school offers a teacher training program with some form of certification. There is no national standard of teacher certification.

REGENERATING ENERGY
Nutrition

16

Abstract

Healthy nutritional and eating patterns are major factors influencing health. However, the promotion of healthy dietary habits has been problematic. Cultural meanings assigned to food, as well as multiple societal factors, influence eating habits and nutritional intake. Additionally, food habits are acquired early in life, and once established, are likely to be long-lasting and resistant to change. After a brief discussion of influences on the meaning of food, the chapter will summarize standard Western dietary guidelines and goals, and present a discussion of essential dietary nutrients, phytonutrients, antioxidants, nutritional medicine supplements, and selected diets, providing a scientific foundation for the development of nutritionally based health promotion interventions.

Learning Outcomes

By the end of this chapter the student will be able to:

- Appreciate that cultural, geographical, social, psychological, religious, economic, and political factors shape food intake

- Discuss meanings of food and appropriate dietary guidelines and goals to provide and conserve energy for health and well-being

- Describe therapeutic considerations of selected essential dietary nutrients, phytonutrients, antioxidants, and nutritional supplements

- Describe essential elements of the macrobiotic, Pritkin, Gerson, Ornish, Atkins, and Ayurvedic diets to prevent or treat various diseases

- Identify individual/family and environmental strategies that can promote healthy nutrition

The Meaning of Food

FOOD AND CULTURE

Food intake is shaped by a wide variety of geographical, social, psychological, religious, economic, and political factors. Food habits are maintained because they are practical or symbolically meaningful behaviors in a particular culture (Fieldhouse, 1995). Food habits are acquired early in life as part of learned culture and tend to be long-lasting and resistant to change. As a result, it is important to develop sound nutritional practices in childhood as a basis for life-long healthy eating (1995). In practice, however, malnutrition remains a significant problem for youth and adolescents worldwide, along with an increasing prevalence of obesity (Schneider, 2000) in all income groups. In developed countries, "social pressures to achieve a distorted body image are creating a malnutrition of affluence among some groups of adolescents" (2000, p. 963).

Food is one of the basic mediums through which adult attitudes and sentiments are communicated. Early eating experiences readily become associated with family sentiments of happiness and warmth or of anger and tension; it is not surprising then that foods may unlock childhood memories when they are encountered in later life. The socialization process teaches social, cultural, and psychological meanings and uses of food.

As children grow older, they are exposed to diverse experiences and viewpoints and to multiple influences. Socializing influences may complement or conflict with one another, but the habits learned earliest are most likely to persist in later life and to be most resistant to change. Thus, when there is a conflict, such as between what is taught at school and what is taught in the home, the latter is most likely to dominate. This reinforces the idea that the creation of early likes and dislikes consistent with healthy eating habits is a desirable nutrition strategy (Fieldhouse, 1995).

Cultural beliefs have the potential to influence most aspects of nutrition and diet intake, including:

- What substances are regarded as food and what are not

- How food is cultivated, harvested, prepared, and served

- The actual manner of eating the food

- Who prepares and serves the food, and to whom

- Which individuals eat together, where, and on what occasions

- The order of dishes within a meal

FOOD AND HUMAN NEEDS

Maslow (1970) proposed that human needs occur hierarchically. Box 16-1 demonstrates how nutrition fits within each stage of Maslow's hierarchy of human needs.

Box 16-1

Nutrition Within Stages of Maslow's Hierarchy of Human Needs

- *Survival.* Food is fundamental for individual survival.
- *Security.* Security needs can be met through storage and hoarding of food.
- *Love-belongingness.* Use of foods as rewards or gifts. "Traditionally, American women have expressed love of family through careful selection, preparation, and service of meals" (Fieldhouse, 1995, p. 23).
- *Self-esteem.* Pride in food preparation. However, advertising stresses success and reliability over individual innovation and experimentation. "As the expanding convenience food industry sought new markets, it offered women self-esteem in a can" (Fieldhouse, 1995, p. 23).
- *Self-actualization.* Expressed by the innovative use of foods, new recipes, and food experimentation. Food becomes a personal trademark—a source of personal satisfaction and achievement.

Source: Adapted from Fieldhouse, P. (1995). *Food and nutrition: Customs and culture* (2nd ed.). London: Chapman & Hall.

FOOD IDEOLOGY

Food ideology is the sum of the attitudes, beliefs, customs, and taboos affecting the diet of a given group. "It is the idea of what is food, as much as the food itself, which evokes both physiological and psychological feelings" (Fieldhouse, 1995, p. 31). Ideology includes symbolic meanings associated with food, such as religious connotations, rewards, prestige, or status. Advertising influences food ideology, in that advertising utilizes powerful symbolic meanings of foods, so that what is being sold is not just a product, but a lifestyle, a dream, and a source of emotional fulfillment (1995). "In the business of selling transformation," advertising perpetuates envy and a sense of dissatisfaction with one's body (Nichter & Nichter, 1991, p. 249). The message is that we are inadequate as we are, but that when beauty (as a commodity) has been purchased at a cost, we are told we are worth it! Advertising has a major impact on food intake.

FOOD CATEGORIZATIONS

With the possible exception of modern Western society, no cultural group evaluates the individual foods and combinations that it ingests in terms of the scientific categories of energy, fat, protein, vitamins, and minerals. Most commonly, foods are assigned values according to their functional role, as well as their perceived nutritional and non-nutritional effects (Fieldhouse, 1995). Fieldhouse (1995, p. 49) points out that "approaches to food classification by nutritional professionals have resulted in a diversity of food guides, which while claiming justification in scientific rationality nevertheless show themselves as cultural constructs with built-in biases." Some of the possible categories in worldwide food classifications (Fieldhouse, 1995; Helman, 1994) are presented in Table 16-1.

Table 16-1

Food Classification Groups

CLASSIFICATION	DESCRIPTION
Cultural superfoods	The dominant staple foods of a society. Much effort is expended in producing and preparing them and they are often involved in the religious rituals and the mythology of the society.
Prestige foods	Reserved for important occasions or for important people. They are characterized by relative scarcity and high price.
Body-image foods	Contribute to good health by maintaining balance in the body. Yin-yang (Chinese medicine beliefs) and hot-cold (allopathic beliefs) food are examples of systems which embody this idea. In Western culture, we hold the idea of fattening and slimming foods.
Sympathetic magic foods	Believed to have special properties that are imparted to those who eat them.
Physiological group foods	Foods restricted to persons of a particular age, sex, or physiological condition.
Core foods	Universal, regular, staple, important, and consistently used foods. Form the mainstay of the diet for most members of the society (e.g., milk, meat, vegetables, cereal).
Secondary foods	Widespread but not universal. Are of less emotional importance and include recently introduced and store-bought foods (e.g., cake mixes).

continued

Table 16-1	**Food Classification Groups (continued)**

CLASSIFICATION	DESCRIPTION
Peripheral foods	Least common and are infrequently consumed. May be new foods or only included through economic necessity (e.g., oysters, sweetbreads).
Food versus nonfood	Definitions of what is considered edible and what is not tend to be flexible, especially under conditions of famine, economic deprivation, and foreign travel. Virtually no human groups in the world define human flesh as food.
Sacred versus profane	"Profane" food is seen as unclean and dangerous to health; taboos forbid physical contact. "Junk" versus whole foods—additives are unclean and dangerous, while vegetarianism is whole and spiritual ("sacred").
Parallel	Health is balance
Food as medicine	Vitamins; food illnesses such as "high blood pressure."
Social foods	Symbolic family meal or religious feast. Expresses relationships and important occasions in the life of the group; can symbolize social status.

Essential Dietary Nutrients

Essential nutrients are those nutrients derived from food that the body is unable to manufacture on its own. These are absolutely necessary for human life and include eight amino acids, at least 13 vitamins, and at least 15 minerals, plus certain fatty acids, water, and carbohydrates:

- Amino acids are the building blocks of protein. The essential amino acids are L-lycine, L-isoleucine, L-leucine, L-valine, L-methionine, L-threonine, L-phenylalanine, and L-tryptophan.

- Essential vitamins are broken up in two groups: fat-soluble and water-soluble. The essential vitamins classified as fat-soluble include vitamins A, D, E, and K. The water-soluble essential vitamins are C (ascorbic acid), B_1 (thiamine), B_2 (riboflavin), B_3 (niacin), B_5 (pantothenic acid), B_6 (pyridoxine), B_{12}, folic acid, and biotin.

- The essential minerals include calcium, magnesium, phosphorus, iron, zinc, copper, manganese, iodine, chromium, potassium, sodium, and a number of trace elements.

- Essential fatty acids required for proper metabolism include linoleic and linolenic acid, found in seafood and unrefined vegetable oils, plus oleic and arachidonic acids, found in most organic fats and oils and peanuts.

- Accessory nutrients that help support metabolism include vitamin C-complex cofactors choline and inositol, as well as coenzyme Q10 (a close relative of the B-vitamins), and lipoic acid. Other accessory nutrients that have demonstrated preventative functions include B-complex cofactor PABA (para-aminobenzoic acid), and substance P or bioflavonoids that work with vitamin C (Burton Goldberg Group, 1995).

FOOD MYTHS

Clark (1996) describes several food myths that nurses should be aware may affect nutritional patterns of clients:

- *Meat contains more protein than other foods.* Actually, meat contains only about 25% protein and is in the middle of the protein quantity scale, ranking below soybeans, fish, milk, soybean flour, and eggs.

- *Large quantities of meat must be eaten to provide sufficient protein to grow and replace body tissues.* In fact, most Americans eat twice the amount of protein their bodies can use; the recommended daily allowance of protein, 50 to 60 grams, can be reached even when all meat, fish, and poultry are eliminated from the diet:

    1. Wheat and beans, milk and rice, milk and peanuts, or beans and rice are complete proteins (all amino acids).
    2. All soybean products (tofu, tempeh) are complete proteins.
    3. Fortifying cornmeal with the amino acid lysine also results in a complete protein.
    4. Vegetarians must fortify their diet with vitamin B_{12}.

- *Meat offers the highest quality protein available.* Actually, eggs and milk are more useable by the body than meat, and soybeans and unrefined rice are as useable.

- *There are "good" and "bad" forms of sugar.* Actually, sugar is sugar. Sugar occurs naturally in milk, fruits, and vegetables, so the sugar is being ingested with fiber, minerals, vitamins, and proteins.

- *Sugar is a good source of energy.* In fact, refined sugar leads to less energy because the food is digested quickly, and the blood glucose level rises, insulin is released, and liver stores of glycogen are used, resulting in fatigue, shakiness, irritability, faintness, and, in some people, violent behavior. Eating refined sugar results in highs and lows. For high energy, frequent, high-protein meals or complex carbohydrates such as grains or vegetables are recommended.

- *Starchy foods lead to weight gain.* Actually, complex carbohydrates such as whole grain pasta, baked potatoes, unrefined rice, and whole grain breads and cereals contain a great deal of fiber that is filling; it is only when butter, margarine, sour cream, or other fillings or toppings are used that calories accrue.

MINERALS AND VITAMINS

The term *nutritional supplementation* refers to the use of vitamins, minerals, and other food factors to support good health and prevent or treat illness. The key function of nutrients like vitamins and minerals in the human body is to serve as essential components in enzymes and coenzymes (Murray, 1996). Nutritional supplementation has become a major business in the United States. Many people believe that all that is needed to make up for a limited diet is to take a multivitamin pill. However, Murray (1996, p. 9) points out that "a person cannot make up for poor dietary habits, a negative attitude, and a lack of exercise by taking pills—whether the pills are drugs or nutritional supplements... For the long-term, it is absolutely essential that individuals devote attention to developing a positive mental attitude, a regular exercise program, and a healthful diet." Safe and toxic levels of vitamins and minerals are listed in Appendix B.

Iron

Iron functions in oxygen transportation from the lungs to body tissues and in carbon dioxide transportation from the tissues to the lungs. Iron also functions in several key enzymes in energy production and metabolism, including DNA synthesis. Iron deficiency may be caused by an increased iron requirement (e.g., pregnancy), decreased dietary intake, diminished iron absorption or utilization, blood loss, or a combination of factors. Some degree of iron deficiency occurs in 35% to 58% of young, healthy women (Murray, 1996).

Heme iron is in animal products and is the most efficiently absorbed form of iron. The absorption rate of heme iron is as high as 35%. Heme iron doesn't have the side effects (nausea, flatulence, and diarrhea) associated with nonheme sources of iron. Although the recommended dietary allowance (RDA) for iron is 10 mg for males and 15 mg for females, the recommended dose of (heme) iron supplement is 30 mg bound to either succinate or fumarate twice daily between meals. If the supplement causes abdominal discomfort, 30 mg can be taken with meals three times a day.

High intakes of other minerals, particularly calcium, magnesium, and zinc, can interfere with iron absorption (Murray, 1996). Iron is best absorbed when taken separately from pancreatic enzymes and should not be taken with vitamin E. Vitamin C taken with iron provides maximum absorption. To enhance absorption, iron supplements should be taken between meals with water or juice.

Zinc

Adequate zinc levels are essential to good health. Zinc is by far one of the most critical minerals for overall immune functioning. Zinc's ability to optimize the immune system works directly and indirectly. "Preventing zinc deficiency can help to ensure that the body manufactures adequate supplies of T cells and thymic hormones and maintains proper white-blood-cell functioning" (Meletis, 1999, p. 45). Zinc supplementation has also been found to improve progressive hearing loss and other related ear problems. When recovering from surgery, a person may need a higher level of zinc than usual.

The average American consumes about 10 mg of zinc per day. The dosage range for zinc supplementation for general health support is 15 to 20 mg. Zinc forms bound to picolinate, acetate, citrate, glycerate, or monomethionine are better absorbed and utilized than zinc sulfate (Murray, 1996). Zinc competes with copper for absorption, and other minerals (most notably calcium and iron) can adversely affect zinc absorption if supplemented at a high dosage. Zinc supplements should be taken apart from high-fiber foods for best absorption. Zinc does not appear to interact in a negative fashion with any drug (Murray, 1996). However, excess zinc intake interferes with the body's use of copper, another essential mineral (Kava, 1995).

Calcium and Magnesium

In addition to its major function in building and maintaining bone and teeth, calcium is important in much of the body's enzyme activity. The contraction of muscles, release of neurotransmitters, regulation of the heart beat, and the clotting of blood all depend on calcium (Murray, 1996). It has been suggested that an intake of 1,500 mg of calcium daily will inhibit age-related bone loss in postmenopausal women (Clark, 1996). This amount usually requires dietary supplementation in the range of 1,000 to 1,200 mg daily.

Calcium citrate and other soluble forms (lactate, aspartate, orotate) are the best supplements available for optimal absorption (Murray, 1996). Both achlorhydric and normal individuals efficiently absorb calcium citrate more than calcium carbonate (Gaby & Wright, 1988). However, a number of other substances can affect calcium blood levels, as, for example:

- A diet high in phosphorus, a mineral found in animal protein, can cause lowered calcium levels

- A diet high in soy protein maintains calcium levels

- A high level of caffeine consumption may increase the risk of calcium deficiency

- High dosages of magnesium, zinc, fiber, and oxalates negatively affect calcium absorption

- Caffeine, alcohol, phosphates, protein, sodium, and sugar increase calcium excretion

- Aluminum-containing antacids ultimately lead to an increase in bone breakdown and calcium excretion

Bone health depends not just on estrogen and calcium, but on a wide range of other nutrients, including vitamins B_6, C, D, K, folic acid, magnesium, manganese, boron, zinc, copper, strontium, and silicon (Gaby & Wright, 1988). When accelerated bone formation is desirable, as in osteoporosis or after a fracture, a greater amount of vitamin K is required. Vitamin D is required for intestinal calcium absorption, and manganese is required for bone mineralization. Zinc is essential for normal bone formation. This mineral also enhances the biochemical actions of vitamin D (Gaby & Wright, 1988).

Magnesium functions in the development, distribution, and function of immune cells and soluble factors that are critical for humoral and cell-mediated immunity. Alterations of potassium, calcium, phosphorus, and sodium metabolism are associated with magnesium deficiency (Kubena & McMurray, 1996). Alkaline phosphatase, an enzyme involved in forming new calcium crystals, is activated by magnesium. Many drugs adversely effect magnesium status, particularly many diuretics, insulin, and digitalis (Murray, 1996).

Excessive calcium prevents the absorption of magnesium. Because magnesium suppresses parathyroid hormone and stimulates calcitonin, it helps move calcium into bones. Dairy products contain nine times as much calcium as magnesium. A magnesium-rich diet contains whole grains like brown rice, millet, buckwheat (kasha), whole wheat, triticale, quinoa, and rye, as well as legumes, including lentils, split peas, and all varieties of beans (Fuchs, 1993).

Magnesium supplementation is as important as calcium supplementation in the treatment and prevention of osteoporosis. However, most Americans do not get the RDA for magnesium of 350 mg per day for adult males and 280 mg for adult females (Murray, 1996). Lactating women need additional magnesium and protein, and post-menopausal women require increased calcium and vitamin D to maintain strong bones.

Vitamin D

"Vitamin D is actually a hormone that is activated by the sunlight. Calciferol, the active form, is needed for the transport of calcium from the intestine into [cells]. Ergocalciferol (D2), which is equally potent, is derived from the diet and is most commonly used for food fortification and supplements" (Kroll, 1995, p. 172). Fat-soluble vitamin D has properties of both hormones and vitamins. It is needed for the absorption and metabolism of calcium and phosphorus from the small intestine for depositing in bones and teeth; for bone mineralization; for improving renal absorption of calcium; for preventing excessive urinary loss of calcium and phosphorus; and for maintaining serum calcium and phosphorus levels. In addition, vitamin D maintains and keeps nerves, skin, heart, and muscles healthy by regulating the level of calcium in the blood. It is also believed to aid in the regulation of normal blood sugar.

Vitamin D deficiency exacerbates osteoporosis and causes the metabolic bone disease osteomalacia. The effectiveness of supplemental vitamin D in treating osteoporosis and preventing bone loss and fractures is not clear (Kroll, 1995). Other conditions that may be prevented or treated by vitamin D are arthritis, acne, alcoholism, herpes simplex and herpes zoster, cystic fibrosis, and hearing loss (lack of vitamin D causes the cochlea to become porous). Hypothyroidism requires very large doses of vitamin D, 50,000 units per day or greater (Kroll, 1995).

Sufficient intake and/or absorption of vitamin D requires 10 to 20 minutes per day of exposure to sunlight and fat equal to at least 10% of total calories. Most milk (400 units per quart), infant feeding formulas, and cereals are fortified. Vitamin D is also present in such fatty foods as egg yolk, butter, milkfat, cheese, liver, beef, shrimp, fatty fish, and cod liver and halibut liver fish oils.

Older patients are more vulnerable because the skin gradually loses its ability to convert vitamin D to the active hormone that is necessary for dietary calcium to be incorporated into bone. The most vulnerable patient groups are the aged, children, and premature infants, dark skinned, and those who cover their skin much of the time. The drugs cholestyramine, Dilantin (Parke-Davis, NY, NY), phenobarbital, and mineral oil all interfere with the absorption and/or metabolism of vitamin D (Murray, 1996).

If the diet is not adequate, a daily multivitamin tablet that contains 200 to 400 units of vitamin D can be taken. The latest U.S. recommendations for vitamin D intake, based on amounts that have retarded the rate of bone loss, are 200 IU/day for men and women 19 to 50 years old, 400 IU for men and women 51 to 70 years old, and 600 IU for men and women more than 70 years old (Abramowicz, 1998). Toxic and adverse effects such as hypercalcemia can result from doses four to five times greater than the RDA. Vitamin D is not readily excreted and is stored in the liver, skin, brain, bones, and other tissues. However, the body self-regulates the development of the vitamin from sunlight, so an accumulation can only come from diet or supplements. An extensive listing of vitamin and mineral supplementation ranges can be found in Appendix B.

FAT

A fat or lipid describes compounds composed of carbon, hydrogen, and oxygen and that are not soluble in water. The three major classes of dietary fats are triglycerides, phospholipids, and sterols (like cholesterol). Approximately 95% of all ingested fats are triglycerides (Murray, 1996). A triglyceride is a saturated fat because the carbon molecules in the fatty acids are "saturated" with all the hydrogen molecules they can carry. If some of the hydrogen molecules were removed, what remains is an unsaturated fatty acid and thus an unsaturated fat. The American Heart Association recommends fewer than 10% of daily calories come from saturated fats and fewer than 10% come from polyunsaturated fats. Monounsaturated fats should make up the rest (Keegan, 1996). A description of categories and effects of fats can be found in Table 16-2.

After digestion of fat, free fatty acids and monoglycerides are absorbed into the body and, along with cholesterol, are transported by special protein-wrapped molecules known as lipoproteins. Cholesterol is a waxy substance made primarily in the liver and in the cells lining the small intestine. It is an essential constituent of cell membranes and nerve fibers, and is a building block of certain hormones. It is found in all body tissues, but the cholesterol that circulates in the blood creates the most concern. The National Cholesterol Education Program designates blood levels less than 200 mg/dL as desirable; levels between 200 and 240 mg/dl as borderline-high; and those over 240 mg/dL as indicative of a greater risk of heart disease. People with blood cholesterol over 265 mg/dL have two and a half times the risk of developing coronary heart disease (CHD) as those with 190 mg/dL or less. However, a low total cholesterol does not guarantee protection against heart disease (Sebastian, 1997). The American Heart Association recommends a reduction in dietary cholesterol to less than 300 mg per day for healthy American adults. For those with CHD, cholesterol intake is usually reduced to less than 200 mg per day.

The major categories of lipoproteins are very low-density lipoprotein (VLDL), low-density lipoprotein (LDL), and high-density lipoprotein (HDL). HDL cholesterol is considered "good" because it is thought to carry cholesterol away from the arteries and to the liver for elimination. HDL can be raised by eating foods containing monounsaturated fats (such as olive oil), and avoiding foods high in unhealthy saturated fat (such as palm or coconut oil), losing weight, exercising, and stopping smoking. LDL cholesterol is considered "bad," because after the cholesterol actually needed by the cells is delivered, any excess is deposited in arterial walls and other tissues. Elevations of either LDL or VLDL are associated with an increased risk for developing atherosclerosis, the primary cause of a heart attack or stroke, and elevations of HDL are associated with a lower risk of heart attacks.

Murray (1996) offers the following practical dietary advice about the consumption of fats:

■ Reduce the amount of saturated fat and total fat in your diet by eating less animal and more plant foods.

Table 16-2	*Categories and Effects of Fat*

CATEGORY	EFFECTS
Saturated fat	Mostly from animal products and lard. Tropical vegetable oils (palm kernel, palm, and coconut). Increase total blood cholesterol, especially LDLs.
Hydrogenated fats (transfatty acids)	Give liquid fat more consistency and stability against rancidity Transfatty acids (hydrogenated margarine) raise LDL cholesterol almost as much as saturated fats (butter) and also lower HDL cholesterol. No more healthy than comparable animal-based saturated fats (butter).
Polyunsaturated fat	When substituted for saturated fat, polyunsaturated fat produces a decline in LDL levels. Includes the omega-6 (vegetable oils such as corn, safflower, and soybean) and omega-3 (cold water fish such as salmon, mackerel, and tuna) fatty acids (Sebastian, 1997, p. 13). Corn, cottonseed, soybean, and safflower oils also contain linoleic acid that may enhance the growth of certain cancers.
Monounsaturated fats	Canola, olive, and high-olein safflower oils. The best oils for cooking and baking are liquid canola and olive vegetable oils. Reduce levels of LDLs while preserving the beneficial HDLs.
Essential fatty acids	Transformed into regulatory compounds known as prostaglandins, which are important in a host of bodily functions. However, according to Murray (1996), approximately 80% of the U. S. population consumes an insufficient quantity of essential fatty acids. The three primary factors contributing to the current essential fatty acid deficiency are: 1. Unavailability of high-quality oils rich in essential fatty acids because of mass commercialization and refinement of fats and oil products. 2. Transformation of healthful omega-3 and omega-6 oils into toxic compounds (hydrogenated and transisomers). 3. Metabolic competition of hydrogenated and transfatty acids with the essential fatty acids.

- Eliminate the intake of margarine and foods containing transfatty acids and partially hydrogenated oils.

- Take 1 or 2 tablespoons of flaxseed oil daily—the world's richest source of omega-3 fatty acids.

- Some dietary fat is necessary, but the total dietary fat intake should be limited to 20 to 30 percent of calories consumed.

FIBER

Since fiber, found mainly in fruits, vegetables, and grains, is not digested, it is not used as an energy source by the body. However, studies associate fiber with normal digestion, control of blood glucose, blood pressure, and cholesterol levels, and protection against cancer and heart disease. Unfortunately, average intake of fiber in the United States is less than half the amounts recommended. The average low-fiber, refined diet provides about 10 to 20 grams of fiber per day; while the suggested optimal amount ranges from 30 to 50 grams per day (Keegan, 1996).

Insoluable Fiber

- Includes cellulose, hemicellulose, and lignin.

- Found in wheat bran, whole grains, fruits, vegetables, and nuts.

- Decreases food transit time and increases the weight and softness of the stool.

- Needs large amounts of water to prevent cramping, flatulence, or constipation.

Soluble Fiber (Nonlaxative)

- Lowers the absorption of cholesterol, regulates blood sugar by slowing the absorption of sugar into the bloodstream, and absorbs and removes toxic materials and carcinogens from the body.

- Oat bran. Refrigerate or store in the freezer for no more than 2 months.

- Flax seeds. The outer walls of the seeds swell and absorb water to form a mucilage coating that provides bulk and lubrication.

- Guar gum (from legumes) and pectin (from apples). Form a jelly-like substance.

- Psyllium seeds. Swell rapidly by absorbing water, so preparations should be used immediately.

The best way to increase fiber in the diet is to eat whole grain foods that are high in complex carbohydrates. However, increasing fiber intake may cause flatulence and bloating, therefore any increase should be gradual in order to give the digestive system time to adjust. Just one serving of a high-fiber food should be added each week, and liquid should be increased to 8 to 10 glasses to account for the extra liquid that will be absorbed by the fiber. Large amounts of dietary fiber may result in impaired absorption and/or negative balance of some minerals and reduce the need for insulin and other medications. Fiber supplements may also inhibit the absorption of certain drugs, so the fiber supplement should be taken hours apart from any medication (Murray, 1996).

PHYTONUTRIENTS

Phytonutrients are biologically active substances in foods that have health-enhancing or possibly curative abilities. "'Non-nutritive' substances, such as fibers and phytochemicals, have been identified as bioactive agents or biological response modifiers (BMRs) from the plant world. These substances modulate key disease-related mechanisms, such as immune function, oxidative stress, homeostasis, inflammatory activity, and hormonal balances" (Block, 1999, p. 490).

Soy

Soy is comprised of plant estrogens (phytoestrogens) such as isoflavones. Genistein is an example of a prominent isoflavone. Estrogen links to both types of estrogen receptors, but alpha- and beta-phytoestrogens may link only to one or the other. When phytoestrogens link to either receptor, they may have the same effect as estrogen or they may act as antiestrogens, linking to the receptor, but failing to initiate the necessary reaction to activate a gene. Phytoestrogens are also weaker than animal estrogens. They are broken down in the body more readily and are not stored in fat. Thus, they are associated with fewer side effects (Harvard Women's Health Watch, 2000).

The role of isoflavones in breast and prostatic cancer is unclear. It has been suggested that soy proteins may promote, but not initiate, breast tumors (Harvard Women's Health Watch, 2000). However, "phytoestrogens have shown promise in alleviating hot flashes… (so has the herb black cohosh, which is marketed as Remifemin)… It [genistein] can reduce many of the risk factors that contribute to cardiovascular disease. In randomized controlled trials, soy-protein supplements have consistently lowered both total cholesterol and LDL (bad) cholesterol in perimenstrual women, and in most cases have increased HDL (good) cholesterol as well. Soy has also been shown to improve the elasticity of blood vessels and to lower systolic blood pressure" (2000, p. 4). Phytoestrogens may relieve symptoms of perimenopause and reduce the risk of heart disease and osteoporosis with fewer adverse effects than hormone replacement therapy. The available information suggests that the beneficial effects of phytoestrogens outweigh the negative effects (2000).

Consuming soy protein, approximately 30 grams (2 scoops) of soy protein or more each day has been shown to lower total and LDL cholesterol in humans (Megna, 1997). The RDA is 1 to 2 cups. Many foods are made from the soybean, such as tofu, soy protein isolate, soy flour textured vegetable protein (TVP), miso, and tempeh. Soy protein is essentially equal in quality to animal protein. In addition, soy foods are rich in other nutrients, including calcium, iron, zinc, and many of the B vitamins.

Garlic and Onions

Allyl sulfide (allicin) and ajoene decrease risk of stomach cancer, lower LDL cholesterol, and reduce blood clotting. If eaten raw, all of the breakdown compounds are available and each has specialized activity. Garlic may encourage the production of gluthathione S-transferase, an enzyme that helps rid the body of carcinogens. Garlic possesses antimutagenic/anticarcinogenic, immune enhancing (raw), antitumor, antifungal, antiparasitic, anticholesterol (cooked), decongestant (cooked), and antiplatlet/ antileukocyte adhesion (cooked) action. It is generally recommended that people eat about two cloves a day, both raw and cooked.

Other Phytonutrients

- *Other beans*. Kidney beans, chickpeas, and lentils have saponins, which may slow cancer-cell production and spread.

- *Tomatoes*. Lycopene is a carotenoid antioxidant (protects against cell damage). P-coumaric acid (also in berries) stops the production of cancer-causing nitrosamines and is anti-inflammatory.

- *Citrus*. Limonene in red grapefruit stimulates cancer-killing immune cells.

- *Orange vegetables and fruits*. Carotenes (squash, sweet potatoes, carrots, mangoes, pumpkins, and cantaloupes). Alpha-carotene increases vitamin A activity and boosts general immunity, beta carotene improves immunity. Other carotenes are lycopene, lutein, zeaxanthin, and cryptoxanthin.

- *Crucifers*. Indoles (broccoli, Brussels sprouts, cabbage) weaken cancer-promoting entrogens and increase general immunity. Sulforphanes inhibit breast-cancer tumor growth. Chemoprotective action on liver, colon, lung (specifically against tobacco nitrosamines), mammary glands, the fundic region of the stomach, and esophagus. RDA is 1 to 2 cups.

- *Grapes and turnips*. Ellagic acid blocks cancer-helper enzymes.

- *Berries*. Polyphenols are found in red grapes and red wine, strawberries and blueberries, artichokes, and yams. They may flush carcinogenic toxins and lower risk of heart disease. Flavonoids interfere with carcinogenic hormones, fight cell damage from oxidation, strengthen blood vessels, decrease capillary permeability, protect skin integrity, and are anti-inflammatory and good for the eyes.

- *Flax seed*. Contains lignin precursors that may help prevent some estrogen-related cancers by binding to estrogen receptors. Also contains omega-3 fatty acids.

- *Leafy greens*. Lutein in spinach, mustard, turnip, and collard greens, as well as yellow squash, are carotenoid antioxidants that appear to protect against some cancers, slow degenerative eye disease, and increase immunity. Dark, leafy greens also contain indoles (see crucifers).

- *Grains*. Supply lignins and vitamin E. RDA is 1 to 2 cups cooked.

It has been suggested that foods containing phytonutrients are best eaten fresh and raw, or lightly steamed. Juicing is also a good way to concentrate nutrients. Canned and frozen fruits and vegetables are probably better than none at all. However, isolated extracts in a pill may not work as well as the whole food (Landis, 1997; Zimmerman, 1995).

ANTIOXIDANTS

Antioxidants are compounds that help protect against free-radical damage. The body's cells use oxygen to produce energy. During these normal metabolic processes, oxygen sometimes reacts with body compounds to produce unstable molecules known as free radicals— molecules with unpaired electrons. An unpaired electron is unstable and highly reactive; it needs to pair with another electron in order to return to a stable state. Free radicals quickly react with other compounds in an attempt to capture that needed electron. Antioxidants neutralize free radicals by donating one of their own electrons.

Free radicals not only arise spontaneously during metabolism, but also are made by cells of the immune system to help inactivate viruses and bacteria. In addition, environmental factors such as radiation, pollution, cigarette smoke, and herbicides can generate free radicals. Free radicals cause cell damage. They commonly attack lipoproteins and unsaturated fatty acids in cell membranes, starting chain reactions called lipid peroxidation. Left uncontrolled, lipid peroxidation damages cell structures and impairs their functions. Free radicals also damage proteins and DNA. Rampant free-radical formation and the resulting damage is referred to as oxidative stress. This stress has been implicated in the aging process and in the development of diseases such as cancer, arthritis, cataracts, and heart disease.

"It appears that a combination of antioxidants will provide greater antioxidant protection than any single nutritional antioxidant" (Murray, 1996, pp. 10-11). Antioxidants (protector nutrients) that prevent or delay degenerative processes, include vitamins E, C, and beta carotene (a close relative of vitamin A) and the minerals zinc, copper, manganese, and selenium.

- Vitamins E, A, and C work together as a team

- There are relationships between low intakes of beta carotene (pro-vitamin A), vitamin E, and vitamin C and higher incidences of cancer

- Vitamin B_3 (niacin) can help combat heart disease, while vitamin B_6 can help prevent atherosclerosis

- Smokers require more vitamin E, C, and beta carotene than nonsmokers, and persons who consume a significant amount of alcohol require more vitamin B_1 and magnesium than the average person

- Women taking oral contraceptives may need to increase their zinc, folic acid, and vitamin B_6 intakes, while pregnant women may require more folic acid for proper fetal development

- Individuals who are exposed to smog or other pollutants require higher levels of the protector nutrients such as selenium, and vitamins E and C

- Anyone who is under heavy emotional or physical stress will need higher intakes of all the B vitamins

The best way to supplement antioxidant nutrients is to eat five generous servings of fruits and vegetables daily, especially citrus fruits and green and yellow vegetables. Supplements should not exceed daily doses of 750 retinol equivalents of vitamin A, 30 mg of vitamin E, and 100 mg of vitamin C from supplements.

Vitamin E

Vitamin E (tocopherol) is the most abundant fat-soluble antioxidant. The principal use of vitamin E is as an antioxidant in the protection against heart disease, cancer, and strokes. It functions as a free radical scavenger, protecting lipids from oxidation, preventing the formation of arterial plaque, and subsequently lowering the incidence of coronary artery disease and fatal myocardial infarction. Individuals taking 100 IU of vitamin E daily for 2 years had a 37% to 41%

reduction in heart disease risk (Massey, 2002). Vitamin E may stimulate wound healing and prevent adhesions, and autoimmune disease may be affected positively. Anecdotally, vitamin E has been reported to be beneficial in reducing the symptoms of restless leg syndrome and nocturnal calf cramps. Large doses of vitamin E have also been found to strengthen immune functioning and reduce the severity of age-related diseases such as Parkinson's disease. It is thought that daily supplements of vitamin E enhance the action of insulin by stabilizing the membranes of responding cells. The result is to improve glucose control in diabetes. The antioxidant properties of vitamin E also provide protection to the thymus gland and to white blood cells (Meletis, 1999).

Vitamin E is found in nuts, vegetable oils, whole grains, egg yolks, and leafy green vegetables. There are no significant toxicities associated with normal amounts of vitamin E. It should be taken with meals to optimize absorption. However, the benefits of taking high doses of vitamin E remain to be established (Abramowicz, 1998), and excessive amounts of vitamin E may cause possible gastrointestinal disturbances and may enhance the anticoagulant effects of drugs.

Vitamin C

Vitamin C is the most abundant water-soluble antioxidant in the body. High intakes and serum concentrations of vitamin C have been associated with low incidences of senile cataract, cancer, coronary artery diseases, and higher high-density lipoprotein (HDL) cholesterol concentrations (Abramowicz, 1998). Some factors that deplete the body of vitamin C include cigarette smoke, stress, birth control pills, alcohol, and the consumption of fast foods (Clark, 1996).

Meletis (1999, p. 45) suggests that "supplementation with 1 to 3 gm per day can enhance immunity." However, Abramowicz (1998) indicates that short-term randomized trials have shown that taking vitamin C does not prevent upper respiratory infections, and there is no convincing evidence that taking supplements of vitamin C prevents any disease.

Vitamin C regenerates oxidized vitamin E in the body and potentiates its antioxidant benefits (Murray, 1996). Therefore, supplemental vitamins C and E might be effective in minimizing the chemotherapy and radiotherapy used for treatment of patients with cancer (Kubena & McMurray, 1996). In addition, long-term supplementation of elderly people with moderate amounts of vitamins C and E can significantly reduce serum peroxide levels and protect against free-radical damage, and thereby, aging and degenerative diseases (Clark, 1996). However, an antagonistic effect between vitamins E and A has been noted in several studies. Although supplements of both vitamin E and A were observed to increase antibody production and phagocytosis, when either one was increased, immune function was less (Kubena & McMurray, 1996). Also of concern is that "vitamin E in supplements is mostly alpha-tocopherol, which in vivo may block the antioxidant activity of gamma-tocopherol and have a pro-oxidant effect" (Abramowicz, 1998, p. 75).

Selenium

"The trace mineral selenium functions primarily as a component of the antioxidant enzyme glutathione peroxidase, which works with vitamin E in preventing free radical damage to cell membranes" (Murray, 1996, p. 223). Supplementation with selenium stimulates leukocyte activity and thymus-gland function (Meletis, 1999).

When selenium and vitamin E are not present in adequate levels, immune function is impaired more severely than when only one is inadequate. Both nutrients are needed for optimal response. However, limited evidence exists about the relationship between supplementation of vitamin E and selenium and the effect on immune response. The adverse effect of excessive intake of selenium on immune function has been documented (Kubena & McMurray, 1996).

For adults, a daily intake of 50 to 200 μg is often recommended (Murray, 1996). Patients receiving chemotherapy drugs may have increased requirements.

Coenzyme Q10

Coenzyme Q10 functions like a vitamin that provides critical energy for proper immune functioning, while conferring antioxidant protection (Meletis, 1999). There are no known significant side effects of a basic level of coenzyme Q10 supplementation at 30 mg daily:

- Biochemically functions much like vitamin E in that it participates in antioxidant and free radical reactions.

- Required for the production of cell energy in the mitochondria and serves as an antioxidant.

- Improves the heart tissue's ability to survive under low oxygen conditions. Also has a stabilizing effect on heart rhythm, and has been effective in normalizing blood pressure.

Vitamin A and Beta Carotene

Vitamin A is critically important to the maintenance and integrity of tissue, normal growth, and healthy immune system function. Epidemiologic studies have revealed that higher levels of carotenoids in the diet and higher serum levels of beta carotene are associated with a lower incidence of cardiovascular disease and cancer, particularly lung cancer (Abramowicz, 1998). Vitamin A nutrition is clearly linked to optimal immune responses (Kubena & McMurray, 1996).

Beta carotene is the most nutritionally active of approximately 50 provitamin A carotenoids. It is found primarily in vegetables such as carrots, other orange and dark green leafy vegetables and tomatoes, and orange-colored fruits such as cantaloupes and mangos. One "large" carrot is estimated to contain 11,000 units of vitamin A in the form of beta carotene. However, Meletis (1999) indicates that supplemental carotenes are absorbed better than those from carrots and other vegetables. Palm oil carotenes appear to give the best antioxidant protection (Murray, 1996).

The most recognizable form of vitamin A deficiency is night blindness. People with chronic vitamin A deficiency have more respiratory illness, dry skin, kidney stones, and diarrhea. Epidemiologic studies have strongly implicated low intake of vitamin A with the development of precancerous cells in the mouth, throat, and lungs. Although vitamin A may be given to counteract any symptom of deficiency, symptoms will not be alleviated unless they are caused by a vitamin A deficiency (McDowell, 1995).

The RDA for vitamin A is 5,000 IU for men and 4,000 IU for women. If necessary, 25,000 IU a day may be used as a long-term supplement. For persons older than 60 years, the dosage may be reduced to 10,000 IU a day, taken shortly following a meal. Small amounts of vitamin E and zinc will increase the capacity of all body tissues to store vitamin A.

Women must avoid vitamin A supplementation during pregnancy (Murray, 1996). In fact, large-dose supplements of vitamin A in its active form cause toxicity. No one should take beta carotene supplements (Abramowicz, 1998).

Dietary Guidelines, Goals, and Obesity

"Optimal diets should provide energy and the full complement of essential nutrients in proportions that maximize health and longevity, prevent nutritional deficiencies as well as conditions related to nutritional excesses and imbalances, and be obtained from foods that are available, palatable, acceptable, and affordable" (Nestle, 1996, p. 193). Large areas of the world still experience widespread famine and starvation. However, ironically in the developed countries, with improvements in economic status, dietary patterns throughout the world have tended to shift from a dependence on plant foods as sources of energy and nutrients to an increasing reliance on animal foods that are higher in fat, saturated fat, and cholesterol. This shift has been accompanied by a decline in the prevalence of health problems related to undernutrition and by an increase in the prevalence of diet-related chronic diseases (Nestle, 1996).

Proper total nutrition is by far the most critical factor in maintaining overall optimal immune function (Meletis, 1999). In the simplest sense, the strategy for strengthening the system is to increase positive life influences and reduce negative life influences as much as possible. Examples of what this would mean is reducing mental stress; consumption of simple sugar, alcohol, saturated, and certain other harmful fats; and eliminating smoking and drug use. It would mean increasing intake of whole grains; legumes, fresh fruits and vegetables; getting plenty of fresh, clean water, rest, relaxation, and sleep; doing moderate exercise; and experiencing as much genuine joy, happiness, and self expression as possible (Landis, 1997). Figure 16-1 displays the "nutrition pyramid" and describes what constitutes a nutritious serving.

Since the 1940s, chronic diseases such as coronary heart disease, certain cancers, diabetes, and stroke have replaced infectious diseases and conditions related to undernutrition as leading causes of death among adults in the United States. The role of diet in chronic disease prevention is well established. Substantial evidence indicates that the typical American diet—high in fat, saturated fat, cholesterol, salt, sugar, and alcohol, but low in starch and fiber—contributes to chronic disease incidence and severity. Some estimates suggest that as much as one-third of coronary heart disease and cancer incidence can be attributed to dietary factors. Diet and physical inactivity account for an estimated 300,000 deaths each year in the United States (Nestle, 1996). Moreover, an estimated 60 million adults have elevated blood cholesterol levels, 60 million have high blood pressure, and 30 million are obese; many of these individuals could benefit from improved dietary intake.

Another major nutritional problem in the United States today is "overconsumptive undernutrition," or too much "junk" food! Foods low in nutrient density are often termed "empty-calorie" or "junk" foods, which refers to the relative ratio of nutrients to calories. Most Americans do not even come close to meeting all their nutritional needs through diet alone (Murray, 1996). Nutritional needs, in terms of specific amounts of nutrients that a healthy individual should receive every day, have been called recommended dietary allowances since the term was introduced in 1973, as a reference value for vitamins, minerals, and protein in

Anatomy of MyPyramid

One size doesn't fit all

USDA's new MyPyramid symbolizes a personalized approach to healthy eating and physical activity. The symbol has been designed to be simple. It has been developed to remind consumers to make healthy food choices and to be active every day. The different parts of the symbol are described below.

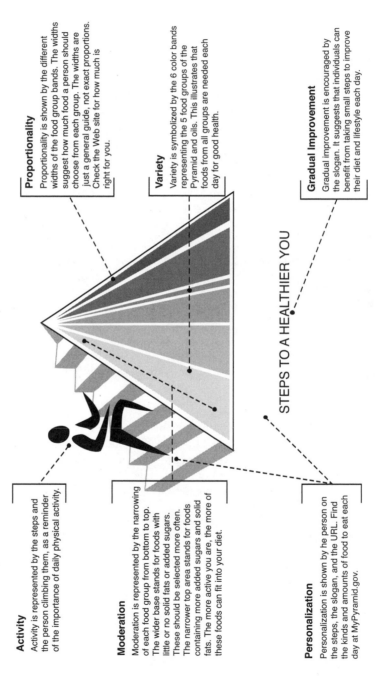

Proportionality

Proportionality is shown by the different widths of the food group bands. The widths suggest how much food a person should choose from each group. The widths are just a general guide, not exact proportions. Check the Web site for how much is right for you.

Variety

Variety is symbolized by the 6 color bands representing the 5 food groups of the Pyramid and oils. This illustrates that foods from all groups are needed each day for good health.

Gradual Improvement

Gradual improvement is encouraged by the slogan. It suggests that individuals can benefit from taking small steps to improve their diet and lifestyle each day.

Activity

Activity is represented by the steps and the person climbing them, as a reminder of the importance of daily physical activity.

Moderation

Moderation is represented by the narrowing of each food group from bottom to top. The wider base stands for foods with little or no solid fats or added sugars. These should be selected more often. The narrower top area stands for foods containing more added sugars and solid fats. The more active you are, the more of these foods can fit into your diet.

Personalization

Personalization is shown by he person on the steps, the slogan, and the URL. Find the kinds and amounts of food to eat each day at MyPyramid.gov.

STEPS TO A HEALTHIER YOU

Figure 16-1. The nutritional pyramid. *Source:* U.S. Department of Agriculture and the U.S. Department of Health and Human Services.

voluntary nutritional labeling. In 1992, the term was renamed reference daily intakes (RDIs). Daily reference values (DRVs) are figures for nutrients such as fat and cholesterol for which no standards previously existed. The figures are based on the number of calories consumed per day. For labeling purposes, 2,000 calories have been established as the reference for calculating percent daily values. The United States Department of Agriculture (USDA) has found that a significant percentage of the U.S. population receives well under 70% of the U.S. recommended daily allowance (U.S. RDA) for vitamin A, vitamin C, B-complex vitamins, and the essential minerals calcium, magnesium, and iron. Most typical diets contain less than 80% of the RDA for calcium, magnesium, iron, zinc, copper, and manganese; the people most at risk are young children and adolescent to elderly women (Burton Goldberg Group, 1995).

"For the most part, we Americans consume more calories than we need. Caloric requirements depend on your size, age, and level of activity" (Keegan, 1996, p. 46). Sedentary women and some older adults need 1,600 calories, whereas teenage boys and most active men need 2,800 calories per day. Whatever the caloric level, DRVs for the energy-producing nutrients are always calculated as follows:

- Fat based on 30% of calories
- Saturated fat based on 10% of calories
- Carbohydrates based on 60% of calories
- Protein based on 10% of calories
- Fiber based on 11.5 grams per 1,000 calories (Keegan, 1996)

"RDAs focus on the prevention of nutritional deficiencies in population groups only; they do not define 'optimal' intake for an individual" (Murray, 1996, p. 9).

DIETARY GUIDELINES

The food guide pyramid recommends that the daily diet contain 6 to 11 portions (1 oz of cereal foods) or (1 slice of bread), 2 to 4 servings (one-half cup) of fruits, 3 to 5 servings (one-half cup) of vegetables, 2 to 3 servings (2 to 3 oz) of meats or meat substitutes, and 2 to 3 servings (1 cup milk) (1.5 oz cheese) of dairy foods. However, "less than 10% of the population consumes the recommended number of fruits and vegetables on any given day" (Nestle, 1996, p. 195). In Box 16-2, the USDA dietary guidelines are presented.

DIETARY GOALS AND OBESITY

Obesity has been proclaimed a major health problem by medicine and the pharmaceutical industries (Kumanyika, 2001). It is alleged that the direct and indirect costs of obesity are 7% of the total health care costs in the United States (Visscher & Seidell, 2001). "Fatness as chronic disease and weight reduction as cure stand as almost universally accepted medical dogma" (Robison, 1999, p. 47) based on medical premises that weights above recommended levels predispose to disease and decreased longevity, and that weight loss increases longevity and improves health. However, these premises are not well supported by existing studies (Robison, 1999). Instead, the common pattern of weight loss followed by weight gain (weight

Box 16-2

Department of Agriculture Dietary Guidelines

- Eat a variety of foods
- Maintain healthy weight, don't starve yourself
- Choose a diet low in fat, saturated fat, and cholesterol
- Choose a diet with plenty of vegetables, fruits, and grain products
- Try to eat as few animal products, especially meats, as possible
- Avoid foods with stimulants, drugs, hormones, and chemicals
- Use sugars only in moderation
- Use salt and sodium only in moderation
- If you drink alcoholic beverages, do so in moderation

Source: U.S. Department of Agriculture. (1995). *Nutrition and your health: Dietary guidelines for Americans* (4th ed.). Washington, DC: US Government Printing Office.

cycling) experienced by most dieters is associated with increased risk for heart disease, hypertension, and diabetes (Robison, 1999).

Body mass index (BMI) is a means of expressing weight relative to height. BMI is calculated by dividing weight in kilograms by height in meters squared (weight in pounds, multiplied by 705, divided by height in inches, and divided again by height in inches). A BMI from 19 to 25 is considered to be a healthy target for adults. However, the majority of American adults has a BMI of 25 to 30 and is considered overweight. Twenty-three percent of American adults have a BMI of 30 or more and are considered obese.

Robison (1999) suggests that health professionals should not prescribe weight loss, because it is ineffective, potentially harmful, and associated with negative psychological effects, guilt, and disordered eating. Instead, he suggests that the goal of interventions should be behavior, lifestyle, and/or attitude change. Instead of weight loss, appropriate outcomes might include decreased reliance on medications, improved quality of life, increased physical activity, decrease in health risks, normalized eating behaviors, and improved quality of food intake. However, the biomedical health care system continues to focus on diet as a treatment for obesity.

Healthy People 2010 (USDHHS, 2000) presents national objectives for health promotion and disease prevention, to be achieved by the year 2010, to address the overarching goal to promote health and reduce chronic disease associated with diet and overweight. These are presented in Table 16-3.

Table
16-3

Healthy People 2010 Nutrition Objectives

GOAL	METHODS
Area 1. Weight status and growth	Increase the proportion of adults who are at a healthy weight. Reduce the proportion of adults who are obese. Reduce the proportion of children and adolescents who are overweight or obese. Reduce growth retardation among low-income children under age 5 years.
Area 2. Food and nutrient consumption	Increase the proportion of persons aged 2 years and older who consume at least two daily servings of fruit. Increase the proportion of persons aged 2 years and older who consume at least three daily servings of vegetables, with at least one-third being dark green or deep yellow vegetables.
Area 2. Food and nutrient consumption (continued)	Increase the proportion of persons aged 2 years and older who consume at least six daily servings of grain products, with at least three being whole grains. Increase the proportion of persons aged 2 years and older who consume less than 10% of calories from saturated fat. Increase the proportion of persons aged 2 years and older who consume no more than 30% of calories from fat. Increase the proportion of persons aged 2 years and older who consume 2,400 mg or less of sodium daily. Increase the proportion of persons aged 2 years and older who meet dietary recommendations for calcium.
Area 3. Iron deficiency and anemia	Reduce iron deficiency among young children and females of childbearing age. Reduce anemia among low-income pregnant females in their third trimester.

continued

<table>
<tr><td>Table 16-3</td><td colspan="2">*Healthy People 2010 Nutrition Objectives (continued)*</td></tr>
<tr><td></td><td>GOAL</td><td>METHODS</td></tr>
<tr><td></td><td>Area 4. Schools, worksites, and nutrition counseling</td><td>Reduce iron deficiency among pregnant females. Increase the proportion of children andadolescents aged 6 to 19 years whose intake of meals and snacks at schools contributes proportionally to good overall dietary quality.

Increase the proportion of worksites that offer nutrition or weight management classes or counseling.
Increase the proportion of physician office visits made by patients with a diagnosis of cardiovascular disease, diabetes, or hyperlipidemia that include counseling or education related to diet and nutrition.</td></tr>
<tr><td></td><td>Area 5. Food security</td><td>Increase food security among U. S. households and in so doing reduce hunger.</td></tr>
</table>

NUTRITIONAL MEDICINE

Nutritional medicine goes beyond the correction of nutrient imbalances toward modulating specific disease processes by nutritional means. "Successful long-range management of chronic disease requires a biologically based approach that is grounded in an understanding of the biochemical synergisms and antagonisms that influence disease progression" (Block, 1999, p. 492). It is estimated that about half the diseases a primary care physician sees have a nutrition-related cause, and at least five of the top 10 causes of death in the United States are linked to diet. Randomized placebo-controlled trials have demonstrated that modest supplementation with vitamins and minerals significantly improves immunity and decreases the risk of infection in old age (Block, 1999).

Nutrigenomics tries to explain how common dietary chemicals (i.e., nutrition) affect health by altering the expression and/or structure of an individual's genetic makeup. The tenets of nutrigenomics are (Hyman, 2004):

- Common dietary chemicals act on the human genome, either directly or indirectly, to alter gene expression or structure.

- Under certain circumstances and in some individuals, diet can be a serious risk factor for a number of diseases.

- Some diet-regulated genes (and their normal, common variants) are likely to play a role in the onset, incidence, progression, and/or severity of chronic diseases.

■ The degree to which diet influences the balance between healthy and disease states may depend on an individual's genetic makeup.

■ Individualized dietary interventions based on knowledge of nutritional requirement, nutritional status, and genotype can be used to prevent, mitigate, or cure chronic disease.

Nutritional medicine involves therapeutic application of dietary and nutritional modifications to reestablish harmony of the body (Block, 1999). Nutritional biotherapy is the clinical use of diet and nutrition to influence host-disease relationships as well as the relationships between nutritional biochemistry and standard treatment (Block, 1999).

Nutritional biotherapy bridges complementary and conventional care. This emergent field consists of three major areas of clinical application:

1. *Prescriptive dietetics.* The selective use of foods and diets specifically designed for different diseases, depending on many individual factors.

2. *Nutritional pharmacology.* The supplemental use of specific vitamins, minerals, phytochemicals, and botanicals (herbal or plant-derived substances), which are tailored to the individual.

3. *Nutrition support.* The use of intravenous or parenteral nutrition when a general diet cannot be consumed (Block, 1999).

Prescriptive dietetics and nutritional pharmacology incorporate therapeutic strategies and prophylactic strategies. Therapeutic strategies address biochemical imbalances or physiological disturbances, while prophylactic strategies "are aimed at preventing the expression of a particular disease-related genotype and enabling patients to enjoy reasonably good health if they select foods and food preparation methods within certain parameters." Noninvasive interventions may be used to "prolong the success of a standard medical therapy by adding a specific biomodulation effect (e.g., reducing serum cholesterol) and thus reducing the relapse rate" (Block, 1999, p. 491). Complementary applications of nutritional biotherapy may translate into considerable reductions in treatment costs as well as reductions in overall disease burden and suffering (Block, 1999).

According to Block (1999), the principal concepts of nutritional medicine include:

1. Core dietary regimen

2. Dietary fat as a separate food

3. Variety and meaningful quantification

4. Individual nutritional tailoring

5. Safe and appropriate supplementation

The first step in effective nutritional medicine is assessment of the patient's current nutritional status, using the ABCDs of nutritional assessment, which stands for anthropometric, biochemical, clinical, and dietary assessment. In anthropometric assessment, weight is considered in relation to height. The body mass index (BMI) can be calculated from this and used in risk factor assessment if needed. Clinical assessment includes consideration of nutrition-related problems and risk factors, such as anorexia and nausea, as well as potential treatment-nutrient interactions.

As part of nutritional assessment, the nurse should ask clients about their diets, including:

- Food and income resources

- Housing

- Employment

- Family and social patterns

- Ethnic and cultural background

- Cooking facilities

- Availability of shopping and transportation

- Food preferences and dislikes

Counseling is most likely to be successful when:
- The client is motivated to change

- Recommendations are consistent with the client's cultural background, food preferences, belief systems, and economic status

- Suggestions are positive

- Changes are made gradually and reinforced over time

USE OF NUTRITIONAL SUPPLEMENTS

Today, an estimated 46% of adult Americans take nutritional supplements, many on a daily basis (Burton Goldberg Group, 1995). Although the quality and number of subjects in blind, controlled clinical trials of nutritional and dietary supplements is variable, and few supplements have been shown to be effective (Fillmore et al., 1999), glucosamine sulfate (1,500 mg) and condroitin sulfate (800 mg) per day "have sufficient controlled trials to warrant their use in osteoarthritis, having less side effects than currently used nonsteroidal anti-inflammatory drugs, and are the only treatment shown to prevent progression of the disease" (Fillmore et al., 1999, p. 693). Improvement may not be evident for 1 to 3 months.

The following are suggested strategies to facilitate absorption and utilization of nutritional supplements:

- Nutritional supplements should be taken with meals to promote increased absorption. Fat-soluble vitamins (such as vitamins A, E, beta carotene, and the essential fatty acids linoleic and alpha linolenic acid) should be taken with the meal that contains the most fat during the day.

- Amino acid supplements should be taken on an empty stomach at least an hour before or after a meal, with fruit juice to help promote absorption. A liquid form, diluted in a beverage, may help if a tablet causes nausea.

- If nauseated or ill within an hour after taking nutritional supplements, the client may need a bowel cleansing program prior to beginning a course of nutritional supplementation.

- If high doses are being taken, the supplements should not be taken all at one time, but divided into smaller doses taken throughout the day.

- Digestive enzymes can be taken with meals to assist digestion. Pancreatic enzymes taken for other therapeutic reasons should be taken on an empty stomach between meals.

- Mineral supplements should be taken separate from the highest fiber meals of the day, as fiber can decrease mineral absorption.

- Whenever an increased dosage of an isolated B vitamin is taken, be sure there is also supplementation with a B-complex.

- When nutrients are taken, an adequate amount of liquid must be taken to mix with digestive juices and prevent side effects.

- Nutritional supplements should never take the place of proper dietary habits or appropriate medical care when warranted.

- Prolonged intake of excessive doses of vitamins A, D, and B_6, for example, may produce toxic effects.

Additives have been suspected as possible cancer causing agents. Therefore, as Kahn and Saulo (1994) suggest, advise clients to stay away from any food containing artificial sweeteners, artificial coloring, flavor enhancers, or sodium nitrite or nitrate.

BASIC DIETS TO AFFECT DISEASE PROCESSES AND WEIGHT LOSS

A number of therapeutic diets have been developed to help to prevent or treat various diseases, or to promote weight loss. In general, there is evidence that regardless of macronutrient composition, diets that reduce caloric intake result in weight loss (Freedman et al., 2001). The moderate-fat balanced nutrient reduction diet is optimal for ensuring adequate nutritional intake, while low-fat, low-calorie diets are most effective for maintenance of weight loss (Freedman et al., 2001). Participation in a therapeutic dietary regimen should be supervised by a health professional. A few selected examples of well-known therapeutic diets (Block, 1999) are discussed in the next section.

High-Fiber, High-Carbohydrate, Low-Fat Diets

The Macrobiotic Diet

The so-called standard macrobiotic diet consists of 50% to 60% whole grains, 20% to 25% vegetables, 5% to 10% beans and sea vegetables (typically combined), and 5% vegetable soups. Other foods such as nuts and seeds, fruits, and fish are consumed on an occasional basis. Red meat, dairy, sugar, and raw fruits are generally avoided. Each person's dietary needs vary according to level of activity, gender, age, climate, season, and various individual factors.

The Pritikin Diet

The Pritikin program is a low-fat, low-cholesterol, low-sodium, and high-complex-carbohydrate diet (5% to 10% fat, 10% to 15% protein, and 80% carbohydrate) combined with regular aerobic exercise. The diet is similar to the macrobiotic diet, but with more rigid emphasis on restricting fat intake, as well as the inclusion of low-fat dairy products and greater variety in choices of animal products. Protein consumption is limited to 3.5 ounces of lean meat a day to reduce total fat and cholesterol intake.

Ayurvedic Diet

The Ayurvedic system is primarily vegetarian, although meat may be prescribed for certain doshas (e.g., one with a predominance of vata). There are limited published reports of the therapeutic effects of Ayurvedic dietary practices per se.

The Ornish Diet

Developed to reverse the development of atherosclerosis and coronary heart disease, this diet is very similar to the Pritikin diet. In terms of total calories, the diet is 10% to 12% fat, 70% to 75% carbohydrates, and 15% to 20% protein. Egg whites, nonfat yogurt, and skim milk are allowed as sources of complementary proteins. Ornish emphasizes the importance of gentle exercises, such as yoga and walking, and of relaxation and visualization techniques to help relieve the body of stress and tension.

Evidence indicates that overweight subjects eat fewer calories, lose weight, and lose body fat related to decreased fat and energy intake, increased energy expenditure, or both. However, the diet is low in vitamins E, B_{12}, and zinc, and the diet often lowers HDL cholesterol in addition to LDL cholesterol (Freedman et al., 2001).

The Gerson Diet

This vegetarian diet consists mainly of raw vegetables and fruit juices, raw calf liver juice (now largely discontinued because of the chemical residues found in calves), and coffee enemas to stimulate bile elimination. The program initially includes a period of juice fasting and enemas, after which patients are placed on a low-sodium, high-potassium diet.

High-Protein, Low-Carbohydrate Diet

The Atkins Diet

There are four stages to the Atkins diet, including the fortnight induction diet, the ongoing weight loss diet, premaintenance, and maintenance. The diet emphasizes the consumption of nutrient-dense, unprocessed foods, avoidance of processed or refined carbohydrate foods, and use of a full-spectrum multivitamin and an essential fatty acid nutrient supplement. Supplementation is necessary because the basic diet is nutritionally inadequate, providing lower than recommended intakes of vitamins E, A, thiamin, B_6, and folate, and calcium, magnesium, iron, zinc, potassium, and dietary fiber (Freedman et al., 2001). The diet is high in saturated fat, cholesterol, and animal protein.

Moderate-Fat, Balanced Nutrient Reduction Diets

Moderate-fat, balanced nutrient reduction diets contain 20% to 30% fat, 15% to 20% protein, and 55% to 60% carbohydrates. Popular diets include commercial weight loss centers such as Weight Watchers, Jenny Craig, and Nutri-Systems, and diets based on the USDA food guide pyramid if calories are reduced. The underlying philosophy of these diets is that weight loss occurs when the body is in negative energy balance. Diets are calculated to provide a deficit of between 500 to 1,000 kcal/day, but a minimum of 1,000 to 1,200 daily calories for women and 1,200 to 1,400 daily calories for men are recommended. Increased energy expenditure through physical activity is also promoted. The goal is to provide a wide range of food choices, allowing for nutritional adequacy and compliance, while still resulting in a slow but steady rate of weight loss (e.g., 1 to 2 lbs/week). Evidence indicates that low-calorie diets (1,000 to 1,200 kcal/day) can reduce total body weight by an average of 8% over 3 to 12 months (Freedman et al., 2001).

Strategies to Promote Healthy Nutrition

According to the American Dietetic Association, "health promotion activities include personal, environmental, organizational, community, policy, and social change interventions that facilitate changing societal and personal behavior to reduce risks to health" (Anderson et al., 1998, p. 205). Behavior change needs to be viewed in the context of social, economic, and cultural considerations, and not as an isolated task controlled by an individual.

One categorization of behavior change strategies based on system level of environmental intervention uses the analogy of a swiftly flowing river. Approaches that target individuals and families are "downstream," local and community approaches are "midstream," and broad-based societal approaches that focus on modifying economic, political, and environmental factors are designated as "upstream" (McKinlay, 1979). In this analogy, physicians and nurses are so caught up rescuing victims with downstream, short-term individual-based interventions that they don't look upstream where the real problems are (to see who is pushing people into the river). It has been suggested that full-spectrum (downstream to upstream) interventions are needed for greatest impact across populations (Butterfield, 1990; McKinlay, 1979, 1995), a premise that is being supported by increasing evidence (Orleans et al., 1999). The following section presents selected downstream, midstream, and upstream interventions that can be applied concurrently to promote healthy nutrition.

INDIVIDUAL AND FAMILY-BASED (DOWNSTREAM) APPROACHES

- Case finding (e.g., cholesterol screening), counseling, group education, and mediated strategies have been effective in reducing dietary fat intake in high-risk persons (Glanz, 1999).

- Therapeutic diets for chronic disease management (e.g., the Ornish diet is effective for primary prevention of cardiovascular disease).

- Minimal-contact interventions such as print guides, tailored messages, and supportive telephone counseling have been found to be effective in promoting healthy eating (Glanz, 1999).

- Targeting stage of readiness for change with appropriate strategies (see Chapter 8).

- Promote lower pricing for low-fat vending machine choices (e.g., fresh fruit).

- Encourage walking and bicycling instead of automobile use for transportation.

- Reduce calorie-dense foods such as regular milk, sugar-sweetened beverages, high-fat foods.

- Reduce the time spent snacking and watching commercials promoting unhealthy food (and limiting energy expenditure through physical activity), particularly for children.

- Modify food preparation to reduce fat or oil in cooking and cream, butter, and high-fat cheeses in recipes.

- Encourage family meals with reduction of eating out at restaurants and fast-food meals. Away-from-home meals have larger portion sizes (French et al., 2001).

- Use nutrition messages that are limited in number, simple, targeted, practical, and reinforced.

- Encourage an interactive process, with client involvement in setting goals and evaluating the effectiveness of the intervention (Sahyoun, Pratt, & Anderson, 2004).

- Goal setting has shown some promise in promoting dietary and physical activity behavior change among adults, but methodological issues still need to be resolved (Shilts, Horowitz, & Townsend, 2004).

- Interventions should use the learner's own experience and expertise, be problem-based, and relevant to the challenges they face (Higgins & Barkley, 2003).

- Use practical application of information rather than facts.

- The nurse should act as a facilitator rather than a "know-it-all."

- Encourage physical activity as part of the daily routine (e.g., walking to school, doing errands with parents, safe outdoor play).

MIDSTREAM APPROACHES

- School-based programs including classroom instruction and modifying food service choices (e.g., vending machines and cafeteria), especially targeted at younger children. Results have been positive but inconsistent (Glanz, 1999).

- Nutrition information programs at point-of-choice (e.g., grocery stores, restaurants).

- Worksite nutrition education programs.

- Increase physical education classes with individualized fitness goals. Only 15% of schools require individualized fitness programs (Dietz & Gortmaker, 2001).

- Small signs near stairways have been effective in increasing their use instead of escalators or elevators (French et al., 2001).

- Increase availability of safe jogging and bike paths.

UPSTREAM APPROACHES

- Change reimbursement policy for nutrition counseling.

- Point-of-purchase nutrition information (e.g., product labeling). Survey data suggest that nutrition information labels are used (French et al., 2001).

- Dietary guidance, nutrition information, and regulatory strategies. For example, chain restaurants and hospitals could be required to provide information about fat and calories of menu choices.

- Tax soft drinks, candy, and high-fat, high-sugar snacks to fund subsidies for fruits and vegetables.

- Add more water drinking fountains in public buildings and outdoor areas.

- Modify the social, physical, and community (home and neighborhood) environments that have an influence on how persons make lifestyle decisions (Sahyoun, Pratt, & Anderson, 2004).

- Address the wider issues of who controls the food supply and thus the influences on the food chain and the food choices of the individual and communities (Caraher & Coveney, 2004).

Food intake is shaped by a wide variety of geographical, social, psychological, religious, economic, and political factors. This chapter has emphasized the importance of meaning of food in shaping dietary intake. An understanding of dietary guidelines and goals, nutrients, and supplements is essential as the basis for teaching clients about healthy nutrition and therapeutic diets. A variety of strategies can be used at individual, community, and policy levels to promote healthy nutrition for health and well-being.

Chapter Key Points

- An understanding of essential dietary nutrients, phytonutrients, and antioxidants is essential as the basis for teaching clients about healthy nutrition.

- Nutritional supplements should never take the place of proper dietary habits or appropriate biomedical care when warranted.

- A number of therapeutic diets, including the macrobiotic, Pritkin, Gerson, Ornish, Atkins, and Ayurvedic diets have been developed to help to prevent or treat various diseases.

- Downstream, midstream, and upstream approaches can be used concurrently to promote healthy nutrition and dietary habits.

References

Abramowicz, M. (Ed.). (1998). Vitamin supplements. *Medical Letters on Drugs and Therapeutics, 40*, 75-77.

Anderson, J. V., Palombo, R. D., & Earl, R. (1998). Position of the American Dietetic Association: The role of nutrition in health promotion and disease prevention programs. *Journal of the American Dietetic Association, 98*, 205-208.

Block, K. I. (1999). Nutritional biotherapy. In W. B. Jonas, & J. S. Levin (Eds.), *Essentials of complementary and alternative medicine*. Philadelphia: Lippincott Williams & Wilkins.

Burton Goldberg Group. (1995). *Alternative medicine: The definitive guide*. Fife, WA: Future Medicine.

Butterfield, P. G. (1990). Thinking upstream: Nurturing a conceptual understanding of the societal context of health behavior. *Advances in Nursing Science, 12*, 1-8.

Caraher, M., & Coveney, J. (2004). Public health nutrition and food policy. *Public Health Nutrition, 7*, 591-598.

Clark, C. C. (1996). *Wellness practitioner* (2nd ed.). New York: Springer.

Dietz, W. H., & Gortmaker, S. L. (2001). Preventing obesity in children and adolescents. *Annual Review of Public Health, 22*, 337-353.

Fieldhouse, P. (1995). *Food and nutrition: Customs and culture* (2nd ed., pp. 1-49, 165-205). London: Chapman & Hall.

Fillmore, C., Bartoli, L., Bach, R., & Park, Y. (1999). Nutrition and dietary supplements. *Physical Medicine and Rehabilitation Clinics of North America, 10*, 673-703.

Freedman, M. R., King, J., & Kennedy, E. (2001). Popular diets: A scientific review. *Obesity Research, 9*(Suppl 1), 1S-40S.

French, S. A., Story, M., & Jeffery, R. W. (2001). Environmental influences on eating and physical activity. *Annual Review of Public Health, 22*, 309-335.

Fuchs, N. K. (1993). Calcium controversy. *Women's Health Letter*.

Gaby, A. R., & Wright, J. V. (1988). *Nutrients and bone health* (pp. 1-4). Baltimore, MD: Wright/Gaby Nutrition Institute.

Glanz, K. (1999). Progress in dietary behavior change. *American Journal of Health Promotion, 14*, 112-117.

Harvard Women's Health Watch. (January, 2000). *Phytoestrogens* (pp. 4-5). Boston: Harvard Health Publications.

Helman, C. G. (1994). *Culture, health, and illness* (3rd ed.). Oxford, UK: Butterworth-Heinemann.

Higgins, M. M., & Barkley, M. C. (2003). Concepts, theories, and design components for nutrition education programs aimed at older adults. *Journal of Nutrition for the Elderly, 23*, 57-75.

Hyman, M. (2004). Paradigm shift: The end of "normal science" in medicine. Understanding function in nutrition, health, and disease. *Alternative Therapies in Health and Medicine, 10*, 10-15, 91-94

Kahn, S., & Saulo, M. (1994). *Healing. A nurse's guide to self-care and renewal*. Albany, NY: Delmar.

Kava, R. (1996). The benefits of vitamin supplements are unproven. In S. Barbour & K. L. Swisher (Eds.), *Health and fitness: Opposing viewpoints* (pp. 44-52). San Diego: Greenhaven Press.

Keegan, L. (1996). *Healing nutrition*. Albany, NY: Delmar.

Kroll, D. (1995). Vitamin D: The easy-to-get vitamin. *Alternative and Complementary Therapies, 1*, 172-176.

Kubena, K. S., & McMurray, D. N. (1996). Nutrition and the immune system: A review of nutrient-nutrient interactions. *Journal of the American Dietetic Association, 96*, 1156-1164.

Kumanyika, S. K. (2001). Minisymposium on obesity: Overview and some strategic considerations. *Annual Review of Public Health, 22*, 293-308.

Landis, R. (1997). *Herbal defense*. New York: Warner Books.

Maslow, A. H. (1970). *Motivation and personality* (2nd ed.). New York: Harper & Row.

Massey, P. B. (2002). Dietary supplements. In Perlman, A. (Ed.), *Complementary and alternative medicine. The medical clinics of North America*. Philadelphia: WB Saunders.

McDowell, B. (1995). Vitamin A and beta carotene: Broad therapeutic applications. *Alternative and Complementary Therapies, 1,* 67-75.

McKinlay, J. B. (1979). A case for refocussing upstream: The political economy of illness. In E. G. Jaco (Ed.), *Patients, physicians, and illness* (3rd ed., pp. 9-25). New York: Free Press.

McKinlay, J. B. (1995). The new public health approach to improving physical activity and autonomy in older populations. In E. Heikkinen et al. (Eds.), *Preparation for aging.* New York: Plenum Press.

Megna, J. (1996). *Nutrition Quarterly, 1,* unpaginated.

Meletis, C. D. (1999). Basic nutrient support for proper immune function. *Alternative and Complementary Therapies, 5,* 43-46.

Murray, M. T. (1996). *Encyclopedia of nutritional supplements.* Rocklin, CA: Prima.

Nestle, M. (1996). Nutrition. In S. Woolf, R. Lawrence, & S. Jonas (Eds.), *Health promotion and disease prevention in clinical practice* (pp. 193-216). Baltimore: Williams & Wilkins.

Nichter, M., & Nichter, M. (1991). Hype and weight. *Medical Anthropology, 13,* 249-284.

Orleans, C. T., Gruman, J., Ulmer, C., Emont, S. L., & Hollendonner, J. K. (1999). Rating our progress in population health promotion: Report card on six behaviors. *American Journal of Health Promotion, 14,* 75-82.

Robison, J. I. (1999). Weight, health, and culture: Shifting the paradigm for alternative health care. *Alternative Health Practitioner, 5,* 45-69.

Sahyoun, N. R., Pratt, C. A., & Anderson, A. (2004). Evaluation of nutrition education interventions for older adults: A proposed framework. *Journal of the American Dietetic Association, 104,* 58-69.

Schneider, D. (2000). International trends in adolescent nutrition. *Social Science and Medicare, 51,* 955-967.

Sebastian, L. A. (1997, December). Fat and cholesterol. *Nursing Spectrum,* 12-14.

Shilts, M. C., Horowitz, M., & Townsend, M. S. (2004). Goal setting as a strategy for dietary and physical activity behavior change: A review of the literature. *American Journal of Health Promotion, 19,* 81-93.

U.S. Department of Agriculture. (1995). *Nutrition and your health: Dietary guidelines for Americans* (4th ed.). Washington, DC: U.S. Government Printing Office.

U.S. Department of Health and Human Services (2000). *Healthy people 2010* (Conference Edition, in two volumes). Washington, DC: Author.

Visscher, T. L. S., & Seidell, J. C. (2001). The public health impact of obesity. *Annual Review of Public Health, 22,* 355-375.

Zimmerman, M. (1995). Phytochemicals and disease prevention. *Alternative and Complementary Therapies, 1,* 154-157.

Additional Information

ASSOCIATIONS AND CREDENTIALING

Two certifying examinations exist for nutritional therapy. Licensing varies greatly from state to state. Advanced training in nutrition is available at many universities.

Certification Board for Nutrition Specialists
Hospital for Joint Diseases
301 E. 17th Street
New York, NY 10003
Tel: (212) 777-1037

The Certification Board for Nutrition Specialists provides certification as a Certified Nutrition Specialist (CNS). Eligibility requires an advanced degree (master's or doctoral level) from a regionally accredited university program in the field of nutrition, nutritional sciences, or a field allied to nutrition and relevant to the practice of nutrition in a professional setting.

Clinical Nutrition Certification Board
5200 Keller Springs Road, Suite 410
Dallas, TX 75248
Tel: (972) 250-2829

The Clinical Nutrition Board provides the title of Certified Clinical Nutritionist (CCN). Eligibility requires a bachelor's degree or equivalent, plus a 900-hour clinical nutrition internship.

American Dietetic Association
216 West Jackson Boulevard
Chicago, IL 60606
Tel: (312) 899-0040
www.eatright.org

RESTORING ENERGY FIELD HARMONY

Energy Patterning

Abstract

Harmonious flow of vital energy is basic to health. Energy healing occurs in the human energy field surrounding, supporting, and interpenetrating the human body. When energy in the human energy field is blocked, deficient, or excessive, illness manifests in the body. Energy healing is a systematic, purposeful intervention aimed to help another person by means of focused intention, hand contact, and/or aligning with the universal energy field. Reiki and prayer are examples of modalities that are based on channeling of a spiritual energy that has innate intelligence or logic, whereas music, color therapy, polarity therapy, therapeutic touch, and thought field therapy pattern the vibrations of the environmental energy field for healing purposes. Additional information about organizational resources and certification is presented at the end of the chapter.

Learning Outcomes

By the end of the chapter, the student will be able to:

- Perform an instant centering technique
- Discuss the 49th vibrational technique for color therapy
- Describe the elements of music therapy that can produce therapeutic outcomes
- Describe the techniques that comprise polarity therapy
- Discuss types of prayer

- Demonstrate hand positions in reiki
- Describe the process of therapeutic touch
- Discuss the components of thought field therapy

Energy Healing

Energy field therapeutics is also known as the laying on of hands, or energy healing. A field is described as "a domain of influence, presumed to exist in physical reality, that cannot be observed directly but that is inferred through its effects. For example, we do not actually see a magnetic field around a bar magnet; but because iron filings arrange themselves in a certain pattern, we know the field exists" (Dossey, 2000, p. 112). The human being is a unitary energy field that is open to and continuously interacting with an environmental energy field (Leddy, 1998), which in turn continuously interacts with the universal energy field. "Self-organization distinguishes the human energy field from the environmental field with which it is inseparable and intermingles" (1998, p. 192). The environment is dynamic, changing through continuous transformation of universal energy field matter and information (1998).

Energy healing is an integrative therapy defined as "a systematic, purposeful intervention aimed to help another person by means of focused intention, hand contact, and aligning with the universal energy field" (Starn, 1998, pp. 209-210). According to Slater (1997, p. 52), energy healing occurs "at the quantum and electromagnetic levels of a person, plant, or animal." Energy varies in quantity and quality (vibration), has polarity (yin and yang), and is arranged in specific patterns. In traditional Chinese medicine, the chi dynamic force of energy is constantly circulating within the body in 12 well-defined channels called meridians, which exist as a series of points following line-like patterns.

The American Nursing Diagnosis Association has classified "energy field disturbance" as a legitimate nursing diagnosis, defining it as "a disruption of the flow of energy surrounding a person's being which results in disharmony of the body, mind, and/or spirit." Disruptions in energy occur as blockages, deficiencies, and excesses. In illness, the energy flow is obstructed, disordered, or depleted. Illness manifests in the human field long before it is obvious in the body (Starn, 1998). "The prevention of disease doesn't so much depend on avoiding pathogens as cultivating a healthy vital chi energy" (Selby, 1997, p. 270). Through augmenting his or her own relatively healthy human energy field, the energetic practitioner can, "through resonance and induction, reinforce the overall resonant field of his or her [client] by identifying diseased resonant patterns of specific organs and 'harmonizing' the energy by 'sending' health qi [chi]" (1997, pp. 274-275). Healing is fundamentally the restoration of harmony from disharmony (Gaynor, 1999).

Energy healing occurs in the human energy field surrounding, supporting, and interpenetrating the human body. The human energy field is composed of seven layers, reaching out to about 3.5 feet beyond the body. The lowest frequency layer, the physical body, contains meridians that circulate chi and chakras, which transmute higher-frequency energy into a form useable by the physical body (Gerber, 1988). Radiating from the chakras are nadis, or channels of electromagnetic energy, that subdivide finally to the cellular level, supporting the concept that healing can affect the cellular level of the physical body (Starn, 1998). "The specific frequency of a particular chakra may modulate a particular emotion, need, drive, and/or organ" (Slater, 1997, p. 54). (See Chapter 4, *Models and Theories* for additional discussion of qi, chakras, and levels of energy fields.)

It is often not necessary for the energy healer to "do" anything. The person heals him or herself, with the healer merely acting as a booster to accelerate the client's healing process (Sharp, 1997). Actual physical touch and "exchange" of energy are not needed for any of the energetic healing modalities discussed in this chapter, because of the outward extension from the body of the field that permeates a physical body. It is assumed that the energy field of the practitioner and that of the client are in constant interaction, or "mutual process" (Rogers, 1990, p. 246). The actual mechanism for energy healing could be a bioelectronic wave that moves between healer and client, initiated by intention or expectation in the therapist's mental energy field (Leddy, 2002). The healer may focus human/environment field energy by placing his or her hands very near, not necessarily touching, the physical body of the person being treated. Energy field interaction may be experienced as:

- A cool breeze

- A tingling or prickling feeling

- A pulsation

- A vibration

- Heat or other changes in temperature

- An expanding force

- Electricity (sensation of light static)

- Pressure or magnetism

There are two alternative beliefs about causation in energetic healing (Berman & Larson, 1994). One belief is that the "healing force" comes from a source other than the practitioner, such as God, the cosmos, or another supernatural entity. For example, reiki and prayer are based on channeling of a spiritual energy that has innate intelligence or logic and knows where and to what extent it is required. A second belief is that a human energy field—directed, modified, or amplified in some fashion by the healer is the operative mechanism. For example, music, color therapy, and therapeutic touch pattern the vibrations of the environmental energy field for healing purposes. As the energy field itself is metaphysical (outside the observable dimensions of space and time), these causal beliefs are currently testable only through manifestations of the energy field.

The lack of a solid research base is one of the major barriers to the acceptance of energetic healing modalities. Until recently, few testable hypotheses have been proposed, an adequate outcomes database has not been available, and accumulation of empirical evidence has not been systematic. In addition, conceptual confusion and conflicting claims as to causal factors, best methods, and procedures have obscured the extent of efficacy of modalities. As a result, many scientists regard energetic healing modalities with disdain.

Despite the lack of empirical evidence, energetic treatment modalities have been used for many conditions:

- Stress relief, improvement of general health and vitality.

- Biologic reduction of inflammation, edema, pain, change in hematocrit and T-cell levels, and acceleration of wound healing and fracture repair.

- Vegetative functions. Improvement of appetite, digestion, and sleep patterns.

- Emotional states. Reduction of anxiety, release of pent-up grief, reduction of recurrent panic attacks, depression, and improved feelings of self-worth.

- Dysfunctions (psychosomatic). Relief of irritable bowel syndrome, premenstrual syndrome, post-traumatic stress disorder, migraine, anorexia and bulimia, nonbiological sexual dysfunction, drug, alcohol, and codependence recovery.

- Pain. Reduction of acute and chronic pain, reduction of the pain of thermal burns and acceleration of healing time, reduction of sunburn pain and coloration.

CENTERING

Essential to energetic healing is the protection and balancing of the healer's energy field. One way that this is accomplished is through the process of centering. Krieger (1986) defines centering "as a sense of self-relatedness that can be thought of as a place of inner being where one can feel truly integrated, unified, and focused." Slater (1997, p. 57) suggests that "centering may be the act of altering one's electromagnetic characteristics through a type of self-referencing meditative-type biofeedback." The nurse should be sure to center the energy field before performing any type of energetic healing modality.

An instant centering technique is the following:

1. Sit comfortably, but in postural alignment.

2. Relax. Check possible tension spots and relax those areas. If there is tension in the neck or shoulder muscles, strongly push your shoulders down so that they are not hunched upward toward your neck.

3. Inhale deeply and gently.

4. Slowly exhale.

5. Inhale again.

Another technique is to stand or sit, with the feet firmly planted flat on the floor. Relax and imagine a line going through the center of your body to connect you to the earth below and the universe above. Inhale and exhale deeply and slowly a few times as you visualize the line.

Energy Healing Modalities

COLOR THERAPY (CHROMATHERAPY)

All of the cells in the body vibrate (Gerber, 1988). Color therapy is based on the concept that a chemical imbalance, a state of disease, and an inappropriate energy vibration in the body are all synonymous. Color deals effectively with disease because it treats the body's etheric field, and the physical, psychological, and spiritual planes or levels are all connected by the mind for an integrated understanding (Klotsche, 1993).

Vibrating colors generate electrical impulses and magnetic currents or fields of energy. Light or color rays are characterized by their specific wavelength (i.e., measurement in space) and frequency (measurement in time). As the rays accelerate (raise their speed or frequency), the wavelengths are shortened. Each color has its own wavelength, which can be attuned to the other colors (or vibrations) to alter a function or balance the system. Particular vibrations raise, lower, or neutralize energy levels. Specific arrays of vibrations are harmonizing, neutralizing, or distorting to each other. In every organ, there is an energetic level at which the organ best functions (Klotsche, 1993).

The colors visible to our eyes are those that are reflected away from an object. Color therapy utilizes different characteristics of the colors: red for its stimulating effects; blue for its sedating effects; and green for its ability to balance. Food colors have the same vibrational effect on our bodies as light therapy, but to a lesser degree. Color also affects the functioning of each system or organ in the body. Thus, color therapy can heal not only the energy body (aura/emotions) by the energy properties of colors, but also the physical body by the colors' chemical properties (Klotsche, 1993). Our bodies are made up of chemical elements consisting of a certain balance of color waves or vibrations. A specific disease thus constitutes a specific imbalance of color waves.

Klotsche (1993) describes a specific color therapy program he calls the 49th vibrational technique. The colors used in the system vibrate in the visible spectrum (the 49th octave) between 397 trillion (red) and 665 trillion (violet) times per second. According to the 49th vibrational technique, the warm colors of the spectrum (red, yellow, orange, and lemon) are stimulating and detoxifying. They are, as a rule, not to be used with fevers or inflammations:

- *Red*, a primary color, is located at one end (the infrared) of the visible spectrum. Red, which has a connotation of heat or fire, is a stimulant, and when used properly activates all five senses, the sensory nervous system, and the liver, as well as the generation of red blood platelets and hemoglobin. Red vibrates at 436 trillion times per second.

- *Orange* is next to red moving toward the center of the visible spectrum. Orange boosts the energy in the lungs and stomach, even assisting vomiting if necessary. It raises the pulse rate but not the blood pressure. This color also stimulates the thyroid and the growth of bone, producing life energy that then radiates throughout the entire body. Orange vibrates at 473 trillion times per second.

- *Yellow*, the third color from the infrared end, is a vibrational combination of red and green. This secondary color is a stimulant for the sensory and motor nervous systems. Yellow tones the muscles, activates the lymph glands (which in turn cleanse the blood) and improves the digestive system, stimulating the intestines, pancreas, and digestive fluids. Yellow, the color of the mind or intellect, can raise low-energy emotional states (depression, apathy, discouragement). Yellow vibrates at 510 trillion times per second.

- *Lemon* is a combination of yellow and green. It stimulates the colon like a mind laxative and activates the thymus gland, an important organ in the immune system. It is a bone builder and an excellent detoxifier of harsh chemicals. It dissolves blood clots often within hours, rejuvenates the body, and stimulates the brain. Lemon vibrates at 547 trillion times per second (Klotsche, 1993).

- *Green* is the master color, the middle of the spectrum. This balancing color builds cells and tissues, and is the stabilizing color for all dysfunctions, whether chronic or acute. Green relieves tension and regulates the etheric body. Green vibrates at 584 trillion times per second.

On the other side of the spectrum toward the ultraviolet end are the colors turquoise, blue, indigo, and violet. They relieve fevers and soothe many types of pains:

- *Turquoise* (a combination of blue and green) is the opposite of the color lemon. It rejuvenates the skin and is useful for the repair and nourishment of cells in acute disorders. When used with green or blue, it is extremely effective for healing infections, burns, and wounds. Turquoise is cerebrally calming and is an effective vibration for sound sleep. It vibrates at 621 trillion times per second.

- *Blue* increases the elimination of toxins through perspiration, stimulates intuitive powers and is a vitality builder. Blue activates the pineal gland; it is the color of the spirit. Blue vibrates at 658 trillion times per second.

- *Indigo* is a cooling color that activates the parathyroid and calms the thyroid. It controls abscesses and relieves or eliminates discharges and bleeding. It also calms the respiratory system, reduces swelling, and has an anesthetic effect. Indigo can improve one's emotional state by its sedative effect, and it has a generally calming, inward-turning energy vibration. It also has contractive characteristics whereby it can firm, tone, and tighten up the flesh and arrest or shrink tumors, swellings, and unhealthy growths. Indigo vibrates at 695 trillion times per second.

- *Violet* has the shortest wavelength of the visible colors. It has the capability to control hunger (and thus weight) through calming the metabolic process. It relaxes muscles and has antibiotic characteristics. Calming the nerves, it is an aid to meditation and sleep. Violet may act as a pain reliever after first trying indigo. Violet vibrates at 731 trillion times per second.

In addition to these nine warm, neutral, and cool colors, there are three more colors in the visible spectrum that further fine-tune the energy for specific healing purposes, especially heart, kidney, and circulatory functions. These three additional colors are magenta, purple, and scarlet:

- *Purple* (a combination of violet and yellow) calms the emotions as well as the activity in the arteries. It stimulates activity in the veins and relieves headaches and excessive pain from pressure by decreasing sensitivity. It lowers blood pressure and induces sleep. Purple can eliminate recurrent high fevers associated with such diseases as malaria and rheumatic fever. Purple vibrates at 621 trillion times per second.

- *Magenta* (a combination of red and violet) balances the emotions. It levels blood pressure, automatically raising or lowering it to normal. Magenta stimulates and nourishes the kidneys, the adrenals, the heart and the circulatory system. It is also an aura builder and is similar to green in that it can be used for most energy disorders. It vibrates at 584 trillion times per second.

■ *Scarlet* (a combination of red and blue) speeds up the heartbeat, stimulates the arteries, and sedates the activity of the veins (the reverse of purple). Scarlet is a general stimulant. It is the strongest of the twelve healing colors and needs to be used with utmost care. Scarlet vibrates at 547 trillion times per second.

Ten of the 12 healing colors have a complementary color or vibration that is used to balance or counterbalance their vibratory effects. It is important, in some cases, to use the exact complementary color for this purpose. The 49th vibrational technique generally establishes a rule of seven: For every six uses of predominantly one color, a color of the opposite side of the spectrum should be used once for balance. The main color for counterbalancing the warm colors is turquoise; lemon counterbalances the cool colors. There is a lack of scientific evidence of the effectiveness of color therapy. The 49th vibrational technique for color therapy (Klotsche, 1993) is presented in Box 17-1.

Box 17-1

The 49th Vibrational Technique for Color Therapy

■ Uses plastic color transparencies (filters or gels). The transparencies are assembled, using tape or staples, with specific combinations of 10 colored sheets. Klotsche (1993, p. 101) specifies that only Roscolene and no other gels should be used.

■ A heat shield is placed between the light source and the filters.

■ Any incandescent lamp (60 to 100 watt) with a single opening for the light can be used.

■ The room should be quiet, totally dark, and at 80 degrees.

■ The client should not eat or bathe at least 1 hour before or after a tonation.

■ The tonation is applied for 1 hour on the bare skin.

■ The individual must be as relaxed as possible for optimal absorption of the colored rays by the aura. The eyes may be closed or open at the individual's option. One can meditate, relax, or sleep.

continued

BOX 17-1 CONTINUED

- The technique is most effective when the individual lies on his or her back or side with the crown of the head toward magnetic north. If for any reason it is undesirable to lie down for the color treatment, an alternative approach is to sit facing south during the treatment (back of the head toward north), to keep the body's polarity in alignment with the earth's magnetic field.
- The lamp should be a meter (or yard) or more above and behind the feet or, alternatively, above or beside the body.
- Tonation time is ideally 1 hour. One should wait at least 1 hour (2 is preferred) after one tonation before staring a second one.
- Light therapy should be used in combination with an appropriate diet.

Source: Adapted from Klotsche, C. (1993). *Color medicine*. Sedona, AZ: Light Technology.

Color therapy can be learned by careful study with an instructional guide and experience with a clinician using this modality. There is no national certification for this modality. The author is not aware of any organized courses. Another energy field modality that is based on vibration theory is music therapy.

MUSIC THERAPY

When music is used for therapeutic purposes it is termed music therapy. Music therapy has been defined as a behavioral science concerned with the systematic application of music to produce relaxation and desired changes in emotions, behavior, and physiology (Guzzetta, 1997). Music therapy may include therapies designed to increase one's social, physical, or mental well-being via such methods as songwriting or lyric analysis, expression of feeling through music, or relaxation through listening to music (Harding, 1999).

Music therapy is based on the physics and physiology of sound. The earth vibrates at a frequency of 8 cycles per second. The body acts as a vibratory transformer that gives off and takes in sound, at an inaudible frequency of approximately 8 cycles per second when it is in a relaxed state. During relaxed meditation, the frequency of brainwaves produced is also about 8 cycles per second (Brewer, 1998). Every human cell has its own frequency, and the frequency of every human organ may be a harmonic of its component cells (Gaynor, 1999). Results with sound are not a function of volume (amplitude, or quantity) but pitch (frequency, quality). The sound waves of vibration are measured in frequencies according to how many waves are formed per second, and these units are called hertz (Hz). Human hearing normally exists within a range of 16,000 to 25,000 Hz, although many people cannot hear sound above 10,000 Hz (Harding, 1999).

Sound is defined as oscillating energy waves within the audible range. The ear is not only the primary organ of hearing (the passive ability to perceive sound), but also has powerful influences on eye movement, the rhythms of the physical body, prebirth brain growth, and general regulation of stress levels in the body. People respond to sound vibrations in two main ways: via rhythm entrainment and resonance (Burton Goldberg Group, 1995).

1. *Entrainment.* There is a tendency in the universe toward harmony, a phenomenon known as entrainment. This is a process whereby two objects vibrating at similar frequencies will tend to cause mutual sympathetic resonance. Part of what promotes healing in a therapy situation is the entrainment that occurs between therapist and client.

2. *Resonance.* The ability of a vibration to set off a similar vibration in another body. "It is vibrational language that helps the body-mind attune itself with its own resonance" (Brewer, 1998, p. 11). Different frequencies of sound (different pitches) stimulate the body to vibrate in different areas.

As the human body vibrates, "some sounds assault the body because they are not in harmony with its fundamental vibratory pattern.... Musical vibrations can help restore regulatory function to a body out of tune (e.g., during times of stress) and help maintain and enhance regulatory function of a body in tune" (Guzzetta, 1997, p. 197).

When considering the use of music as an intervention, there are several things to keep in mind. The type of music and personal preferences of the client are critical. Other choices include active versus passive involvement (listening via cassette tape or compact disc), use in a group or on an individual basis, and length of time to use music. An argument can be made for group therapy as a way to foster social interaction in the elderly and in persons with psychiatric disorders. However, diversity in the preferences of individuals in a group or the lack of an appropriate site for a group session may necessitate implementing music on an individual basis (Chlan, 1998). Left and right ears may have different thresholds in different frequency ranges (Campbell, 2001). There are cultural differences in music preference (Good et al., 2000). A minimum of 20 minutes is probably necessary to induce relaxation, with some form of relaxation exercise, like deep breathing, before initiating the music intervention.

Music is most commonly used as a relaxation technique, utilizing a pleasant stimulus to block out sensations of anxiety, fear, and tension, and to divert attention from unpleasant thoughts. Guzzetta (1997) suggests that the healing capabilities of music are intimately related to the personal experience of inner relaxation. Music that contains many changes of mood and tempo can stimulate the listener, whereas music that stays on a steady and predictable course can be used as a sedative (Harding, 1999).

Four necessary elements have been suggested for promoting relaxation: a quiet environment, a comfortable position, a passive attitude, and focused concentration on the music (Chlan, 1998). "Slow-moving music lengthens our perception of time because our memory has more time to experience the events (tensions and resolutions) and the spaces between the events. So, the time clock becomes distorted and clients can actually lose track of time for extended periods, enabling them to reduce anxiety, fear, and pain" (Brewer, 1998, p. 10).

As illness is viewed as a manifestation of disharmony within the body, healing can be achieved by restoring the normal vibratory frequency of the disharmonious (Gaynor, 1999) through music therapy. "Music therapy evokes psychophysiologic responses because of its influence on the limbic system. This system is influenced by musical pitch and rhythm, which, in turn, affect emotions and feelings. Our emotional reaction to music may occur because the limbic system is the seat of emotions, feelings, and sensations" (Brewer, 1998, p. 10). By enhancing melatonin release via pineal gland stimulation, music may unlock and restore "the expression of emotional connections with our deeper self, whether in a state of health or disease" (Kumar et al., 1999, p. 56).

The elements of music that can influence therapeutic outcomes (Chlan, 1998) are presented in Box 17-2.

Box 17-2

Elements of Music That Can Affect Therapeutic Outcomes

- *Pitch.* Produced by the number of sound vibrations per second. Rapid vibrations (high-pitched sounds) tend to act as a stimulant, whereas slow vibrations bring about relaxation.

- *Intensity.* Refers to the volume of the sound. It is related to the amplitude of the vibrations. Intensity can be used to produce effects such as intimacy (soft music), protection (loud music), and power. Emotions are affected by the intensity of the music.

- *Tone color* (or timbre). A nonrhythmical, purely sensuous property that results from the harmony present or the characteristics of a voice or instrument.

- *Interval.* The distance between two notes. It is related to pitch. The sequence of intervals results in the melody and harmony of a piece.

- *Duration.* Refers to the length of sounds.

- *Rhythm.* A time pattern fitted into a certain speed. Musical tempos may be used to harmonize, synchronize, or entrain the physiological state. The pitch and rhythm of music affect the limbic system, which is integrally involved in emotions and feelings.

Source: Adapted from Chlan, L. (1998). Music therapy. In M. Snyder & R. Lindquist (Eds.), *Complementary/alternative therapies in nursing* (3rd ed., pp. 243-257). New York: Springer.

Harding (1999) discusses the idea of patterning alpha and theta brainwaves through entrainment via rhythm and sound (e.g., drumming). "An alpha-level drum frequency (7 to 13 cycles per second sustained for at least 13 to 15 minutes) stimulates an alpha-wave cycle in the brain. High alpha states are associated with meditation and holistic modes of consciousness" (1999, p. 88). Another apparent benefit from drumming is a higher state of brain hemispheric synchronicity, in which both hemispheres cooperate in harmonic resolution. Bittman and colleagues (2001) found that group drumming altered stress-related hormones and enhanced immunologic measures associated with natural killer-cell activity and cell-mediated immunity.

In music therapy, it is essential to choose the appropriate music for the desired response. Gaynor (1999) suggests a number of categories and specific music selections from which to choose depending on the purpose for the therapy.

Chlan (1998) suggests several basic steps for utilizing music intervention to promote relaxation:

1. Ascertain the client has adequate hearing

2. Ascertain the client's like or dislike for music

3. Assess music preferences and previous experience with music for relaxation; assist with tape selection as needed

4. Determine mutually agreed upon goals for music intervention with the client

5. Complete all nursing care prior to the intervention; allow at least 20 minutes of uninterrupted listening time

6. Gather equipment and ensure it is in good working order. Provide the client a choice of soothing selections for relaxation

7. Assist the client to a comfortable position as needed; ensure call-light is within easy reach

8. Assist the client with equipment as needed

9. Enhance environment to suit the client (draw blinds, close door, turn off overhead lights, etc.)

10. Post a "do not disturb" sign to minimize unnecessary interruptions

11. Encourage and provide the client with opportunities to practice relaxation with music

The goal of music therapy is the reduction of psychophysiological stress, pain, and anxiety (Brewer, 1998). The rhythmicity, melody, and harmony of music are often effective in alleviating emotional conflict (1998). There are many desired outcomes of music therapy (Chlan, 1998; Guzzetta, 1997; Kumar et al., 1999), including minimizing disruptive behaviors; decreasing anxiety; managing pain; reducing stress; relaxing; stimulation; decreasing isolation; developing self-awareness and creativity; improving learning; clarifying personal values; improving alertness, recall memory, and motor and verbal skills (in clients with Alzheimer's disease); coping with a variety of psychophysiologic dysfunctions; and coping with dying. Music therapy for people with Alzheimer's disease can promote interactions with other patients, foster communication with caregivers, and may enhance retention and recall, and effectively manage behavior problems, reducing the need for restraints or medications (Brotons et al., 1997).

Box 17-3 presents a music therapy study abstract.

Box 17-3

Music Therapy Study

Twenty male inpatients with Alzheimer's disease received 30 to 40 minute morning sessions of music therapy five times per week for 4 weeks. Blood samples were obtained before initiating the therapy, immediately at the end of 4 weeks of music therapy sessions, and at 6 weeks follow-up after cessation of the sessions. Melatonin concentration in serum increased significantly after music therapy and was found to increase further at 6 weeks follow-up. The authors concluded that increased levels of melatonin following music therapy may have contributed to patients' relaxed and calm mood.

Source: Adapted from Kumar, A. M., Tims, F., Cruess, D. G., Mintzer, M. J., Ironson, G., Loewenstein, et al. (1999). Music therapy increases serum melatonin levels in patients with Alzheimer's disease. *Alternative Therapies in Health and Medicine, 5*(6), 49-57.

Although music therapy is generally safe and effective, there may be a lack of effectiveness after 3 minutes of continuous exposure (due to neural adaptation), music may increase intracranial pressure following head injury, and decibels (volume) higher than 90 dB can cause discomfort (Chlan, 1998).

Like color therapy, music therapy lacks organized instructional courses, as well as national certification. The modality is best learned through careful study of instructional guides and experimental study with practitioners using this modality. In contrast, practice of the integrated therapeutic system called *polarity therapy*, requires extensive organized study and certification by the American Polarity Therapy Association.

POLARITY THERAPY

Polarity therapy was developed in the mid 1900s by Randolph Stone, a chiropractor, naturopath, and osteopathic physician. According to Polarity Therapy, the process of life, or "becoming" as the Buddhists would say, is a flow of energy. However, physical form is better visualized as pulsations of light in specific patterns, rather than as moving energy in channels. For any energy to arise or for physical form to come into being, there must be movement. Movement of energy is based on or due to a relationship (polarity) that sets up two opposing fields. Yang is the positive, outgoing pole, and yin is the negative, receptive pole. According to polarity theory, "energy flows via a positive outward movement from a neutral source, through a neutral field, to some form of completion. It is then drawn back to the source by a negative, receptive pull" (Sills, 1989, p. 11). "The bonding, balancing force between and within all forms of energy and matter is clearly the polarity of positive and negative" (Klotsche, 1993, p. 29).

An "energy anatomy" that precedes and creates physical anatomy exists in several layers. Polarity theory predicts that the relative freedom and balance of the energetic and physical movement patterns in mental, emotional, and physical fields create differences between health and disease. The free flow of energy is needed for health. When energy is not moving in a fluid and balanced way, vitality is low.

Polarity therapy supports the healing process by promoting cleansing, building, and toning, on physical and energetic levels (Olsen, 1990). Polarity balances subtle or electromagnetic energy through:

- Touch or working with polarity trigger points.

- Stretching exercises called polarity yoga or polar energetics that give clients tools to use to work with their physical contractions and patterns without a dependency on the clinician.

- An approach to eating and nutrition based on the discipline's principles. Cleansing and health-building diets not only help to clean the body of toxicity and waste products but also promote an exploration of relationships to food and nourishment. Knowledge of both the cleansing and energetic properties of food are used as therapeutic tools (Sills, 1989).

- Attitude or mental-emotional balancing (Olsen, 1990).

The main focus of much of polarity work is bodywork. Polarity therapy does not manipulate muscles or bones but works through the body's own energy system by placing hands on the body's energy centers and poles to redirect the flow (Olsen, 1990). In the bodywork, the imbalances are literally "touched on," with the clinician's hands used to reflect patterns back for client awareness. The clinician is not only a guide, but a facilitator (Sills, 1989). The purpose of polarity manipulation is to locate blocked energy and release it. When energy is blocked, it manifests itself as soreness, tenderness, or pain (Sharp, 1997). When energy is released, healing can take place naturally, and organs and systems can regain normal function.

"All this focus on body energy needs the support of positive thinking.... Thoughts are vibrations of energy that move faster than light or sound. Thoughts and emotions as vibrations affect the flow of energy in the body" (Olsen, 1990, p. 240). See Chapter 4, *Models and Theories*, for a discussion of energy anatomy.

The techniques of polarity therapy are very simple and gentle. They involve simple touching using bipolar contacts (use of two contacts on the patient's body simultaneously). For example, a positive contact (right hand or fire—middle—finger) pushes energy and is stimulating while a negative contact (left hand or air—second—finger) is relaxing and receives energy. These contacts balance the chakras to each other and the energy flowing through the longitudinal and horizontal energy currents. Once the appropriate contacts have been made, the clinician should concentrate on feeling energy, which is usually experienced as a tingling or warmth between the hands and the client's body. After stimulating for a couple of minutes, the nurse should hold and feel the energy for 30 to 60 seconds and then move to another manipulation. If after 2 minutes energy is not felt, the nurse should hold for another minute and then move on (Sharp, 1997).

The treatment session is concluded by chakra balancing to produce overall relaxation and facilitate deep energy flow. The chakra balance is performed by placing the client supine, with the clinician standing on the right side of the body. With loose fists the right thumb is used to touch the umbilicus and the left thumb to touch between the eyebrows. When these positions are held for 2 minutes, the energy flow through the body can be felt (Sharp, 1997).

Polarity therapy includes multiple hands-on techniques including manipulation of pressure points and joints, massage, breathing techniques, hydrotherapy, exercise, reflexology, and even simply holding pressure points (acupressure) on the body. These techniques, combined with dietary and nutritional counseling, as well as the emotional balancing work that is also part of polarity therapy, help clients achieve a heightened level of well-being. In addition to an enhanced sense of well-being, the benefits of polarity therapy can include improvement in physical health, increased energy, and a deeper understanding of oneself (Burton Goldberg Group, 1995).

Box 17-4 presents a polarity therapy study abstract.

Box 17-4

Polarity Therapy Study

In order to assess the fluctuation (but not the effectiveness) of extremely high-frequency electromagnetic fields, or gamma rays, during polarity therapy treatment, 30 volunteers were divided among 10 treatment and 20 control (10 sham and 10 standing-observer) subjects. Marked decreases in gamma counts were found at every anatomical site location for all subjects during polarity therapy, with less change noted during the standing-observer and sham sessions. Gamma radiation decreased in 100% of subjects during therapy sessions. The authors strongly recommend "the collection of additional data, especially on subjects with cancer, whose long-term survival might be enhanced as a result of the radiation hormesis effects of alternative energy therapies."

Source: Adapted from Benford, M. S., Talnagi, J., Doss, S., Boosey, S., & Arnold, L. E. (1999). Gamma radiation fluctuations during alternative healing therapy. *Alternative Therapies in Health and Medicine, 5*(4), 51-56.

PRAYER

Prayer has been described as a form of distant healing through the act of communing with God, the divine, the supernatural, or the universal mind. Sicher and colleagues defined distance healing as "a conscious, dedicated act of mentation attempting to benefit another person's physical and emotional well-being at a distance" (cited in Koopman & Blasband, 2002, p. 100). "The essence of prayer is faith" (Thomson, 1997, p. 95).

There are basically two kinds of prayer: meditative/worshipful and supplicative. In the former, one prays for faith, understanding, and a state of grace. Examples include prayers of thanksgiving, adoration, confession, lamentation, contemplation, and surrender, in which nothing is asked and any outcome is accepted. Supplicative prayer, by contrast, is the more selfish version, in which one prays for rain, to pass an examination, to recover from an illness (or, less selfishly, for someone else to recover from an illness). The result prayed for is direct divine intervention—a miracle (Thomson, 1997). Examples of supplicative prayer include:

1. *Petition*. Individuals ask for something for themselves, generating a mental request for a particular outcome of God's will.

2. *Intercession*. Individuals ask for help for another person. Intercessory is derived from the Latin *inter*, "between," and *cedere*, meaning "to go." Intercessory prayer is therefore a go-between—an effort to mediate on behalf of, or plead the case of, someone else. Intercessory prayer is often called distant prayer, because the individual being prayed for is often remote from the person who is praying (Dossey, 2000).

Feelings that are central to prayer include love, empathy, compassion, and a sense of connectedness, oneness, and unity with the object that the client is attempting to influence

(Dossey, 1997). The key issue in understanding distant healing is the separation of the distant effect from effects that may be due to other causes. Factors such as hope, expectation, or relaxation can influence or bias results if they are not controlled. "It is possible that so-called psychic healing effects may in fact represent a synergistic effect of distant healing intention and the nonparanormal, psychological benefit of the presence or knowledge of the attention of a caring person" (Targ, 1997, pp. 74, 77).

Distant mental intentions require a model of consciousness that recognizes a nonlocal quality of mind, in which consciousness cannot be completely localized or confined to specific points in space (such as brains or bodies), or to discrete points in time (such as the present moment). "Quantum-scale events share three salient characteristics: they are said to be immediate (i.e., they occur simultaneously), they are unmediated (i.e., they do not depend on any known form of energy for their 'transmission'), and they are unmitigated (i.e., their strength does not diminish with increasing spatial separation). Distant, intercessory prayer bears a strong resemblance to these events" (Dossey, 1997, pp. 116-117).

Dossey (1997, p. 118) states that "there are a sufficient number of well-designed, well-executed studies demonstrating statistically significant effects to support an assertion that healing is a potent intervention.... Our major difficulty is that we seem to be suffering from a failure of the imagination. Unable to see how prayer could work, too many people insist that it cannot work." For example, in a meta-analysis of 30 studies, "single-mean t-tests produced independently significant evidence for the remote intentionality or remote observation effect (i.e., an associated p of .05 or less) in 14 of the possible 30 cases, yielding an experiment-wide success rate of 47%, compared with a success rate, expected on the basis of chance alone, of 5%.... Results across the experiments showed a significant and characteristic variation during distant intentionality periods, compared with randomly interspersed control periods (the average effect size was +.25)" (Schlitz & Braud, 1997, p. 62).

In a coronary care unit (CCU), 201 clients in a control group required ventilatory assistance, antibiotics, and diuretics more frequently than the 192 clients in the intercessory prayer group. "The data suggest that intercessory prayer to the Judeo-Christian God has a beneficial therapeutic effect in [clients] admitted to a CCU" (Byrd, 1997, p. 87). However, no published studies have yet replicated this study. In a randomized trial of nearly 1,000 hospitalized heart clients, half of the clients were prayed for daily by volunteers for 4 weeks, while the other half did not have anyone assigned to pray for them. None of the clients were aware of the study. After 4 weeks, the prayed-for-clients had experienced 11% fewer complications—a small but statistically significant difference (Weil, 2000). Koopman and Blasband (2002, p. 101) conclude that "distant healing is real and transcends chance occurrence. The full range of its applicability and longitudinal effect has yet to be explored."

REIKI

The National Institutes of Health Center for Complementary and Alternative Medicine (NCCAM) has classified energy medicine therapies into two basic categories: bioelectromagnetic-based therapies and biofield therapies that include reiki, qigong, and therapeutic touch (Miles & True, 2003). Reiki has its roots in Tibetan scriptural narratives (sutras) and was reintroduced by Japanese physician, Mikau Usui, in the 19th century. It means free passage of the universal (rei) life force energy (ki) (Nield-Anderson & Ameling, 2001). Following the Eastern concept of balancing energies, a reiki healer is initiated into the art of a gentle placing of hands in specific positions on the body through energy attunement by a reiki master. The healer's energy field is attuned to enable him or her to act as a conduit to facilitate another or the self in balancing energies or healing. "The reiki practitioner is a facilitator, not a provider.... There is no attempt made to evaluate the recipient's energy field or condition. There is no manipulation of the recipient's body or energy field" (Nield-Anderson & Ameling, 2000, p. 22). Reiki can be used for mental, emotional, physical, or spiritual balancing (Olsen, 1990).

Engebretson (1996) emphasizes that the act of healing is not an intellectual rational activity but a spiritual intuitive activity that uses human touch as the medium for healing. This touch is gentle, expressive, and compassionate, and involves feelings of lightness and love. Physical sensations associated with reiki include warmth, tingling, pulling, drawing, and energy transfer. "Reiki is not intrusive, does not demand any technology, can be practiced anywhere at any time, and does not require a practitioner or recipient to engage in verbal exchange. Reiki is not for diagnosing disease conditions and therefore does not require a practitioner to collect information, and there are no body manipulations in a reiki treatment (p. 26).... The healing of self and others is viewed as reciprocal and integral to the practice of reiki" (Nield-Anderson & Ameling, 2000, p. 27). Both the clinicians and the client are mutually healed. Clinicians are not depleted during sessions and rarely reported aftereffects (e.g., heightened symptoms of pain, stiffness, or headache) subside quickly.

Reiki requires no particular spiritual practice, discipline, or faith requirements. A reiki clinician does not provide nor direct energy. It is believed that energy goes naturally to the places where it is needed. "A reiki master links a student to a cosmic, radiant energy, opens chakras, or 'attunes' that individual as a receiver for universal life energy vibrations or unconditional love" (Olsen, 1990, p. 252).

The reiki energy is drawn in and focused through the hands to make a link between two living beings. The first degree training or attunement is for physical healing and can be taught in a weekend. Hand positions are taught and experienced in hands-on practice sessions. Four attunements (initiations), spiritual, sacred, and confidential rituals involving symbols and mantras "activate the chakras and heighten a practitioner's abilities to self-heal and to serve in the healing process" (Nield-Anderson & Ameling, 2001, p. 46). The second degree focuses on absent or distant healing, plus amplification of the initiate's energy. It can be taught in a day. Two attunements are administered that "deepen the practitioner's own healing and increase their energy vibrations" (2001, p. 46). The third degree, the master level, prepares the practitioner to teach reiki as well as heal with reiki and involves several stages. The higher the degree of initiation, the more power that is available to channel. "This, the most intense attunement process, provides the life force vibration for personal growth on all levels" (2001, p. 46).

Clients usually start with a series of three or four full treatments lasting about an hour each. Hand positions are each held for 3 to 5 minutes. A session can be as long or short as needed. Full treatments typically last 45 to 75 minutes. The receiver need not be conscious so reiki can be offered during surgery (Miles & True, 2003). The experience can range from feeling more calm and centered to more energized, or both. Reiki can be applied to anybody or to any condition to enhance a treatment program, help relieve pain, or as a general energy "tune-up" (Olsen, 1990).

Each treatment begins at the client's head as the clinician proceeds through a series of 13 to 16 hand positions that are designed to cover all body systems. The clinician holds each position for 5 minutes or until the flow of energy is perceived in the targeted tissues (Van Sell, 1996). Hand positions in reiki therapy are depicted in Figure 17-1.

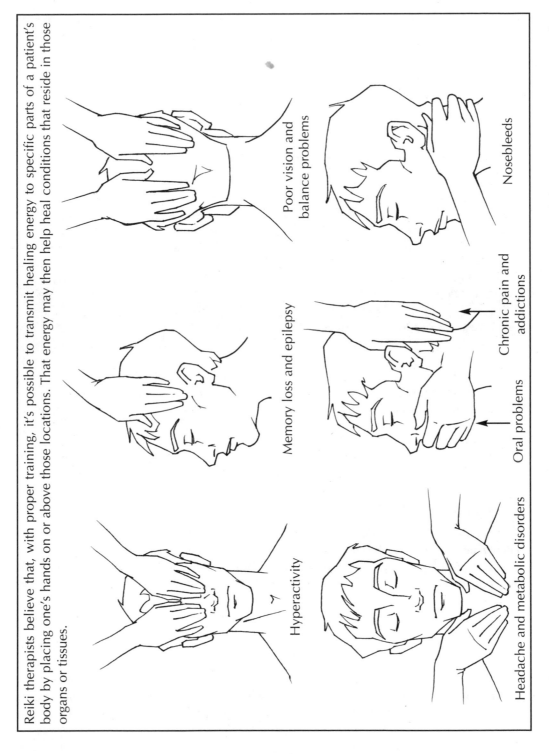

Reiki therapists believe that, with proper training, it's possible to transmit healing energy to specific parts of a patient's body by placing one's hands on or above those locations. That energy may then help heal conditions that reside in those organs or tissues.

Poor vision and balance problems

Nosebleeds

Memory loss and epilepsy

Chronic pain and addictions

Oral problems

Hyperactivity

Headache and metabolic disorders

Figure 17-1. Hand positions in reiki therapy (reprinted from Sell, S. L. (1996). Reiki: An ancient touch therapy. *RN, 59*, 58. ©1996 Medical Economics. Montvale, NJ with permission).

Little controlled research has been done with reiki. The preponderance of reiki studies reported in the literature to date consists of a limited number of case reports, descriptive studies, or randomized controlled studies conducted with a small number of participants (Miles & True, 2003). Box 17-5 presents a more recent study abstract.

Box 17-5

Reiki Study

In a study of outpatients with HIV/AIDS at an inner hospital clinic, 30 subjects experienced either 20 minutes of reiki self-treatment or treatment by a reiki student. The first degree reiki training was given in 4-hour sessions on consecutive weekdays. Evaluation indicated a decline in reported pain and anxiety after the reiki treatment. There was no significant difference in pain or anxiety reduction as a function of whether the reiki was self-administered or administered by another (Miles, 2003).

Source: Adapted from Wardell, D. W., & Engebretson, J. (2001). Biological correlates of reiki touch healing. *Journal of Advanced Nursing, 33,* 439-445.

Nield-Anderson and Ameling (2001) recommend that regular self-Reiki be performed daily during the first 21 days "cleansing period" to enhance clinician balance and centering, and continued increase in confidence in and mastery of ability. Practice research is needed to answer questions of how much, how often, for how long (Nield-Anderson & Ameling, 2001). Some examples include: which hand positions are most appropriate for specific conditions, how long certain hand positions should be held for maximum benefit, and how many treatments are needed and for what length of time for specific conditions?

THERAPEUTIC TOUCH

Therapeutic touch (TT), developed by Dolores Krieger (a nurse) and Dora Kunz (an energy healer), proposes that "in an orderly universe, when conscious intent to help or to heal is guided by compassion, it can have a powerful healing influence" (Meehan, 1998, p. 118). The primary experience of TT is opening to the flow of the universal life energy and involves three key concepts: compassion, intention, and nonattachment.

"Compassion is described as pure caring such that the person wants to help, but is without expectations for the outcome. Intentionality is the intent to help or heal and is the conscious direction of the energy to the patient with a deficit of energy. Compassion serves as the catalyst for the energy exchange process and intentionality serves as the means of transmitting energy" (Egan, 1998, p. 51). Nonattachment is a deliberate detachment from personal feelings or emotions.

Meehan (1998) insists that a specific procedure must be followed for TT. "Significant changes from the standard practice of TT can result in practices which may or may not involve the therapeutic use of touch, but they are not TT" (p. 120). The five-step technique consists of (Horowitz, 1999; McCormack & Galantino, 1997):

1. *Centering*, physically and psychologically, on the intent to help the client. This is a process by which the nurse finds a calm, focused state of being. This is done by conscious direction of attention inward. It can be achieved by various methods, such as deep breathing, visualization, and focusing.

2. *Assessing the client's energy field.* This is a process by which the nurse notes areas of balance and imbalance in the client's energy field by using the hands to scan the client's energy field from head to toe. Perception of heat, cold, tingling, congestion, or pressure indicates imbalances or obstructions in the field.

3. *"Unruffling" the client's energy field.* This is a process by which the client's energy field congestion, sluggishness, or static is removed or lessened. This is performed by making slow brushing sweeps with the nurse's hand over the client's body without touching the body itself, sweeping from head to toe. This allows the energy to move freely.

4. *Directing or modulating that energy.* Once the field has been cleared, areas that have been blocked or congested are treated. The nurse lets the hands rest on or near the body where the block or congestion was detected or in other areas of energy imbalance. Energy is directed to the area in order to balance or correct the "blockage" or modulate energy by changing the outflow to meet the client's needs. This is performed as an act of consciousness as the nurse images a flow or movement of particles, color, fluid, or whatever visualization is clearly formulated in the mind.

5. *Scanning or recognizing when the process is complete and it is time to stop.* Stop when there are no longer any cues, when the body is symmetrical and there are no perceivable differences bilaterally, such as magnetic-like repulsions, heat, cold, static electricity, emptiness, or fullness.

Meehan (1998, pp. 119-120) integrates these steps in her description of TT process. Preparation for TT is begun by achieving an inner focus on a center of calm, quiet, and balance (centering). While the nurse remains quite aware of the physical environment, this is not the primary focus of attention. The nurse "attunes to the universal healing energy so she may become an instrument for its healing influence. Her attitude becomes one of clear, gentle, and compassionate attention to the patient and of focused intent to help facilitate the patient's own natural healing tendency." The nurse remains detached from any personal feelings or emotions. For the experienced clinician, centering takes about 10 seconds. The nurse remains centered throughout the process.

"The assessment is done in relation to two principles: openness and symmetry. In a state of health, the [client] as an energy field is perceived as a gentle, symmetrical, open flow from head to feet. In a state of illness, the flow is perceived as congested, asymmetrical, and impeded." The hands are moved in a smooth, gentle movement, with the palms facing toward the client, about 1 to 2 inches over client's clothed body, from head to feet. The nurse perceives the pattern of the energy flow through differences in sensory cues in her hands. These subtle cues are typically described as "warmth, coolness, tightness, heaviness, tingling, or emptiness" (Meehan, 1998, pp. 119-120). The overall pattern of the energy flow and any area of imbalance or impeded flow are noted. The initial assessment takes about 30 seconds, but assessment also continues throughout the process.

During the treatment phase, the focus is on the specific repatterning of areas of imbalance and impeded flow, with the hands as focal points. The nurse's intention is to dissipate areas of imbalance and facilitate a gentle, symmetrical, and open flow. The process begins with the nurse moving her hands in gentle sweeping movements from head to feet. Attention is then focused on areas of imbalance or congestion. For example, if an area of heat is felt over the left side of the client's abdomen, the nurse will project an image of coolness as she moves one hand repeatedly through that area. Simultaneously, she will move the other hand over the right side of the abdomen, bringing the left and right side into balance. If areas of heaviness or tingling are perceived over the client's chest, the nurse will project an image of a flowing or smoothing movement as she moves her hands repeatedly through the area until she begins to feel the quality of the energy flow change. To complete the treatment, the hands are placed over the area of the solar plexus (just below the sternum) and the nurse focuses specifically on facilitating the flow of universal healing energy in the client. Physical touch can be incorporated into the treatment.

Subjective observations following TT include generalized feelings of warmth expressed, spontaneous verbal response, a sigh or comment ("I feel relaxed"), or description of change in pain levels. Objective observations include lowering of the client's voice; slowing and deepening of the client's respiration; peripheral flush of the skin, especially in areas treated; physiological changes in the relaxation response, such as decreased pulse, lowered blood pressure. "TT not only alleviates pain, but produces a relaxation response which is known to ameliorate levels of state anxiety or the situational occurrences of anxiety" (McCormack & Galantino, 1997, p. 88). Among the outcomes of TT are a relaxation response, relief of pain, and accelerated healing (Egan, 1998). However, Engle and Graney (2000) unexpectedly found evidence of vasoconstriction in a short-term study of 11 adults as evidenced by decreased total pulse amplitude (large effect size of .57 to 1.32) and decreased time perception (time passing faster) (medium effect size of .40) after a standardized protocol of TT. The authors concluded that TT may have adverse and positive outcomes.

There is increasing research evidence that purports to support the effectiveness of TT. Twenty-three articles in 14 refereed journals from 1981 to 1996 indicated "positive regard for the use of TT" (Easter, 1997). A meta-analytic review of 9 out of 36 studies published between 1986 and 1996 indicated that TT has a positive, medium effect on physiological and psychological variables (Peters, 1999). A meta-analysis of 13 of 38 studies performed between 1975 and 1997 had an average effect size of .39, which is described as moderate (Winstead-Fry & Kijek, 1999).

However, as Peters (1999) states, "it is impossible to make any substantive claims at this time because there is limited published research and because many of the studies had significant methodological issues that could seriously bias the reported results.... It appears that TT can produce a medium effect for physiological outcomes and psychological outcomes within treated subjects. It also appears that TT produces a medium effect on physiological outcomes when comparing treatment with control groups.... There is not enough empirical data to support TT as more effective than control measures in improving psychological well-being" (pp. 52, 59).

Winstead-Fry and Kijek (1999) also indicate concerns with the quality of the research literature. "The review demonstrated that there are many approaches to TT research, samples are described incompletely, and the TT practices vary in the studies" (p. 58). Concerns identified by Winstead-Fry and Kijek include:

- Use of healthy persons as a sample. It is possible that persons with diseases or illnesses have different responses.

- The use of 5-minute research TT treatments, even though clinicians allow an average of 20 minutes for a treatment.

- Inadequate sample size.

- Lack of sophisticated statistical analysis.

- Researcher also serving as healer.

Mathuna (2000) goes even further in her critique of reviews of TT literature published in nursing journals between 1994 and 1998. She found that literature reviews often cited only research with favorable findings and only mentioned the favorable findings even in research with contradictory findings. Of concern, many reviews actually indicated that TT was ineffective, but the research was cited as indicating the efficacy of TT. "Every review examined had at least one significant mistake concerning how research studies were represented" (p. 279).

However, "there appear to be no risks to [clients] associated with TT when it is used appropriately as a nursing intervention.... In extrapolating from data on placebo effectiveness, it could even be suggested that for a [client] in a stress-related situation where the physician, nurse, and patient believe in TT, it could have at least a positive effect 70% of the time and an excellent effect 40% of the time.... It seems clear that TT is intrinsically interrelated with the powerful placebo effect" (Meehan, 1998, p. 123).

Several precautions for TT have been proposed. As a general rule, the client will take the amount of energy that is needed and then will stop drawing from the energy source, however, in some instances precautions must be taken. Infants and children are very sensitive to treatments. Energy should be given slowly and gently in small amounts by an experienced clinician. Aged, extremely ill, or dying individuals may require modifications in treatment or gentle energy input. The head is also very sensitive and only cooling, sweeping motions are used in the head area. Patients with cancer are treated in such a way that energy is not concentrated in a particular area (Egan, 1998).

TT should be learned through an apprenticeship with a mentor over 1 to 2 years to perfect a knowledgeable practice. The supporting organization for TT is the Nurse Healers Professional Organization, Inc. (see Additional Information at the end of the chapter). Nurse Healers provide a three-step process: beginning, intermediate, and advanced. The Nurse Healers Association does not provide certification. The Holistic Nursing Association, which incorporates TT into a process they call healing touch, provides an extensive program leading to certification as a healing touch practitioner. However, the Nurse Healers-Professional Associates International (NH-PAI) does not endorse the Healing Touch Program as a suitable source of training for therapeutic touch practitioners (Bonadonna, 2002).

Thought field therapy is an integrated, meridian-based, mind-body-energy psychotherapy that includes diagnostic and therapeutic procedures performed while patients are attuned to their problem. The goal is to enhance one's bioenergetic level of functioning while a specific problem is being attuned, so that the subtle energetic codes associated with the perturbations in the field can be removed. The negative emotions are alleviated through gentle activation of designated acupuncture points, which neutralizes or eliminates the energetic cause of the problem (Diepold, 2002). Treatment procedures have primarily involved tapping the beginning or end points of the designated meridians or vessels to reversal, g-gamut, collarbone breathing, thought recognition, the healing energy light process, and the eye roll (Gallo, 2002).

Energy healing is based on a view of person-environment process as unitary and open. It is theorized that intentional focus by the healer can foster harmonious entrainment of energy field vibration. Restoration of energy field harmony is associated with healthiness and healing. The emphasis in this chapter has been on patterning of the energy field through non-invasive therapeutic modalities such as color, music, polarity therapy, prayer, reiki, therapeutic touch, and thought field therapy. These modalities are accepted by many states as legitimate components of the professional nurse's scope of practice.

Chapter Key Points

- Energy healing is also known as the laying on of hands or biofield therapeutics.

- Energy healing is a systematic, purposeful intervention aimed to help another person by means of focused intention, hand contact, and aligning with the universal energy field.

- Reiki and prayer are based on channeling of a spiritual energy that has innate intelligence or logic, while music, color therapy, polarity therapy, TT, and TFT pattern the vibrations of the environmental energy field for healing purposes.

References

Benford, M. S., Talnagi, J., Doss, D. B., Boosey, S., & Arnold, L. E. (1999). Gamma radiation fluctuations during alternative healing therapy. *Alterntive Therapies in Health and Medicine*, 5, 51-56.

Berman, B. M., & Larson, D. B. (Eds.). (1994). *Alternative medicine: Expanding medical horizons*. Washington, DC: U.S. Government Printing Office.

Bittman, B. B., Berk, L. S., Felten, D. L., Westengard, J., Simonton, O. C., Pappas, J., et al. (2001). Composite effects of group drumming music therapy on modulation of neuroendocrine-immune parameters in normal subjects. *Alterntive Therapies in Health and Medicine*, 7, 38-47.

Bonadonna, J. R. (2002). Therapeutic touch. In S. Shannon (Ed.), *The handbook of complimentary & alternative therapies in mental health* (pp. 231-248). San Diego: Academic Press.

Brewer, J. F. (1998). Healing sounds. *Complementary Therapies in Nursing & Midwifery*, 4, 7-12.

Brotons, M., Koger, M., & Pickett-Cooper, P. (1997). Music and dementias: A review of literature. *Journal of Music Therapy*, 24, 204-245.

Burton Goldberg Group. (1995). *Alternative medicine: The definitive guide*. Fife, WA: Future Medicine.

Byrd, R. C. (1997). Positive therapeutic effects of intercessory prayer in a coronary care unit population. *Alterntive Therapies in Health and Medicine*, 3, 62-73.

Campbell, D. (2001). Do you hear what I hear? *Alterntive Therapies in Health and Medicine*, 7, 34-35.

Chlan, L. (1998). Music therapy. In M. Snyder & R. Lindquist (Eds.), *Complementary/alternative therapies in nursing* (3rd. ed., pp. 243-257). New York: Springer.

Diepold, J. H. Jr. (2002). Thought field therapy: Advancements in theory and practice. In F. P. Gallo (Eds.), *Energy psychology in psychotherapy* (pp. 3-34). New York: Norton.

Dossey, L. (1997). The return of prayer. *Alterntive Therapies in Health and Medicine, 3,* 10-17, 113-120.

Dossey, L. (2000). Creativity: On intelligence, insight, and the cosmic soup. *Alterntive Therapies in Health and Medicine, 6,* 12-17, 108-117.

Easter, A. (1997). The state of research on the effects of therapeutic touch. *Journal of Holistic Nursing, 15,* 158-175.

Egan, E. C. (1998). Therapeutic touch. In M. Snyder & R. Lindquist (Eds.), *Complementary/alternative therapies in nursing* (3rd ed., pp. 49-62). New York: Springer.

Engebretson, J. (1996). Urban healers: An experiential description of American healing touch groups. *Qualitative Heath Research, 6,* 526-541.

Engle, V. F., & Graney, M. J. (2000). Biobehavioral effects of therapeutic touch. *Journal of Nursing Scholarship, 32,* 287-293.

Gallo., F. P. (2002). Energy diagnostic and treatment methods. In F. P. Gallo (Ed.), *Energy psychology in psychotherapy* (pp. 35-51). New York: Norton.

Gaynor, M. L. (1999). *Sounds of healing.* New York: Broadway Books.

Gerber, R. (1988). *Vibrational medicine: New choices for healing ourselves.* Santa Fe, NM: Bear & Co.

Good, M., Picot, B. L., Salem, S. G., Chin, C., Picot, S. F., & Lane, D. F. (2001). Cultural differences in music chosen for pain relief. *Journal of Holistic Nursing, 18,* 245-260.

Guzzetta, C. A. (1997). Music therapy. In B. M. Dossey (Ed.), *Core curriculum for holistic nursing* (pp. 196-204). Gaithersburg, MD: Aspen.

Harding, S (1999). More noise or sound theory? *Alternative and Complementary Therapies, 5,* 85-92, 164-174.

Horowitz, S. (1999). Rehabilitation medicine. The mainstreaming of a more holistic approach. *Alternative and Complementary Therapies,* 12-17.

Klotsche, C. (1993). *Color medicine.* Sedona, AZ: Light Technology.

Koopman, B. G., & Blasband, R. A. (2002). Distant healing revisited: Time for a new epistemology. *Alterntive Therapies in Health and Medicine, 8,* 100-101.

Krieger, D. (1986). *The therapeutic touch: How to use your hands to help or to heal.* New York: Prentice-Hall.

Kumar, A. M., Tims, F., Cruess, D. G., Mintzer, M. J., Ironson, G., Loewenstein, D., et al. (1999). Music therapy increases serum melatonin levels in patients with Alzheimer's disease. *Alterntive Therapies in Health and Medicine, 5,* 49-57.

Leddy, S. K. (1998). *Leddy and Pepper's conceptual bases of professional nursing* (4th ed.). Philadelphia: Lipppincott.

Leddy, S. K. (2002). A practice theory of energy. Manuscript submitted for publication.

Mathuna, D. P. (2000). Evidence-based practice and reviews of therapeutic touch. *Journal of Nursing Scholarship, 32,* 279-285.

McCormack, G. L., & Galantino, M. L. (1997). Non-contact therapeutic touch. In C. M. Davis (Ed.), *Complementary therapies in rehabilitation* (pp. 83-97). Thorofare, NJ: SLACK Incorporated.

Meehan, T. C. (1998). Therapeutic touch as a nursing intervention. *Journal of Advanced Nursing, 28*, 117-125.

Miles, P. (2003). Preliminary report on the use of reiki for HIV-related pain and anxiety. *Alternative Therapies in Health and Medicine, 9*, 36.

Miles, P., & True, G. (2003). Reiki- Review of a biofield therapy. History, theory, practice, and research. *Alternative Therapies in Health and Medicine, 9*, 62-72.

Nield-Anderson, L., & Ameling, A. (2000). The empowering nature of reiki as a complementary therapy. *Holistic Nursing Practice, 14*, 21-29.

Nield-Anderson, L., & Ameling, A. (2001). Reiki: A complementary therapy for nursing practice. *Journal of Psychosocial Nursing and Mental Health Services, 39*, 42-49.

Olsen, K. G. (1990). *The encyclopedia of alternative health care.* New York: Pocket Books.

Peters, R. M. (1999). The effectiveness of therapeutic touch: A meta-analytic review. *Nursing Science Quarterly, 12*, 52-61.

Rogers, M. E. (1990). Nursing: Science of unitary, irreducible human beings. Update 1990. In E. A. M. Barrett (Ed.), *Visions of Rogers' science-based nursing* (pp. 5-11). New York: National League for Nursing.

Schlitz, M., & Braud, W. (1997). Distant intentionality and healing: Assessing the evidence. *Alterntive Therapies in Health and Medicine, 3*, 62-73.

Selby, P. (1997). Subtle energy manipulation and physical therapy. In C. M. Davis (Ed.), *Complementary therapies in rehabilitation* (pp. 267-278). Thorofare, NJ: SLACK Incorporated.

Sharp, M. B. (1997). Polarity, reflexology, and touch for health. In C. M. Davis (Ed.), *Complementary therapies in rehabilitation* (pp. 235-255). Thorofare, NJ: SLACK Incorporated.

Sills, F. (1989). The polarity process: Energy as a healing art. Longmead, Dorset: Element Books Ltd.

Slater, V. E. (1997). Energetic healing. In B. M. Dossey (Ed.), *Core curriculum for holistic nursing* (pp. 52-58). Gaithersburg, MD: Aspen.

Starn, J. R. (1998). The path to becoming an energy healer. *Nurse Practitioner Forum, 9*, 209-216.

Targ, E. (1997). Evaluating distant healing: A research review. *Alterntive Therapies in Health and Medicine, 3*, 74-78.

Thomson, K. S. (1997). Miracles on demand: Prayer and the causation of healing. *Alterntive Therapies in Health and Medicine, 3*, 92-96.

Van Sell, S. L. (February, 1996). Reiki: An ancient touch therapy. *RN, 59*, 57-59.

Wardell, D. W., & Engebretson, J. (2001). Biological correlates of reiki touch healing. *Journal of Advanced Nursing, 33*, 439-445.

Weil, A. (2000, January). Can spirituality heal? *Self healing,* 8. Retrieved January 2, 2002, from http://www.drweilselfhealing.com/show_document.asp?iDocumentID=120&iBDC=1440&iPageNumber=1

Wetzel, W. S. (1989). Reiki healing: A physiologic perspective. *Journal of Holistic Nursing, 7*(1), 47-54.

Winstead-Fry, P., & Kijek, J. (1999). An integrative review and meta-analysis of therapeutic touch research. *Alterntive Therapies in Health and Medicine, 5*, 58-67.

Additional Information

ASSOCIATIONS AND CREDENTIALING

Music Therapy

> American Music Therapy Association
> 8455 Colesville Road, Suite 1000
> Silver Spring, MD 20910
> Tel: (301) 589-3300
> www.musictherapy.org

For new music therapists, the MT-BC (music therapist-board certified) is the only available credential. The Certification Board for Music Therapists requires education, clinical training, and a national examination. Continuing education is required for recertification.

Prayer

> American Association of Pastoral Counselors
> 9504-A Lee Highway
> Fairfax, VA 22031
> Tel: (703) 385-6967
> www.aapc.org

Provides certification for pastoral counselors.

Light (Color) Therapy

> College of Syntonic Optometry
> 21 E. 5th Street
> Bloomsburg, PA 17815
> Tel: (717) 387-0900
> www.syntonicphototherapy.com

Training is achieved by attending seminars and continuing education in the field. The annual Conference of Light and Vision, sponsored by the College of Syntonic Optometry, provides basic and advanced courses with certification. There is no regulation of practitioners.

Polarity Therapy

> American Polarity Therapy Association (APTA)
> 2888 Bluff Street #149
> Boulder, CO 80301
> Tel: (303) 545-2080
> www.polaritytherapy.org

There are no states that license polarity therapy by itself. The APTA oversees the development of standards for training at two levels and for continuing education. Currently, the first level of associate practitioner (155 required course hours) provides a basis for beginning to practice, with an additional 460 hours required for achieving the status of Registered polarity practitioner.

Reiki

Center for Reiki Training
Tel: (800) 332-8112
www.reiki.org

The therapy is not regulated anywhere in the world and there are no registration processes. An apprenticeship to a reiki master is a common way in which the teachings are passed on.

Therapeutic Touch

The Nurse Healers and Professional Associates Cooperative
175 Fifth Avenue, Suite 2755
New York, NY 10010
(212) 886-3776

Practitioners of TT may receive certificates of completion of classes.

American Holistic Nurses' Association
PO Box 2130
Flagstaff, AZ 86003-2130

APPENDIX

Leddy Healthiness Scale

Directions:

Circle the number that best indicates your degree of agreement with each of the following statements. Please answer all of the questions the way you feel **right now**.

	Completely Agree	Mostly Agree	Slightly Agree	Slightly Disagree	Mostly Disagree	Completely Disagree
1. I think that I function pretty well.	6	5	4	3	2	1
2. I have goals that I look forward to accomplishing in the next year.	6	5	4	3	2	1
3. I am part of a close and supportive family.	6	5	4	3	2	1
4. I don't feel there is much that is meaningful in my life.	6	5	4	3	2	1
5. I have more than enough energy to do what I want to do.	6	5	4	3	2	1
6. I feel I can accomplish anything I set out to do.	6	5	4	3	2	1

	Completely Agree	Mostly Agree	Slightly Agree	Slightly Disagree	Mostly Disagree	Completely Disagree
7. There is very little that I value in my life right now.	6	5	4	3	2	1
8. Having change(s) in my life makes me feel uncomfortable.	6	5	4	3	2	1
9. I have rewarding relationships with people.	6	5	4	3	2	1
10. I enjoy making plans for the future.	6	5	4	3	2	1
11. I feel free to choose actions that are right for me.	6	5	4	3	2	1
12. I feel like I have got little energy.	6	5	4	3	2	1
13. I am pleased to find that I am getting better with age.	6	5	4	3	2	1
14. I don't communicate much with family or friends.	6	5	4	3	2	1
15. I get excited thinking about new projects.	6	5	4	3	2	1
16. I feel good about my ability to influence change.	6	5	4	3	2	1
17. I'm not what you would call a goal-oriented person.	6	5	4	3	2	1
18. I feel energetic.	6	5	4	3	2	1
19. I feel good about my freedom to make choices for my life.	6	5	4	3	2	1
20. I have a goal that I am trying to achieve.	6	5	4	3	2	1

	Completely Agree	Mostly Agree	Slightly Agree	Slightly Disagree	Mostly Disagree	Completely Disagree
21. I don't expect the future to hold much meaning.	6	5	4	3	2	1
22. I like exploring new possibilities.	6	5	4	3	2	1
23. I feel full of zest and vigor.	6	5	4	3	2	1
24. I feel fine.	6	5	4	3	2	1
25. I feel pretty sure of myself.	6	5	4	3	2	1
26. I feel isolated from people.	6	5	4	3	2	1

The Leddy Healthiness Scale is scored by reversing items 4, 7, 8, 12, 14, 17, 21, and 26 (positive responses are scored higher). The summative score can range from 26 to 156, with higher scores indicating higher healthiness.

APPENDIX

Nutritional Supplements

Vitamin and Mineral Supplement Ranges

Fat-Soluble Vitamins

Supplement	Description	U.S. RDA Adult*	Adult Daily Supplement Range	Side Effects
Beta carotene pro-vitamin A	Converted by the body to vitamin A as needed. Primary antioxidant that helps protect the lungs and other tissue.	Not established	10,000-50,000 IU	Prolonged ingestion of relatively high doses may cause a non-harmful yellowing of the skin especially palms and soles. Avoid beta carotene supplement while taking the prescription drug Accutane (Roche USA, Nutley, NJ), especially during pregnancy.
Vitamin A (preformed retinol)	Essential for growth and and development, maintenance of healthy skin, hair, and eyes. Involved in wound healing.	4,000-5,000 IU	5,000-10,000 IU	Prolonged ingestion of excess vitamin A (50,000 IU+/day) may be toxic. Avoid vitamin A supplement while taking the prescription drug Accutane, especially during pregnancy.
Vitamin D (cholecalferol)	Essential for calcium and phosphorus metabolism, required for strong bones and teeth.	400 IU	200-400 IU	Prolonged ingestion of excess vitamin D (1,000 IU+/day) may be toxic and cause hypercalcemia (excess of calcium in blood).
Vitamin E	Primary antioxidant that protects the red blood cells and is essential in cellular respiration.	12-15 IU	200-800 IU	Prolonged ingestion of vitamin E may produce adverse skin reactions and upset stomach.

continued

Vitamin and Mineral Supplement Ranges (continued)

Fat-Soluble Vitamins

Supplement	Description	U.S. RDA Adult*	Adult Daily Supplement Range	Side Effects
Vitamin K (phylloquinone)	Integrally involved in the blood clotting mechanism.	65 μ	50-500 μ	Unlike other fat-soluble vitamins, vitamin K is not stored in significant quantity in the liver. Synthetic vitamin K (menadione) is toxic in excess dosages.

Water-Soluble Vitamins

Supplement	Description	U.S. RDA Adult*	Adult Daily Supplement Range	Side Effects
Vitamin C (ascorbic acid)	Primary antioxidant, essential for tissue growth, wound healing, absorption of calcium and iron, and utilization of the B vitamin-folic acid. Involved in neurotransmitter biosynthesis, cholesterol regulation, and formation of collagen.	60 mg	300-3,000 mg	Essentially nontoxic in oral doses. However, excessive ingestion may cause abdominal bloating, gas, flatulence, and diarrhea. Acid-sensitive individuals should take buffered ascorbate form of vitamin C supplement.
Vitamin B$_1$ (thiamine)	Essential for food metabolism and release of energy for cellular function.	1.2-1.5 mg	5-100 mg	Essentially nontoxic in oral doses.

continued

Vitamin and Mineral Supplemental Ranges (continued)

WATER-SOLUBLE VITAMINS

SUPPLEMENT	DESCRIPTION	U.S. RDA ADULT*	ADULT DAILY SUPPLEMENT RANGE	SIDE EFFECTS
Vitamin B_2 (riboflavin)	Essential for food metabolism and release of energy for cellular function. Important in the formation of red blood cells and activation of other B vitamins.	1.4-1.8 mg	5-100 mg	Essentially nontoxic in oral doses. Moderate to high doses of vitamin B_2 may cause nonharmful bright yellow coloration of urine.
Vitamin B_3 (niacin)	Essential for food metabolism and release of energy for cellular function. Vital for oxygen transport in the blood, and fatty acid and nucleic acid formation. A major constitute of several important coenzymes.	16-20 mg	20-100 mg	Essentially nontoxic in oral doses. High doses (100 mg+) may cause transient flushing and tingling in the upper body area, as well as stomach upset. Prolonged ingestion of excess vitamin B_3 (1,000-2,000 mg+/day) may elevate liver enzymes and cause liver damage.
Vitamin B_5	Involved in food metabolism and release of energy. Vital for biosynthesis of hormones and support of adrenal glands.	4-7 mg	10-1,000 mg	Essentially nontoxic in oral doses. Extremely high doses (10,000 mg+) will produce diarrhea.

continued

Vitamin and Mineral Supplemental Ranges (continued)

WATER SOLUBLE VITAMINS

SUPPLEMENT	DESCRIPTION	U.S. RDA ADULT*	ADULT DAILY SUPPLEMENT RANGE	SIDE EFFECTS
Vitamin B_6 (pyroxidine)	Involved in food metabolism and release of energy. Essential for amino acid metabolism and formation of blood proteins and antibodies. Helps regulate electrolytic balance.	2.0-2.5 mg	5-200 mg	Prolonged high doses (500 mg+/day) may be toxic and cause neurological damage. Prescription oral contraceptives may cause deficiency of vitamin B_6.
Vitamin B_{12} (cobalamin)	Essential for normal formation of red blood cells. Involved in food metabolism, release of energy and epithelial cells (cells that form the skin's outer layer and the surface layer of mucous membranes), and the nervous system.	3.0-4.0 μ	10-500 μ	Essentially nontoxic in oral doses.
Folate (folic acid, folicin)	Essential for blood formation, especially red blood cells and white blood cells. Involved in the biosynthesis of nucleic acids including RNA and DNA.	400 μ	200-800 μ	Essentially nontoxic in oral doses. An excess intake of folate can mask a vitamin B_{12} deficiency.

continued

Vitamin and Mineral Supplemental Ranges (continued)

WATER SOLUBLE VITAMINS

SUPPLEMENT	DESCRIPTION	U.S. RDA ADULT*	ADULT DAILY SUPPLEMENT RANGE	SIDE EFFECTS
Biotin	Essential for food metabolism and release of energy. Assists in the biosynthesis of amino acids, nucleic acid, and fatty acids. Utilization of other B vitamins.	150-300 μ	300-600 mg	Essentially nontoxic in oral doses.

B vitamins should also be taken in a B-complex form because of their close interrelationship in the metabolic process.

MINERALS

The function of minerals are highly interrelated to each other and to vitamins, hormones, and enzymes. No mineral can function in the body without affecting others.

Calcium (Ca++)	Essential for strong bones and teeth. Serves as a vital cofactor in cellular energy production and nerve and heart function.	800-1,200 mg	200-1,200 mg	Prolonged ingestion of excess calcium, along with excess vitamin D, may cause hypercalcemia of bone and soft tissue (such as joints and kidneys) and may also cause a mineral imbalance.

continued

Vitamin and Mineral Supplemental Ranges *(continued)*

MINERALS

SUPPLEMENT	DESCRIPTION	U.S. RDA ADULT*	ADULT DAILY SUPPLEMENT RANGE	SIDE EFFECTS
Magnesium (Mg++)	Essential catalyst for food metabolism and release of energy. A cofactor in the formation of RNA/DNA, enzyme activation, and nerve fuction.	300-350 mg	150-600 mg	Extremely high doses (30,000 mg+) may be toxic in certain individuals with kidney problems. Doses of 400 mg+ may produce a laxative effect, causing diarrhea.
Potassium (K+)	A primary electrolyte, important in regulating pH (acid/base) balance and water balance. Plays a role in nerve function and cellular integrity.	Not established	1,875-5,625 mg (*A typical healthy diet contains adequate K. Very active individuals may require additional electrolytes.*)	Extremely high doses (25,000 mg+/day) of K chloride may be toxic in instances of kidney failure.
Sodium (Na+)	A primary electrolyte, important in regulating pH (acid/base) balance and water balance. Plays a role in nerve function and cellular integrity.	Not established	Limit daily intake to 1,500 mg	Prolonged ingestion of excess sodium has been linked to high blood pressure and increased incidence of migraine headaches. Extremely high intakes of sodium can result in swelling of tissues (edema).

continued

Vitamin and Mineral Supplemental Ranges (continued)

MINERALS

SUPPLEMENT	DESCRIPTION	U.S. RDA ADULT*	ADULT DAILY SUPPLEMENT RANGE	SIDE EFFECTS
Phosphorus (P)	Constituent of the molecule phosphate, which plays a major role in energy production and activation of B vitamins. Component of RNA/DNA, bones, and teeth.	900-1,200 mg	300-600 mg	Although essentially nontoxic, a disproportionately large amount of phosphorus relative to calcium intake may cause a deficiency in calcium and mineral imbalance.
Zinc (Zn++)	Cofactor in numerous enzymatic processes and reactions. Structural constituent of nucleic acids and insulin. Involved in taste, wound healing, and digestion.	15 mg	15-30 mg	Extremely high doses (2,000 mg/day) can be toxic. Excess zinc intake (50 mg+/day) may cause copper deficiency and mineral imbalance.
Iron (FE++ or FE+++)	Combines with other nutrients to produce vital blood proteins.	10-18 mg	10-30 mg	Prolonged ingestion of excess iron can be toxic, affecting the liver, pancreas, heart, and nucleus, also increasing susceptibility to infection. Poorly utilized forms of iron (FE sulfate or FE gluconate) may cause constipation and/or stomach upset. Iron supplements should be taken with food and supplemental vitamin C.

continued

Vitamin and Mineral Supplemental Ranges (continued)

MINERALS

SUPPLEMENT	DESCRIPTION	U.S. RDA ADULT*	ADULT DAILY SUPPLEMENT RANGE	SIDE EFFECTS
Manganese (Mn++)	Important catalyst and co-factor in many enzymatic processes and reactions. Helps maintain skeletal and connective structural tissue, as well as cellular integrity.	2.5-5.0 mg	2-10 mg	Prolonged ingestion of excess manganese may result in non-harmful elevated concentrations in the liver and may cause a mineral imbalance.
Copper (Cu++)	Essential for production of red blood cells. Involved in the maintenance of skeletal and cardiovascular systems. Works with vitamin C in the biosynthesis of collagen and elastin.	2-3 mg	2-3 mg	Prolonged ingestion of excess copper may be toxic, especially with Wilson's disease, a rare metabolic disorder resulting in an excess accumulation of copper in the liver, red blood cells, and the brain.
Iodine (I-)	Essential component of thyroid hormones, which regulate growth and rate of metabolism.	150 µ	50-300 µ	Prolonged ingestion of excess iodine may cause "iodine goiter," an enlargement of the thyroid gland. May also induce acne-like skin lesions or aggravate pre-existing acne conditions.

continued

Vitamin and Mineral Supplemental Ranges (continued)

MINERALS

SUPPLEMENT	DESCRIPTION	U.S. RDA ADULT*	ADULT DAILY SUPPLEMENT RANGE	SIDE EFFECTS
Chromium (Cr+++)	Vital as a cofactor of GTF (glucose tolerance factor), which regulates the function of insulin. Involved in food metabolism, enzyme activation, and regulation of cholesterol.	50-200 μ	200-500 μ	Essentially nontoxic in oral doses.
Selenium	Important constituent of the antioxidant enzyme gluathione peroxidase, which is contained in white blood cells and blood platelets. Synergistic nutritional partner of vitamin E.	55-200 μ	100-200 μ	Prolonged ingestion of excess selenium may be toxic.

*Because the current U.S. RDA's are an inadequate guide to the therapeutic benefits of nutritional supplements, research should be made to develop an accurate guide to the ranges of supplementation.

Reprinted with permission from Burton Goldberg Group. (1995). *Alternative medicine: The definitive guide*. Tiburon, CA: Future Medicine.

INDEX